T0075124

BASIC MEDICAL LANGUAGE

SEVENTH EDITION

Danielle LaFleur Brooks, MEd, MA

Faculty, Allied Health and Science
Faculty Co-Chair, Advising and Teaching
Excellence Curriculum Committee
Community College of Vermont
Montpelier, Vermont

Dale Levinsky, MD

Clinical Associate Professor, Family, Community,
& Preventative Medicine
University of Arizona College of Medicine
Phoenix, Arizona
Clinical Associate Professor, Family, and Community Medicine
University of Arizona College of Medicine
Tucson, Arizona

Myrna LaFleur Brooks, RN, BEd

Founding President
National Association of Health Unit Coordinators
Faculty Emeritus
Maricopa Community College District
Phoenix, Arizona

ELSEVIER

Elsevier
3251 Riverport Lane
St. Louis, Missouri 63043

BASIC MEDICAL LANGUAGE, SEVENTH EDITION   ISBN: 978-0-323-87638-4
Copyright © 2024 by Elsevier Inc. All rights reserved.

No part of this publication may be reproduced or transmitted in any form or by any means, electronic or mechanical, including photocopying, recording, or any information storage and retrieval system, without permission in writing from the publisher. Details on how to seek permission, further information about the Publisher's permissions policies and our arrangements with organizations such as the Copyright Clearance Center and the Copyright Licensing Agency, can be found at our website: www.elsevier.com/permissions.

This book and the individual contributions contained in it are protected under copyright by the Publisher (other than as may be noted herein).

Although for mechanical reasons some pages of this publication are perforated, only those pages imprinted with an Elsevier Inc. copyright notice are intended for removal.

Notice

Practitioners and researchers must always rely on their own experience and knowledge in evaluating and using any information, methods, compounds or experiments described herein. Because of rapid advances in the medical sciences, in particular, independent verification of diagnoses and drug dosages should be made. To the fullest extent of the law, no responsibility is assumed by Elsevier, authors, editors or contributors for any injury and/or damage to persons or property as a matter of products liability, negligence or otherwise, or from any use or operation of any methods, products, instructions, or ideas contained in the material herein.

Previous editions copyrighted 2019, 2016, 2013, 2010, 2004, and 1996.

Content Development Director: Laurie Gower
Senior Content Strategist: Luke Held
Senior Content Development Specialist: Elizabeth McCormac
Publishing Services Manager: Julie Eddy
Senior Project Manager: Abigail Bradberry
Design Direction: Renee Duenow

Printed in India

Last digit is the print number: 9 8 7 6 5 4 3 2 1

Working together
to grow libraries in
developing countries

www.elsevier.com • www.bookaid.org

For our students, who continue to inspire us with their dedication to learning while balancing life's other demands. Every page is for you.

Contents

Anatomy of a Lesson

Let's take a look at the structure of body systems lessons using Lesson 4 on the respiratory system as an example.

CASE STUDY

ANATOMY
- Anatomic Structures of the Respiratory System
- Functions of the Respiratory System
- How the Respiratory System Works

CAREER FOCUS

MEDICAL TERMS

OBJECTIVE 1
Terms Built from Word Parts
- Word Parts
- Build and Translate Terms
- Table of Terms
- Pronounce and Spell

OBJECTIVE 2
Terms NOT Built from Word Parts
- Table of Terms
- Label terms pictured and defined
- Learn Medical Terms NOT Built from Word Parts
- Pronounce and Spell

ABBREVIATIONS

OBJECTIVE 3
- Table of Abbreviations
- Abbreviate Medical Terms

CLINICAL CATEGORIES

OBJECTIVE 4
- Signs and Symptoms
- Diseases and Disorders
- Diagnostic Tests and Equipment
- Surgical Procedures
- Specialties and Professions
- Medical Terms Related to the Respiratory System

PRACTICAL APPLICATION

OBJECTIVE 5
- Use Medical Terms in Clinical Statements
- Apply Medical Terms to the Case Study
- Use Medical Terms in a Document
- Use Medical Language in Online Electronic Health Records

REVIEW

OBJECTIVE 6
- Online Review of Lesson Content
- Lesson Content Quiz
- Lesson at a Glance

Preface

WELCOME TO THE NEW EDITION OF *BASIC MEDICAL LANGUAGE*

The seventh edition offers a learning system designed for quick and lasting acquisition of medical language needed for entry into health professions. Word parts, medical terms, and abbreviations are introduced in manageable amounts, followed by immediate practice. Illustrations and narrative passages using medical terms in context weave between written exercises to reveal the medical concepts the terms represent. Bridging new learning with practical application remains a priority. In this new edition of the book, lesson content has been closely revised to focus on frequently used terms in clinical settings and in billing and coding. We have also included several **new features**:

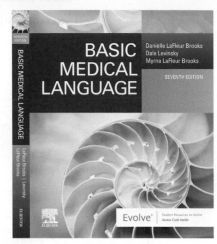

- Introduction to Laboratory Tests and addition of laboratory terms in Lesson 1
- Introduction to Radiology with a new term list in Lesson 2
- Numbered Tables featuring additional content
- Additional exercises to practice Medical Terms NOT Built from Word Parts
- New Medical Records Exercises
- FYI Boxes appearing in term lists with additional information on usage and current trends
- Expanded Lesson Content Quizzes
- Online Resources: Gradable Exercises and Practice Exams

Since 1994, we have dedicated ourselves to creating quality learning opportunities accessing the **multiple intelligences** and **learning styles** of our students. As such, the book and online resources continue to offer numerous and varied ways to interact with lesson content:

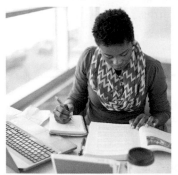

- Flashcards
- Interactive illustrations
- Career focus sections
- Pronunciation and spelling with audio
- Case studies with corresponding medical records
- Online EHR modules, games, and animations
- Lesson At a Glance review of word parts, terms, and abbreviations

Basic Medical Language offers a hybrid of print and electronic materials. Students have the opportunity to hold the book, pencil, and flashcards in their hands. They also have the opportunity to hear terms pronounced, practice spelling with immediate feedback, play games, view animations, and much more using the book's online resources. We believe we have reached an optimal balance of hands-on and virtual opportunities to support long-term learning.

We wish you the best as you begin your study of medical language and invite you to contact us at:

danielle.lafleurbrooks@ccv.edu   *dale.levinsky@gmail.com*   *myrnabrooks@comcast.net*

Warmly,
Danielle, Dale, and *Myrna*

FEATURES

Case Studies

Each lesson begins with a case study depicting a possible experience of a medical condition. Students apply medical terms presented in the lesson to the context of the case study.

CASE STUDY   Roberta Pawlaski

Roberta is experiencing difficulty breathing. She notices it gets worse when she tries to do chores around the house. This has been going on for about four days. She also has a cough and a runny nose. Today when she woke up she noticed that her throat was very sore. She also thinks that she might have a fever because she feels hot all over. She tried taking some over-the-counter cough medicine but this didn't seem to help. She notices when she coughs that a thick yellow mucus comes out. She hasn't had a cough like this since before she quit smoking about 10 years ago. She remembers that her grandson who stays with her after school has missed school because of a cold. She decides to call her doctor's office for advice.

■ *Consider Roberta's situation as you work through the lesson on the respiratory system. At the end of the lesson, we will return to this case study and identify medical terms used to document Roberta's experience and the care she receives.*

Objectives

Lesson introductions list objectives and corresponding page numbers. Exercises, quizzes, and exams correlate directly with the objectives.

OBJECTIVES

1 ■ Build, translate, pronounce, and spell medical terms built from word parts (p. 90).

2 ■ Define, pronounce, and spell medical terms NOT built from word parts (p. 108).

3 ■ Write abbreviations (p. 114).

4 ■ Identify medical terms by clinical category (p. 116).

5 ■ Use medical language in clinical statements, the case study, and a medical record (p. 119).

6 ■ Recall and assess knowledge of word parts, medical terms, and abbreviations (p. 123).

Anatomy

Body system lessons briefly introduce related anatomy and physiology, including anatomic structure term tables with phonetic spelling, illustrations, and labeling exercises, which connect word parts with pictures of the anatomic structures they name.

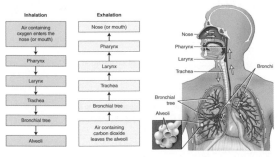

Figure 4.1 Flow of air.

Career Focus

Health professions related to the body system and lesson content are highlighted.

CAREER FOCUS   Professionals Who Work with the Respiratory System

• **Respiratory Therapists (RTs)** treat, evaluate, and maintain function of the heart and lungs. RTs are highly skilled and perform pulmonary function tests, provide treatments, such as oxygen therapy and intermittent positive pressure breathing (IPPB), draw blood for an arterial blood gas (ABG) to monitor carbon dioxide and oxygen in the blood, and assist with ventilation of seriously ill patients.

• **Respiratory Therapy Technicians** provide respiratory care under the supervision of respiratory therapists and physicians.

• **Sleep technologists**, also called **registered polysomnographic technologists (RPSGTs)**, perform polysomnography and other tests to diagnose and monitor sleep disorders. RPSGTs work under the guidance of a physician.

Figure 4.2 Respiratory therapist assisting a patient.

Word Parts

Word part tables present combining forms, suffixes, and prefixes related to lesson content as well as those introduced in previous lessons. Exercises, paper and electronic flashcards, and online activities reinforce learning.

5. LABEL: *Write word parts to complete Figure 4.7.*

Figure 4.7 The nurse anesthetist inserts a(n) _____/_____/_____ tube with a
    within   trachea   pertaining to

_____/o/_____ to guide the tube into place.
    larynx   instrument used for visual examination

Medical Terms Built from Word Parts

Students build, translate, and read medical terms in context. Learning may be extended through practice with online resources, including animations, games, exercises, and quizzes.

23. TRANSLATE: *Complete the definitions of the following terms by using the meaning of word parts to fill in the blanks. Remember, the definition usually starts with the meaning of the suffix. Terms built using the prefix* **endo-**:

a. endo/scope   _____ used for _____ examination _____
(a hollow organ or body cavity)

b. endo/scopic   _____ to visual examination _____ (a hollow organ or body cavity)

c. endo/scopy   visual _____ within (a hollow organ or body cavity)

> **FYI**   The medical terms **endo/scope**, **endo/scopic**, and **endo/scopy** appear to be made up of a prefix and a suffix. The word root **scop**, meaning "to view," is embedded in the suffixes **-scope**, **-scopic**, and **-scopy**.

24. READ: **Endoscopy** (en-DOS-ko-pē), the visual examination within a hollow organ or body cavity, is performed using an **endoscope** (EN-dō-skōp). **Endoscopic** (en-dō-SKOP-ik) surgery is used for diagnosis and treatment. A small incision is made to accommodate a specialized endoscope fitted with a video camera. Other small incisions are made to hold the surgical instruments. The surgeon uses images displayed on a monitor to perform the surgery. Endoscopic surgery, which causes less pain and reduces recovery time, has replaced many large incision surgeries.

25. BUILD: *Write word parts to build terms using the combining form* **thorac/o**, *meaning chest, chest cavity.*

a. pertaining to the chest   _____/_____
                                wr   s

b. visual examination of the chest cavity   _____/ o /_____
                                wr   cv   s

c. instrument used for visual examination of the chest cavity   _____/ o /_____
                                wr   cv   s

d. pertaining to visual examination of the chest cavity   _____/ o /_____
                                wr   cv   s

Medical Terms NOT Built from Word Parts

Lessons present tables of Medical Terms NOT Built from Word Parts with corresponding illustrations and exercises. Practice with online resources, including animations, games, exercises, and quizzes, reinforces learning.

NEW—FYI Boxes appearing in term lists with additional information on usage and current trends.

MEDICAL TERMS NOT BUILT FROM WORD PARTS	
TERM	**DEFINITION**
1. **asthma** (AZ-ma)	respiratory disease characterized by coughing, wheezing, and shortness of breath; caused by constriction and inflammation of airways that is reversible between attacks
2. **chronic obstructive pulmonary disease (COPD)** (KRON-ik) (ob-STRUK-tive) (PUL-mŏ-nar-ē) (di ZĒZ)	progressive lung disease blocking air flow, which makes breathing difficult. Chronic bronchitis and emphysema are two main components of COPD. Most COPD is a result of cigarette smoking.
3. **computed tomography (CT)** (knm-PU-ted) (tŏ-MOG-re-fē)	diagnostic imaging test producing scans composed from sectional radiographic images, which can be taken in any of the anatomic planes for a multidimensional view of internal structures. Chest computed tomography is often performed to follow up on abnormalities identified on previous chest radiographs. (Figure 4.14, *B*)
4. **coronavirus disease (COVID-19)** (kŏ-RŌ-na-vī-rus) (di-ZĒZ)	respiratory illness caused by a newly discovered virus with symptoms that include fever, cough, fatigue, difficulty breathing, and digestive upset; the disease course can range from mild to severe with the possibility of acute respiratory distress syndrome and multi-system organ failure
FYI Several strains of **coronavirus** exist, including those that cause severe acute respiratory syndrome (SARS), Middle East respiratory syndrome (MERS), and coronavirus disease (COVID-19).	
5. **culture and sensitivity (C&S)** (KUL-cher) (sen-si-TIV-i-tē)	laboratory test performed on a collected sample to determine the presence of pathogenic bacteria or fungi and to identify the most effective antimicrobial treatment. The test may be performed on sputum, throat cultures, blood, urine, and other fluids. Sputum culture and sensitivity tests are frequently used in the diagnosis of lower respiratory tract infections such as bronchitis and pneumonia.
6. **emphysema** (em-fi-SĒ-ma)	loss of elasticity of the alveoli results in distension, causing stretching of the lung. As a result, the body does not receive enough oxygen. (component of COPD)
7. **influenza (flu)** (in-flū-EN-za)	highly contagious and often severe viral infection of the respiratory tract

EXERCISE E   Match

Match the terms in the first column with their correct descriptions in the second column.

_____ 1. asthma

_____ 2. tuberculosis

_____ 3. sputum

_____ 4. influenza

_____ 5. coronavirus disease

_____ 6. chronic obstructive pulmonary disease

a. highly contagious and often severe viral infection of the respiratory tract

b. respiratory illness caused by a newly discovered virus, which ranges from mild to severe with the possibility of acute respiratory distress syndrome and multisystem organ failure

c. chronic bronchitis and emphysema are two main components of this progressive lung disease

d. infectious bacterial disease, most commonly spread by inhalation of small particles and usually affecting the lungs (may spread to other organs)

e. caused by constriction and inflammation of airways that is reversible between attacks

f. mucous secretion from the lungs, bronchi, and trachea expelled through the mouth

NEW—Matching Exercise for Terms NOT Built from Word Parts for additional practice.

Pronunciation & Spelling

Pronunciation and spelling exercises may be completed on paper or online. Students may hear terms pronounced and practice spelling using online resources.

Abbreviations

Tables introduce abbreviated medical terms related to lesson content. Exercises, electronic flashcards, and online activities provide practice for new learning. Additional abbreviations and an error-prone list are provided in Appendix B.

ABBREVIATIONS RELATED TO THE RESPIRATORY SYSTEM			
Use the online **flashcards** to familiarize yourself with the following abbreviations.			
ABBREVIATION	TERM	ABBREVIATION	TERM
ABG	arterial blood gas	P	pulse
BP	blood pressure	PFTs	pulmonary function tests
CO₂	carbon dioxide	PSG	polysomnography
COPD	chronic obstructive pulmonary disease	R	respiration
COVID-19	coronavirus disease	RT	respiratory therapist
CPAP	continuous positive airway pressure	SOAP	subjective, objective, assessment, plan (note format)
C&S	culture and sensitivity	SOB	shortness of breath
CT	computed tomography	T	temerature
CXR	chest radiograph (chest x-ray)	TB	tuberculosis
ET	endotracheal	URI	upper respiratory infection

Clinical Categories

Students practice recall of all the terms, built from word parts and NOT built from word parts, presented in the lesson. Exercises group terms in clinical categories, such as signs and symptoms, to give a sense of how terms are used in the field.

 OBJECTIVE 4

Identify medical terms by clinical category.

Now that you have worked through the respiratory system lesson, review and practice medical terms grouped by clinical category. Categories include signs and symptoms, diseases and disorders, diagnostic tests and equipment, surgical procedures, specialties and professions, and other terms related to the respiratory system.

EXERCISE J   **Signs and Symptoms**

Write the medical terms for signs and symptoms next to their definitions.

1. _____ absence of breathing
2. _____ difficult breathing
3. _____ excessive breathing
4. _____ deficient breathing
5. _____ condition of excessive oxygen
6. _____ condition of deficient oxygen
7. _____ condition of deficient carbon dioxide
8. _____ condition of excessive carbon dioxide
9. _____ discharge from the nose

Practical Application

Students apply medical terms to case studies, corresponding medical records, clinical statements, and in electronic health records online.

NEW—Medical Records Exercises for the Urinary System and Endocrine System Lessons.

Electronic Health Record (EHR) Modules

Lessons 4-12 offer Electronic Health Record modules with three related medical records online. Students apply terms from the lesson within electronic medical records.

EXERCISE S   Use Medical Language in Online Electronic Health Records

Select the correct medical terms to complete three medical records in one patient's electronic file.

🌐 Access online resources at evolve.elsevier.com > Evolve Resources > Practice Student Resources > Activities > Lesson 4 > Electronic Health Records

Topic: COPD
Record 1: Progress Note
Record 2: Radiology Report
Record 3: Pulmonary Function Department Note

❏ Check the box when complete.

Lesson Content Quiz

NEW—Expanded end of lesson content quizzes in the worktext and online in Gradable Student Resources allow students to quickly assess their understanding of medical terms and abbreviations.

EXERCISE U   Lesson Content Quiz

Test your knowledge of the terms and abbreviations introduced in this lesson. Circle the letter for the medical term or abbreviation related to the words in italics.

1. After weeks of experiencing a hoarse voice, the patient underwent a *visual examination of the larynx* performed by an otolaryngologist to determine the cause.
   a. laryngoscope
   b. laryngoscopy
   c. laryngectomy

2. The breathing disorder involving the *absence of spontaneous respiration* is called:
   a. apnea
   b. hypopnea
   c. dyspnea

4. A polysomnography test was ordered to rule out *repetitive pharyngeal collapse during sleep* or:
   a. OSA
   b. SOB
   c. C&S

5. During evaluation of the patient presenting with dyspnea, the *condition of excessive carbon dioxide* was discovered.
   a. hyperoxia
   b. hypercapnia
   c. hypoxia

Lesson at a Glance

Lessons conclude with a concise review of word parts, terms, and abbreviations presented.

LESSON AT A GLANCE RESPIRATORY SYSTEM MEDICAL TERMS AND ABBREVIATIONS

SIGNS AND SYMPTOMS
apnea
dyspnea
hypercapnia
hyperoxia
hyperpnea
hypocapnia
hypopnea
hypoxia
rhinitis

DISEASES AND DISORDERS
asthma
bronchitis
bronchopneumonia
chronic obstructive pulmonary disease
 (COPD)
coronavirus disease (COVID-19)
emphysema
influenza (flu)
laryngitis
nasopharyngitis
obstructive sleep apnea (OSA)
pharyngitis
pneumonia
pneumothorax
rhinorrhagia
rhinorrhea
sinusitis
tuberculosis (TB)
upper respiratory infection (URI)

**DIAGNOSTIC TESTS
AND EQUIPMENT**
bronchoscope
bronchoscopy
capnometer
computed tomography (CT)
culture and sensitivity (C&S)
endoscope
endoscopic
endoscopy
laryngoscope
laryngoscopy
oximeter
polysomnogram
polysomnography (PSG)
radiograph
spirometer
thoracoscope
thoracoscopic
thoracoscopy

SURGICAL PROCEDURES
laryngectomy
pneumonectomy
sinusotomy
thoracentesis
thoracotomy
tracheostomy
tracheotomy

SPECIALTIES AND PROFESSIONS
pulmonologist
pulmonology

RELATED TERMS
endotracheal (ET)
laryngeal
mucous
nasal
pharyngeal
pulmonary
sputum
thoracic

ABBREVIATIONS

ABG	CXR	R
BP	ET	RT
CO₂	flu	T
COPD	O₂	SOAP
COVID-19	OSA	SOB
C&S	P	TB
CPAP	PFTs	URI
CT	PSG	V/Q scan

Online Learning Resources at evolve.elsevier.com

Evolve content online provides activities, exercises, quizzes, and exams. Practice Student Resources are available to supplement your learning and scores are for student use only. Gradable Student Resources may populate your class' gradebook if your instructor has set it up to do so. Gradable Student Resources are available to all students whether or not your instructor chooses to record scores.

Practice Student Resources

- Word Part and Abbreviation Flashcards
- Pronunciation and Spelling
- Electronic Health Record Modules
- Games
- Practice Quizzes
- Career Videos
- Animations
- Additional Appendices on Pharmacology, Health Information Technology, and Integrative Medicine

Gradable Student Resources

- Exercises: Terms Built from Word Parts and Terms NOT Built from Word Parts
- Lesson Practice Exams

APPENDIX D

Pharmacology Terms

Topics include:

General Drug Categories, p. e11.
General Pharmacy Terms, p. e12.
Routes of Administration, p. e14.

GENERAL DRUG CATEGORIES	
analgesic	an agent that reduces pain
anesthetic	an agent that reduces sensation locally or systemically and may cause loss of consciousness
antibacterial	a drug that targets bacteria to kill or halt growth or replication
antibiotic	a drug that targets bacteria, fungi, or protozoa to kill or halt growth or replication; commonly used as a synonym for antibacterial
anticholinergic agent	a drug that blocks the neurotransmitter acetylcholine to suppress the parasympathetic

GENERAL DRUG CATEGORIES	
antiretroviral	a drug that suppresses the replication of retroviruses, such as the human immunodeficiency virus (HIV); highly active antiretroviral therapy (HAART) is the combination of three or more of these drugs to treat HIV infection
antiviral	a drug that targets viruses to kill or halt growth or replication
anxiolytic	a drug that calms anxiety
bactericidal	the designation for an antimicrobial agent that kills or destroys bacteria

Create an Account and Register for Evolve Resources

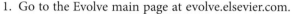 Use the following instructions to request Evolve Student Resources for *Basic Medical Language 7ᵗʰ Edition*. Technical help may be reached by calling 1-800-222-9570.

1. Go to the Evolve main page at evolve.elsevier.com.
2. Click *Sign In* on the upper right corner of the screen.
3. Click Create account and select Student.
4. Enter your personal details and provide a new password of at least 7 characters.
5. Click Submit. After completing these steps: A pop-up appears with your automatically generated username and your provided password; an email with your login details will be sent to the email address you gave at registration, then you can log in to Evolve with your username and password.
6. Select the Catalog near the top of the screen. Use the search box and enter Basic Medical Language, 7th Edition.
7. Click on Evolve Resources for Basic Medical Language, 7th Edition.
8. Click Checkout/Redeem and follow the prompts to finish the process.
9. After completing these steps there are two ways to access Evolve Resources content:
   - My Content tab at evolve.elsevier.com. See the menu to the left of the screen; click on Student Resources.
   - Evolve Links on your course site if your instructor has made them available. Links will take you to the activities, exercises, and quizzes your instructor has chosen.

Note: Gradable Student Resources will upload to the course gradebook if your instructor has set it up as such, otherwise the exercises and exams are for practice only.

FYI   Registration Steps may change as the Evolve website is updated. If difficulties arise, please:
- Call technical support at 1-800-222-9570.
- Type "evolve support center" in your browser and follow the links for help in accessing Evolve.

HOW WILL I LEARN?

The worktext and companion online resources hosted on the Evolve website offer a variety of ways to learn chapter content. The paper and online learning activities are coordinated and designed to cultivate long-term learning.

Word Parts

Worktext
- Read word parts and definitions
- Label anatomic diagrams
- Complete exercises and check responses
- Practice with paper flashcards

Online Resources
- Practice with online Flashcards
- Complete the Pair It Activity for Word Parts
- Take the Word Part Practice Quiz

Medical Terms Built From Word Parts

Worktext
- Build terms
- Translate terms
- Label illustrations
- Read terms in context
- Pronounce and spell

Online Resources
- Listen to and repeat terms aloud using the Audio Glossary
- Complete the Spell Terms Activity
- Complete the Terms Built from Word Parts Activity
- Watch Animations

Medical Terms NOT Built From Word Parts

Worktext
- Read terms with definitions
- Label illustrations
- Complete in-context exercise
- Pronounce and spell

Online Resources
- Listen to and repeat terms aloud using the Audio Glossary
- Complete the Spell Terms Activity
- Complete the Terms NOT Built from Word Parts Activity
- Watch Animations

Abbreviations

Worktext
- Read abbreviations with definitions
- Complete exercises grouped by clinical category
- Reference Appendix B with common abbreviations and an error-prone list

Online Resources
- Practice with online Flashcards
- Complete the Pair It Activity for Abbreviations
- Take Abbreviation Practice Quiz

Practical Application

Worktext
- Define terms grouped by clinical category
- Identify correct terms used in clinical statements
- Apply medical terms to the case study
- Write medical terms within a medical health record and answer related questions

Online Resources
- Apply medical terms to three related medical records in EHR modules

Review

Worktext
- Take lesson content quiz
- Practice recall with Lesson at a Glance

Online Resources
- Review word part and abbreviation flashcards
- Play Games
- Take the Medical Term Practice Quiz
- Take the Practice Exam

DEAR INSTRUCTOR

Thank you for choosing *Basic Medical Language*! We hope you find our learning system supportive of your teaching methods and effective for your students' learning styles. With the purchase of a new worktext, students receive paper flashcards for word parts and access to Evolve Resources for students. You may find the flashcards and online resources, such as pronunciation for term lists and games, useful for class activities and exam preparation.

Additional teaching materials are available online at **evolve.elsevier. com** within Evolve Resources for Instructors. All resources are objective based, and we recommend beginning with the TEACH Lesson Plans for an overview of the various teaching tools. The first step in accessing teaching materials is to register for the *Basic Medical Language 6th Edition* Evolve Resources. Please visit evolve.elsevier.com or call **1-800-222-9570** to register.

We welcome your comments and questions by email. Danielle, who currently teaches medical terminology in the traditional classroom, online, and in hybrid formats, is also happy to share ideas and materials. Contact us at danielle.lafleurbrooks@ccv.edu, dale.levinsky@gmail.com, and myrnabrooks@comcast.net. We also invite you to visit Myrna's Medical Terminology Blog found at https://medical-terminologyblog.com to keep up with trends in teaching medical terminology and emerging medical language.

Looking forward to hearing from you,

Danielle, Dale, and Myrna

Online Teaching Resources at evolve.elsevier.com

Instructor Resources

- Image Collection
- Sample Course Syllabus and Outline
- TEACH Handouts
- TEACH Lesson Plans
- TEACH PowerPoint Slides
- Test Bank

Assessment

- Formative and summative assessment plan for each lesson, TEACH Lesson Plans in Evolve Instructor Resources
- Pretest and Posttest, TEACH Lesson Plans in Evolve Instructor Resources
- Practice Quizzes, Evolve Student Resources
- Practice Exams, Evolve Student Resources
- Test Bank to build quizzes and exams, Evolve Instructor Resources

---

FYI For assistance in registering for Evolve Resources, call **1-800-222-9570** or visit **https://evolve.elsevier.com/education/contact-us**.

Also Available

Elsevier Adaptive Learning

Corresponding lesson-by-lesson to *Basic Medical Terminology*, seventh Edition, **Elsevier Adaptive Learning** combines the power of brain science with sophisticated, patented Cerego algorithms to help you learn faster and remember longer. It's fun, it's engaging, and it constantly tracks your performance and adapts to deliver content precisely when it's needed to ensure core information is transformed into lasting knowledge.

Reviewers and Advisors

REVIEWERS

Nicole J. Boardman
Medical Student
University of Arizona College of Medicine
Phoenix, Arizona

Rachel Farmer
Registered Nurse
AdventHealth
Overland Park, Kansas

PREVIOUS EDITION REVIEWERS/ ADVISORS

Cynthia A. Bjerklie, MEd
Medical Assisting Instructor
Community College of Vermont
Montpelier, Vermont

Richard K. Brooks, MD, FACP, FACG
Internal Medicine and Gastroenterology
Mayo Clinic (retired)
Scottsdale, Arizona

Ruth Buchner
Family and Consumer Science/Health Science
    Educator
Chippewa Falls Senior High School
Chippewa Falls, Wisconsin

Christine Costa, BS, GCM, HUC
Geriatric Care Manager
Tempe, Arizona

Heather Drake, RN, BSN
Instructor, Nursing
Southern West Virginia Community & Technical
    College
Mt. Gay, West Virginia

Erin Hayes, MS, MAT
Foundations of Medicine Instructor
Medicine & Healthcare Strand Leader
Blue Valley Center for Advanced Professional Studies
Overland Park, Kansas

Denise M. Hellman, RN, BN, MN
Nursing Instructor
Medicine Hat College
Division of Health Studies
Medicine Hat, Alberta

Melody Miller, LPN, VOC II
Medical Assistant Instructor
Lancaster County Career & Technology Center
Willow Street, Pennsylvania

Suezette Musick-Hicks, MEd, RRT, CPFT
Director, Respiratory Care Program
Black River Technical College
Pocahontas, Arkansas

Charlene Thiessen, MEd
Program Director Emeritus, Medical Transcription
GateWay Community College
Phoenix, Arizona

Ann Vadala
Professor, Office Administration – Health Services
Coordinator, Health Care Administration
School of Business
St. Lawrence College
Kingston, Ontario

Tiffani Walker, MSRS, RT(R)
Clinical Coordinator, Radiology
North Central Texas College
Gainesville, Texas

Dokagari Woods, PhD, RN
Assistant Professor and Undergraduate Program
    Director, Nursing
Tarleton State University
Stephenville, Texas

Introduction to Medical Language, Body Structure, Oncology, and Laboratory Tests

CASE STUDY Tova Katz

Tova has been having diarrhea. Even worse, she notices blood in it. She had this before when she was younger, and the disease process was identified, but she couldn't remember the name. She was put on medicine and got better. It looked like a positive outcome. Now it's been going on for 3 weeks. She has pain in her belly with cramps and feels kind of full all the time. She notices she is losing weight, even though she isn't trying. She also feels more tired than usual. Tova makes an appointment with her family doctor to see if she needs to go back on medicine.

■ *Consider Tova's situation as you work through the lesson on body structure and oncology. We will return to this case study and identify medical terms used to document Tova's experience and the care she receives.*

OBJECTIVES

1 ■ Identify the origins of medical language, the four word parts, and the combining form (p. 1).

2 ■ Build, translate, pronounce, and spell medical terms built from word parts (p. 6).

3 ■ Define, pronounce, and spell medical terms NOT built from word parts (p. 18).

4 ■ Write abbreviations (p. 23).

5 ■ Identify body structure, oncology, and laboratory terms (p. 24).

6 ■ Use medical language in clinical statements, the case study, and medical records (p. 26).

7 ■ Recall and assess knowledge of word parts, medical terms, and abbreviations (p. 30).

OBJECTIVE 1

Identify the origins of medical language, the four word parts, and the combining form.

The vocabulary of medical language reflects its development over time, starting with the ancient Greeks, who were among the first to study and write about medicine. The Romans continued this practice, adapting elements of the Greek language to use alongside Latin. Today, we can see the historical roots of medical language in the use of **terms built from Greek and Latin word parts**. As medical language evolved with scientific advancements, **eponyms**, **acronyms**, and terms from **modern language** have also come into use (Figure 1.1).

Greek and Latin
Terms built from Greek and Latin word parts, such as **arthritis**.

Eponyms
Terms named after a person or place; examples include **Apgar score**, named after the physician who invented it; **Alzheimer disease**, named after the first person to identify the disease; and **West Nile virus**, named after the first geographical location at which the virus was identified.

Acronyms
Terms formed from the first letters of the words in a phrase that can be spoken as a whole word. Such terms usually contain a vowel. An example is **laser** (light amplification by stimulated emission of radiation).

Modern language
Terms derived from the English language, such as **nuclear medicine scanner**.

Figure 1.1 Origins of medical language.

> **FYI**   **Alzheimer disease vs. Alzheimer's disease**
> The need for clarity and consistency in medical language has resulted in the modern trend to eliminate the possessive form of eponyms and instead use the nonpossessive form, which omits the apostrophe "s." The nonpossessive form is observed by the Association for Healthcare Documentation Integrity, the American Medical Association's Manual of Style, in most medical dictionaries, and in this textbook. With either use, the noun that follows is not capitalized.

EXERCISE A   Identify Origins of Medical Language

For questions 1-4, write the letter of the origin of a medical term next to its description. Check responses using the Answer Key in Appendix C.

_____ **1.** Terms formed from the first letters of the words in a phrase that can be spoken as a whole word

_____ **2.** Terms derived from the English language reflecting scientific advancement and new technologies

_____ **3.** Terms built from word parts

_____ **4.** Terms named for a person or place

a. acronym
b. eponym
c. modern language
d. Greek and Latin

5. *Draw a line matching the origin of medical language with its example.*

    a. acronym   posttraumatic stress disorder
    b. eponym   LASIK
    c. modern language   arthritis
    d. Greek and Latin   Parkinson disease

Categories of Medical Terms and Learning Methods

For the purpose of our studies, medical terms are categorized as *built from word parts* and as *NOT built from word parts*. Specific learning methods will be used for each category.

TABLE 1.1   CATEGORIES OF MEDICAL TERMS AND LEARNING METHODS

CATEGORY	ORIGIN	EXAMPLE	LEARNING METHODS
Terms Built from Word Parts (can be translated to find their meaning)	1. Word parts of Greek and Latin origin put together to form terms that can be translated to find their meanings	1. arthr/itis	1. Translating terms 2. Building terms
Terms NOT Built from Word Parts (cannot be easily translated to find their meaning)	1. Eponyms, terms named for a person or place	1. Alzheimer disease	1. Memorizing terms
	2. Acronyms, terms formed from the first letters of a phrase that can be spoken as a whole word and usually contain a vowel	2. LASIK (laser-assisted in situ keratomileusis)	
	3. Modern language, terms from the English language	3. complete blood count with differential	
	4. Terms of Greek and Latin word parts that cannot be easily translated to find their meanings	4. orthopedics	

Terms Built from Word Parts

Terms built from word parts may be easily understood by learning the meaning of the individual word parts. The four types of word parts that may be used in forming a medical term are **word root, suffix, prefix,** and **combining vowel**.

TABLE 1.2   USING WORD PARTS TO BUILD MEDICAL TERMS

WORD PART	DESCRIPTION	ABBREVIATION
word root	core of the term; fundamental meaning. All medical terms have one or more word roots.	wr
suffix	attached to the end of the word root and provides additional information; modifies meaning. Not all medical terms have a suffix.	s
prefix	attached to the beginning of the word root and provides additional information; modifies meaning. Not all medical terms have a prefix.	p
combining vowel	vowel, usually an **o,** placed between two word roots and between a word root and a suffix (if the suffix does not begin with a vowel); eases pronunciation	cv

EXAMPLE 1: INTRAVENOUS

	WORD PART	MEANING
prefix	intra-	within
word root	ven	vein
suffix	-ous	pertaining to
term = p + wr + s	intra/ven/ous	pertaining to within a vein

> **FYI** Usually, the **meaning of the suffix** will initiate the definition of a medical term categorized as built from word parts.

EXAMPLE 2: OSTEOARTHRITIS

	WORD PART	MEANING
word root	oste	bone
combining vowel	o	none; eases pronunciation
word root	arthr	joint
suffix	-itis	inflammation
term = wr + cv + wr + s	oste/o/arthr/itis	inflammation of the bone and joint

Combining Form

A combining form is a word root with the combining vowel attached, separated by a slash. *For learning purposes, word roots are presented with their combining vowels as combining forms.*

EXAMPLES
arthr/o
oste/o
ven/o

> **FYI** **Word roots** are presented as **combining forms** throughout the text.

Terms NOT Built from Word Parts

Basic Medical Language would not be complete without including commonly used terms, such as **heart failure,** that are not built from word parts. Although there is less emphasis on these terms, they are important in the development of a medical vocabulary. While memorization is the primary method for learning terms not built from word parts, textbook exercises incorporate related information to help remember definitions and to develop a sense of how the terms are used in context.

Some terms containing recognizable word parts are categorized as *NOT Built from Word Parts* because they are difficult to translate. For example, orth/o/ped/ic is made up of three word parts: **orth**, meaning "straight"; **ped**, meaning "child" or "foot"; and **-ic**, meaning "pertaining to." Translated literally, *orthopedic* would seem to mean **pertaining to a straight child or foot**; however, the current use of the term *orthopedic* refers to the **branch of medicine dealing with the study and treatment of diseases and abnormalities of the musculoskeletal system**. Because the term *orthopedic* cannot be translated from word parts to understand its meaning, it is categorized as *NOT Built from Word Parts* in this textbook.

| **EXERCISE B**   Define Word Parts, Combining Forms, and Categories of Medical Terms |

Check your responses using the Answer Key in Appendix C.

A. *Match the phrases in the first column with the correct terms in the second column.*

_____1. Core of the term

_____2. Attached at the end of a word root

_____3. Definitions can be easily understood by knowing meanings of word parts.

_____4. Word root presented with its combining vowel

_____5. Used to ease pronunciation; usually an "o"

_____6. Definitions **cannot** be easily understood by knowing meanings of word parts.

_____7. Attached at the beginning of a word root

a. terms built from word parts
b. terms NOT built from word parts
c. word root
d. prefix
e. suffix
f. combining vowel
g. combining form

B. *Fill in the blanks to complete the following sentences.*

1. There are four types of word parts used to build medical terms. The fundamental meaning of a term may be understood by knowing the meaning of the core of the term or the _____ _____.

2. To modify the meaning of a term, a suffix may be added at the _____ of a word root or a prefix may be added at its _____.

3. Most often, when translating the meaning of a term built from word parts, begin with the definition of the word part attached to the end of the term, or the _____. The next step is to translate the word part attached to the beginning of the term, or the _____. Finally, add the definition of the word root to discern the full meaning of the term. For example, the term **intra/ven/ous** can be translated literally in this way to find its meaning, _____ to _____ a _____ (see Example 1 in Table 1.2).

4. To ease pronunciation, a term may have a vowel placed between two word roots or between a word root and a suffix; use of a vowel in this way is known as a _____ _____. The term **oste/o/arthr/itis** has the combining vowel **o** inserted between the word roots **oste** and **arthr** to ease pronunciation. A combining vowel is not inserted between the word root **arthr** and the suffix **-itis** because the suffix begins with the vowel **i**. Osteoarthritis can be translated literally by defining the suffix and then word roots to mean _____ of the _____ and _____ (See Example 2 in Table 1.2).

OBJECTIVE 2

Build, translate, pronounce, and spell medical terms built from word parts.

Body Structure, Oncology, and Laboratory Tests

The structure of the human body falls into four categories: cells, tissues, organs, and systems. Each structure is a highly organized unit of smaller structures (Figure 1.3). **Oncology** is the study of tumors. Tumors develop from excessive growth of cells. Oncology terms are introduced in this lesson because of their relationship to cells and cell abnormalities. Oncology terms naming tumors of specific organs and body systems are introduced in subsequent lessons.

Laboratory tests provide information that helps diagnose diseases, including cancer. Diagnostic laboratories, or labs, are located in hospitals, providers' offices, and stand-alone facilities. These physical labs are divided into sections according to specialization, such as cytology for the study of cells, or histology for the study of tissues. Additional laboratory terms measuring aspects of specific body systems are introduced in subsequent lessons.

BODY STRUCTURE

STRUCTURE	DESCRIPTION
cell	basic unit of all living things; the human body is composed of trillions of cells that vary in size and shape according to function
tissue	group of similar cells that perform a specific function
organ	two or more kinds of tissues that together perform special body functions
system	group of organs that work together to perform complex body functions

Body Tissues

Tissues can be grouped into four main categories, each having a specific function (Figure 1.4).

BODY TISSUES

TISSUE	DESCRIPTION
muscle tissue	composed of cells that have a special ability to contract, usually producing movement
nerve tissue	found in the nerves, spinal cord, and brain; coordinates and controls body functions
connective tissue	connects, supports, penetrates, and encases various body structures; forms bones, fat, cartilage, and blood
epithelial tissue	the major covering of the external surface of the body; forms membranes that line body cavities and organs and is the major tissue in glands; (also called **epithelium**)

Body Cavities and Organs

The body is not a solid structure, as it appears on the outside, but has cavities containing an orderly arrangement of the internal organs (Figure 1.6).

BODY CAVITIES AND ORGANS

CAVITY	ORGANS
cranial cavity	brain
spinal cavity	spinal cord
thoracic cavity	heart, aorta, lungs, esophagus, trachea, and bronchi
abdominal cavity	stomach, intestines, kidneys, liver, gallbladder, pancreas, spleen, and ureters
pelvic cavity	urinary bladder, certain reproductive organs, parts of the small and large intestines, and rectum

FYI   **Abdominopelvic cavity** refers to the abdominal cavity and the pelvic cavity. See Figure 1.6.

Body Systems

Each system is made up of organs that work together to perform specific tasks. Although body systems play individual roles, they are interrelated, working together to maintain life.

BODY SYSTEMS

BODY SYSTEM	ORGANS, GLANDS, AND TISSUES	BASIC FUNCTIONS
integumentary system	skin, hair, nails, and sweat and oil glands	covers and protects body, regulates body temperature, and helps manufacture vitamin D
respiratory system	nose, pharynx, larynx, trachea, bronchi, and lungs	exchanges oxygen and carbon dioxide between blood and external environment
urinary system	kidneys, ureters, urinary bladder, and urethra	removes waste material (urine), regulates fluid volume, and maintains electrolyte concentration
reproductive system	female: ovaries, uterus, uterine (fallopian) tubes, and vagina; male: testes, vas deferens, prostate gland, and penis	produces offspring, secretes hormones that produce feminine and masculine physical traits
cardiovascular system	heart and blood vessels	pumps and transports blood throughout the body
lymphatic system	lymph, lymph nodes, lymphatic vessels, spleen, and thymus	provides defense against infection and other diseases and drainage of extracellular fluid
digestive system	mouth, pharynx, esophagus, stomach, intestines, gallbladder, liver, and pancreas	prepares food for use by the body's cells and eliminates waste
musculoskeletal system	muscles, bones, cartilage, ligaments, and tendons	provides movement and framework for the body, protects vital organs, stores calcium, and produces blood cells
nervous system	brain, spinal cord, and nerves	regulates specific body activities by sending and receiving messages
endocrine system	pituitary, thyroid, thymus, adrenal glands, and pancreas	secretes hormones that regulate specific body activities

CAREER FOCUS — Professionals Who Work with Body Structure, Oncology, and Laboratory Terms

- **Laboratory technologists and technicians** collect samples and perform tests to analyze body fluids such as blood and urine. Both technicians and technologists perform tests ordered by physicians; however, technologists perform more complex tests and laboratory procedures than technicians.

- **Pharmacy technicians** work under the supervision of a licensed pharmacist to prepare and dispense prescriptions. Tech duties also include answering the phone, data entry, and customer service.

- **Radiation therapists** administer high doses of radiation to treat cancer and other disease. They work closely with radiation oncologists, oncology nurses, and medical physicists.

Figure 1.2 Laboratory technologist working with collection samples.

WORD PARTS — Use the paper or online **flashcards** to familiarize yourself with the following word parts.

COMBINING FORM (WR + CV)	DEFINITION	COMBINING FORM (WR + CV)	DEFINITION
carcin/o	cancer	onc/o	tumor(s)
cyt/o	cell(s)	organ/o	organ
epitheli/o	epithelium, epithelial tissue	path/o	disease
hist/o	tissue(s)	radi/o	x-rays (ionizing radiation)
lip/o	fat, fat tissue	sarc/o	flesh, connective tissue
my/o	muscle(s), muscle tissue	system/o	system
neur/o	nerve(s), nerve tissue	viscer/o	internal organs

Word roots are the core of the word (fundamental meaning). Each medical term contains one or more word roots. *Combining forms* are word roots with their combining vowels.

SUFFIX (S)	DEFINITION	SUFFIX (S)	DEFINITION
-al	pertaining to	-megaly	enlargement
-genic	producing, originating, causing	-oid	resembling
-ic	pertaining to	-oma	tumor
-logist	one who studies and treats (specialist, physician)	-plasm	growth (substance or formation)
-logy	study of	-stasis	control, stop

Suffixes are attached to the end of the word root to modify its meaning. Not all medical terms have a suffix.

Continued

WORD PARTS	Use the paper or online **flashcards** to familiarize yourself with the following word parts—cont'd		
PREFIX (P)	**DEFINITION**	**PREFIX (P)**	**DEFINITION**
meta-	beyond	**neo-**	new

Prefixes are attached to the beginning of the word root to modify its meaning. Not all medical terms have a prefix.

COMBINING VOWEL (CV)

A *combining vowel*, usually an o, is used to ease pronunciation:
- between two word roots
- between a word root and a suffix (if the suffix does not begin with a vowel)

Refer to Appendix A for an alphabetized list of word parts and their meanings.

Pronunciation

Use the following Pronunciation Key to read the phonetic spellings of terms aloud. Phonetic spellings are provided with medical terms in the READ exercises and in term tables.

TABLE 1.3	**PRONUNCIATION KEY**	
GUIDELINES		EXAMPLES
1. Words are distorted minimally to indicate proper phonetic sound.		doctor (dok-tor), gastric (gas-trik)
2. Capital letters indicate the primary accent.		doctor (DOC-tor), gastric (GAS-trik)
3. The macron (¯) indicates the long vowel sound.		donate (dō-nāte)
		ā as in say **ō** as in no
		ē as in me **ū** as in cute
		ī as in spine
4. Vowels with no markings should have the short sound.		medical (med-i-cal)
		a as in sad **o** as in top
		e as in get **u** as in cut
		i as in sit

EXERCISE C	**Build and Translate Terms Built from Word Parts**

*Use the **Word Parts Table** to complete the following questions. Check your responses with the Answer Key in Appendix C.*

1. **MATCH:** Suffixes are attached to the end of word roots to provide additional information. *Draw a line to match the suffix with its definition.*

    a. -al   tumor

    b. -logy   pertaining to

    c. -oma   study of

2. LABEL: The word root is the core of a term. All medical terms built from word parts have one or more word roots. The combining form is the word root presented with its combining vowel. The structure of the human body falls into four categories: cells, tissues, organs, and systems.

Write the combining forms for structures of the human body in Figure 1.3.

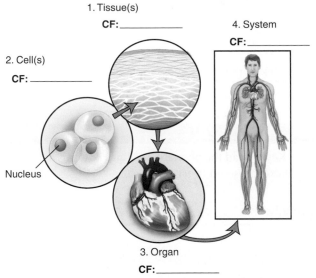

1. Tissue(s)
   CF:_____

4. System
   CF:_____

2. Cell(s)
   CF:_____

Nucleus

3. Organ
   CF:_____

Figure 1.3 Structure of the human body.

3. TRANSLATE: *Complete the definition of the following term by using the meaning of word parts to fill in the blanks. The definition of a term usually starts with the meaning of the suffix, and then moves to the beginning of the term.*

Example: cyt/o/logy   <u>study</u> of <u>cell</u> (s)

            hist/o/logy   _____ of _____(s)

> **FYI**   **Translate** exercises ask you to define medical terms using the meaning of combining forms and word parts. Begin the definition of the term with the meaning of the suffix, and then move to the beginning of the term and apply the meaning of the next word part (prefix) or combining form. **Check your answers using Appendix C.**

4. READ: Knowing the meaning of even a few combining forms and word parts will unlock the meaning of many medical terms. The term **cytology** (sī-TOL-o-jē) contains the combining form **cyt/o**, which means cell. The suffix -**logy** means study of. The medical term cyt/o/logy means study of cells. In the term **histology** (his-TOL-o-jē), **hist/o** means tissue(s). Hist/o/logy means study of tissues. Cytology and histology take place in a medical laboratory and involve microscopic examination of biopsied specimens.

> **FYI**   The **o** in the terms cyt/o/logy and hist/o/logy is a **combining vowel**, which is used between word parts to ease pronunciation.

5. **LABEL:** Tissues are groups of cells that perform specific tasks. Four types of tissues are nerve, connective, muscle, and epithelium.

Write the combining forms for tissues of the human body to complete Figure 1.4.

1. Nerve(s), nerve tissue
   CF: _____

2. Epithelium, epithelial tissue
   CF: _____

3. Flesh, connective tissue
   CF: _____

4. Muscle(s), muscle tissue.
   CF: _____

Figure 1.4 Types of tissue.

---

6. **BUILD:** Tumors may develop from tissues. Medical terms for specific types of tumors are often built with a combining form for the related anatomic structure and the suffix **–oma**.

Write the combining forms and word parts to build the terms defined. The definition of the term usually begins with the meaning of the suffix, followed by the meaning of the prefix or combining form at the beginning of the term.

> **FYI**   **Build**
> exercises ask you to write the components of a medical term using its definition and the meanings of combining forms and word parts. Check your answers using Appendix C.

Example: tumor (composed of)   _____neur___ / ___oma___
      nerve tissue   **wr**   **s**

a. tumor (composed of) muscle   _____/_____
      tissue   **wr**   **s**

b. tumor (composed of)   _____/_____
      epithelial tissue   **wr**   **s**

c. tumor (of) connective tissue _____/_____
                                            wr   **s**

> **FYI**   The definition of the medical term **sarcoma** does not contain the word "composed" because it grows in connective tissue rather than being made up of connective tissue.

7. READ: Definitions of medical terms built from Greek and Latin word parts may contain additional words that are not a part of the literal translation. For example, the definition of **neur/oma** is tumor (composed of) nerve tissue. You will become familiar with these variations as you learn the medical terms. Tumors may be considered benign (nonrecurring) or malignant (tending to become progressively worse). **Neuroma** (nū-RŌ-ma) and **myoma** (mī-Ō-ma) are benign tumors. An **epithelioma** (ep-i-thē-lē-Ō-ma) may be benign or malignant. **Sarcoma** (sar-KŌ-ma) usually indicates a highly malignant tumor arising from connective tissue, such as bone or cartilage.

8. MATCH: *Draw a line matching the word part with its definition.*

   a. lip/o   tumor
   b. carcin/o   fat, fat tissue
   c. -oma   resembling
   d. -oid   cancer

9. TRANSLATE: *Complete the definitions of the following terms by using the meaning of word parts to fill in the blanks. The definition of a term usually starts with the meaning of the suffix, and then moves to the beginning of the term.*

   a. lip/oma   _____ (composed of) _____ tissue
   b. lip/oid   _____ fat
   c. carcin/oid   resembling _____

10. READ: **Lipoma** (li-PŌ-ma) refers to a benign tumor composed of fat tissue (a type of connective tissue). Lipomas are commonly found below the skin of the neck and trunk. **Lipoid** (LIP-oid) describes a fatlike substance. **Carcinoid** (KAR-si-noyd) describes a type of slow-growing tumor that can emit hormones.

11. LABEL: *Write word parts to complete Figure 1.5.*

Figure 1.5 _____/_____.
                          fat   tumor

12. **LABEL:** The body is not a solid structure as it appears on the outside. It has five cavities: cranial, spinal, thoracic, abdominal, and pelvic. Sometimes the abdominal and pelvic cavities are referred to as the abdominopelvic cavity. Body cavities contain internal organs and other anatomic structures.

Write the combining form for internal organs in the space provided in Figure 1.6.

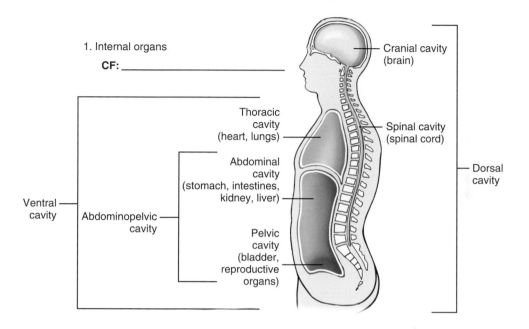

1. Internal organs

   CF: _____

Cranial cavity
(brain)

Thoracic
cavity
(heart, lungs)

Spinal cavity
(spinal cord)

Abdominal
cavity
(stomach, intestines,
kidney, liver)

Dorsal
cavity

Ventral
cavity

Abdominopelvic
cavity

Pelvic
cavity
(bladder,
reproductive
organs)

Figure 1.6 Body cavities.

> **FYI** The five body cavities may be grouped into more general categories known as the **dorsal cavity** and the **ventral cavity**. The ventral cavity, located in the anterior (front) portion of the body, is made up of the thoracic and abdominopelvic cavities. The dorsal cavity, located in the posterior (back) portion of the body, is made up of the cranial and spinal cavities.

13. **MATCH:** *Draw a line matching the word part with its definition.*

    a. -al   organ
    b. -megaly   pertaining to
    c. -ic   epithelium
    d. organ/o   enlargement
    e. epitheli/o   system
    f. system/o

14. BUILD: *Write the combining forms and word parts to build the following terms. Hint: Use **-al** to build the first two descriptive terms.*

a. pertaining to internal organs _____ / _____
                                                 wr   s

b. pertaining to epithelium _____ / _____
                     wr   s

c. pertaining to a (body) system (or the body as a whole) _____ / _____
                     wr   s

d. enlargement of an organ _____ / o / _____
                     wr   cv   s

15. READ: Visceral (VIS-er-al) is an adjective describing internal organs such as those found in the thoracic and abdominal cavities. **Epithelial** (ep-i-THĒ-lē-al) tissue covers the external surface of the body, the surfaces of internal organs, and the linings of body cavities. A **systemic** (sis-TEM-ik) infection occurs when a local infection moves into the bloodstream, where it may then spread to other areas. **Organomegaly** (or-ga-nō-MEG-a-lē) may be discovered during physical examination when the provider applies pressure to the body surface with the fingertips (palpation).

16. MATCH: *Draw a line matching the word part with its definition.*

a. path/o   study of
b. -genic   one who studies and treats (specialist, physician)
c. -logy   disease
d. -logist   producing, originating, causing

FYI The suffix **-logist** may indicate a specialist such as a **psychologist, who is not a physician,** or a specialist such as an **oncologist, who is a physician.** For learning purposes in the text, if the specialist is a physician, it will be indicated in the definition, such as: **oncologist … a physician who studies and treats tumors.**

17. TRANSLATE: *Complete the definitions of the following terms by using the meaning of word parts to fill in the blanks. Hint: Use **producing** for the definition of **-genic**.*

a. path/o/logist   physician who studies _____
b. path/o/genic   _____
c. path/o/logy   _____ of disease

18. READ: A **pathologist** (pa-THOL-o-jist) studies cell, tissue, and organ specimens and performs autopsies to determine the presence and cause of disease. A pathologist is commonly employed in the **pathology** (pa-THOL-o-jē) department of a hospital or healthcare center and does not directly treat patients. Pathology, abbreviated as **PATH**, is a branch of medicine focused on the study of the causes of disease and death. **Pathogenic** (path-ō-JEN-ik), an adjective, describes a substance that produces disease.

19. BUILD: *Write the combining forms and word parts to build the following terms.*

a. study of x-rays

_____ / o / _____
        wr   cv   s

b. physician who studies and treats using x-rays

_____ / o / _____
        wr   cv   s

20. READ: Radiology (rā-dē-OL-o-jē) is the branch of medicine concerned with the use of radiation to diagnose and treat diseases. While literally translated as the study of x-rays, radiology includes other diagnostic imaging procedures, such as computed tomography, magnetic resonance imaging, sonography, and nuclear medicine. A **radiologist** (rā-dē-OL-o-jist) is a physician who interprets images generated by diagnostic imaging procedures and who performs treatments using imaging modalities.

21. MATCH: *Draw a line matching the word part with its definition.*

a. carcin/o   beyond
b. -oma   control, stop
c. -genic   growth (substance or formation)
d. meta-   cancer
e. neo-   producing, originating, causing
f. -plasm   new
g. -stasis   tumor

> **FYI**   The suffixes **-plasm** and **-stasis** are considered to have embedded word roots, which means that they may appear in terms with a prefix and no other combining form. In these instances, suffixes with embedded word roots will be noted as **s(wr)**.

22. BUILD: *Write the combining forms and word parts to build the following terms related to cancer.*

a. new growth

_____ / _____
        p   s(wr)

b. beyond control

_____ / _____
        p   s(wr)

c. producing cancer

_____ / o / _____
        wr   cv   s

d. cancerous tumor
    Hint: In this instance the definition of the term starts with the combining form rather than the suffix.

_____ / _____
        wr   s

23. READ: A **neoplasm** (NĒ-ō-plazm) is a new growth, which may also be called a tumor. Tumors may be either malignant (cancerous) or benign (noncancerous). **Carcinoma** (kar-si-NŌ-ma), abbreviated as **CA**, is a term used to describe a malignant new growth. **Carcinogenic** (kar-sin-ō-JEN-ik), an adjective, describes a substance that produces cancer.

24. LABEL: *Write word parts to complete Figure 1.7.*

Figure 1.7 Mammogram demonstrating _____/_____ of the breast.

                                       cancer   tumor

25. READ: Metastasis (me-TAS-ta-sis), abbreviated as **METS**, indicates the transfer of disease beyond the tissue or organ of origin. Metastasis often describes the spread of cancer from the place it developed to another site in the body. Variations of the term are **metastases** (me-TAS-ta-sēz), which is its plural form, indicating more than one site of metastasis, and **metastatic** (MET-a-stat-ik), which is its adjective form, used to describe a noun (e.g., metastatic cancer).

26. LABEL: *Write word parts to complete Figure 1.8, which illustrates the transfer of breast cancer cells from the tissue of origin to the brain.*

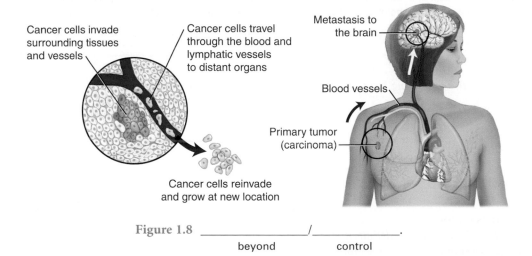

Figure 1.8 _____/_____.

                                     beyond   control

27. MATCH: *Draw a line to match the word part with its definition.*

    a. onc/o   one who studies and treats (specialist, physician)
    b. -logy   tumor(s)
    c. -logist   study of

28. TRANSLATE: *Complete the definitions of the following terms by using the meaning of word parts to fill in the blanks.*

a. study of tumors   _____ / o / _____

                                                 wr   cv   s

b. physician who studies and treats tumors   _____ / o / _____

                                                 wr   cv   s

29. READ: **Oncology** (ong-KOL-o-jē) is the medical specialty devoted to the treatment and care of cancer patients. An **oncologist** (ong-KOL-o-jist) is a physician who treats patients diagnosed with cancer.

30. REVIEW OF BODY STRUCTURE AND ONCOLOGY TERMS BUILT FROM WORD PARTS: The following is an alphabetical list of terms built and translated in the previous exercises.

MEDICAL TERMS BUILT FROM WORD PARTS

TERM	DEFINITION	TERM	DEFINITION
1. **carcinogenic** (kar-sin-ō-JEN-ik)	producing cancer	13. **neuroma** (nū-RŌ-ma)	tumor composed of nerve tissue
2. **carcinoid** (KAR-si-noyd)	resembling cancer	14. **oncologist** (ong-KOL-o-jist)	physician who studies and treats tumors
3. **carcinoma (CA)** (kar-si-NŌ-ma)	cancerous tumor (Figure 1.7)	15. **oncology** (ong KOL-o-jē)	study of tumors
4. **cytology** (sī-TOL-o-jē)	study of cells	16. **organomegaly** (or-ga-nō-MEG-a-lē)	enlargement of an organ
5. **epithelial** (ep-i-THĒ-lē-al)	pertaining to epithelium	17. **pathogenic** (path-ō-JEN-ik)	producing disease
6. **epithelioma** (ep-i-thē-lē-Ō-ma)	tumor composed of epithelial tissue	18. **pathologist** (pa-THOL-o-jist)	physician who studies disease
7. **histology** (his-TOL-o-jē)	study of tissues	19. **pathology (PATH)** (pa-THOL-o-jē)	study of disease
8. **lipoid** (LIP-oid)	resembling fat	20. **radiologist** (rā-dē-OL-o-jist)	physician who studies and treats using x-rays (and other diagnostic imaging procedures)
9. **lipoma** (li-PŌ-ma)	tumor composed of fat tissue (Figure 1.5)	21. **radiology** (rā-dē-OL-o-jē)	study of x-rays (and other diagnostic imaging procedures)
10. **metastasis (pl. metastases) (METS)** (me-TAS-ta-sis) (me-TAS-ta-sēz)	beyond control (transfer of cells from one organ to another, as in malignant tumors); (Figure 1.8)	22. **sarcoma** (sar-KŌ-ma)	tumor of connective tissue
11. **myoma** (mī-Ō-ma)	tumor composed of muscle tissue	23. **systemic** (sis-TEM-ik)	pertaining to a (body) system (or the body as a whole)
12. **neoplasm** (NĒ-ō-plazm)	new growth	24. **visceral** (VIS-er-al)	pertaining to internal organs

EXERCISE D   Pronounce and Spell Terms Built from Word Parts

Practice pronunciation and spelling on paper and online.

1. **Practice on Paper**

    a. **Pronounce**: Read the phonetic spelling and say aloud the terms listed in the previous table, Review of Terms Built from Word Parts. Refer to Table 1.3 Pronunciation Key as needed.

    b. **Spell**: Have a study partner read the terms aloud. Write the spelling of the terms on a separate sheet of paper.

2. **Practice Online** 🌐

    a. **Access** online learning resources. Go to evolve.elsevier.com > Evolve Resources > Practice Student Resources.

    b. **Pronounce**: Select Audio Glossary > Lesson 1 > Exercise D. Select a term to hear its pronunciation and repeat aloud.

    c. **Spell**: Select Activities > Lesson 1 > Spell Terms > Exercise D. Select the audio icon and type the correct spelling of the term.

❏ Check the box when complete.

OBJECTIVE 3

Define, pronounce, and spell medical terms NOT built from word parts.

The terms listed below may contain word parts, but are difficult to translate literally.

MEDICAL TERMS NOT BUILT FROM WORD PARTS

TERM	DEFINITION
1. benign (be-NĪN)	not malignant, nonrecurring
2. biological therapy (bī-ō-LOJ-i-kel) (THER-a-pē)	treatment of cancer with biological response modifiers (BRM) that work with the immune system; (also called **biotherapy** or **immunotherapy**)
3. biopsy (Bx) (BĪ-op-sē)	removal of living tissue to be viewed under a microscope for diagnostic purposes
4. chemistry panel (KEM-is-trē) (PAN-el)	series of laboratory tests performed on a blood sample that gives information regarding multiple systems, including the kidneys, liver, and lungs, and provides glucose and protein levels; (also called **comprehensive metabolic panel**)
5. chemotherapy (chemo) (kē-mō-THER-a-pē)	treatment of cancer with pharmaceuticals that target all cells reproducing at a fast rate; destroys both tumor cells and healthy cells that have rapid production rates
6. complete blood count with differential **(CBC with diff)** (com-PLĒT) (blud) (kownt) (with) (dif-er-EN-shal)	laboratory test for basic blood screening that measures various aspects of red blood cells (erythrocytes), white blood cells (leukocytes), and platelets; this automated test quickly provides a tremendous amount of information about the blood
7. diagnosis (Dx) (dī-ag-NŌ-sis)	identification of a disease

Continued

MEDICAL TERMS NOT BUILT FROM WORD PARTS—cont'd

TERM	DEFINITION
8. **genetic testing** (je-NET-ik) (TEST-ing)	laboratory test usually performed on a blood sample or cheek swab to examine DNA, the chemical database that carries instructions for the body's functions; can reveal changes in genes that may cause illness or disease. Other types of specimens used for testing are amniotic fluid, saliva, skin, and hair.
9. **infection** (in-FEK-shun)	invasion of pathogens in body tissue
10. **inflammation** (in-fla-MĀ-shun)	localized, protective response to injury or tissue destruction characterized by redness, swelling, heat, and pain

FYI **Inflammation** is a natural response that generally assists in the recovery from infection or injury, but it may also cause damage if it occurs inappropriately or is abnormally prolonged.

TERM	DEFINITION
11. **malignant** (ma-LIG-nant)	tending to become progressively worse, possibly resulting in death
12. **prognosis (Px)** (prog-NŌ-sis)	prediction of a possible outcome of a disease
13. **radiation therapy (XRT)** (rā-dē-Ā-shun THER-a-pē)	treatment of cancer with radioactive substances, x-rays, and other forms of radiation; types include external beam, internal placement, and systemic administration of pharmaceuticals; (also called **radiation oncology** and **radiotherapy**)
14. **remission** (rē-MISH-un)	lessening or absence of signs of disease
15. **specimen** (SPES-i-men)	sample of blood, urine, or body tissue that is taken for laboratory testing; (also called **collection sample**)
16. **staphylococcus** **(pl. staphylococci) (staph)** (staf-il-ō-KOK-us) (staf-il-ō-KOK-sī)	bacterium that grows in a pattern resembling grapelike clusters and can cause infections
17. **streptococcus** **(pl. streptococci) (strep)** (strep-tō-KOK-us) (strep-tō-KOK-sī)	bacterium that grows in a pattern resembling twisted chains and can cause infections

---

EXERCISE E   **Label**

Write the medical terms pictured and defined using the previous table of Medical Terms NOT Built from Word Parts. Check your work with the Answer Key in Appendix C.

---

1. _____(singular)

_____(plural)

bacterium that grows in a pattern resembling grapelike clusters and can cause infections

2. _____(singular)

_____(plural)

bacterium that grows in a pattern resembling twisted chains and can cause infections

3. _____

invasion of pathogens in body tissue

4. _____

removal of living tissue to be viewed under a microscope for diagnostic purposes

5. _____

treatment of cancer with pharmaceuticals that target all cells reproducing at a fast rate

6. _____

treatment of cancer with a radioactive substance, x-rays, and other forms of radiation

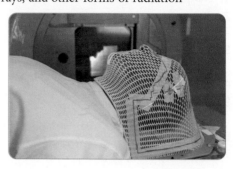

7. _____

tending to become progressively worse

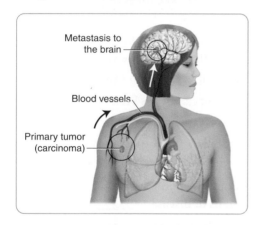

8. _____

series of laboratory tests performed on a blood sample that gives information regarding multiple systems and provides glucose and protein levels

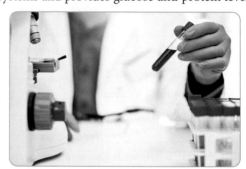

9. _____

laboratory test usually performed on a blood sample or cheek swab to examine DNA

10. _____

sample of blood, urine, or body tissue that is taken for laboratory testing

EXERCISE F   **Match**

Match the terms in the first column with their correct definitions in the second column.

_____	**1.** complete blood count with differential	**a.** not malignant, nonrecurring
_____	**2.** diagnosis	**b.** treatment of cancer with biological response modifiers that work with the immune system
_____	**3.** benign	**c.** laboratory test for basic blood screening that measures various aspects of red blood cells, white blood cells, and platelets
_____	**4.** prognosis	**d.** identification of a disease
_____	**5.** remission	**e.** localized, protective response to injury or tissue destruction characterized by redness, swelling, heat, and pain
_____	**6.** inflammation	**f.** prediction of a possible outcome of a disease
_____	**7.** biological therapy	**g.** lessening or absence of signs of disease

EXERCISE G   **Learn Medical Terms NOT Built from Word Parts**

Fill in the blanks with medical terms defined in bold using the Medical Terms NOT Built from Word Parts table on the previous pages. Check your work with the Answer Key in Appendix C.

1. Neoplasms are classified as either **nonrecurring** _____ or **tending to become progressively worse** _____. A **removal of living tissue to be viewed under a microscope** _____ of a neoplasm may be performed and sent to the lab to make a diagnosis.

2. Once the **identification of disease** _____ of cancer has been made, a **prediction of a possible outcome of a disease** _____ is considered.

3. A Px may be improved with treatments such as **treatment of cancer with pharmaceuticals** _____, **radioactive substances** _____, or **biological response modifiers that work with the immune system** _____. The course of the disease may improve, and the patient may have a **lessening or absence of signs of disease** _____.

4. **Localized, protective response to injury or tissue destruction characterized by redness, swelling, heat, and pain** _____ results from a wound or injury. After surgery, inflammation accompanied by a fever may be an indication of infection.

5. Many common bacterial **invasion of pathogens in body tissue** _____s are caused by **bacterium that grows in grapelike clusters (singular)** _____ and **bacterium that grows in twisted chains (singular)** _____.

6. Two common laboratory tests performed on blood samples are **series of tests that give information regarding multiple systems and provides glucose and protein levels** _____ and **basic blood screening that measures various aspects of red blood cells, white blood cells, and platelets** _____, abbreviated as _____.

7. **Laboratory test performed to examine DNA** _____ may be used to guide cancer prevention or treatment plans. Types of **samples taken for laboratory testing** _____s used include blood, cheek swab, amniotic fluid, saliva, skin, and hair.

Pronounce and Spell Terms NOT Built from Word Parts

Practice pronunciation and spelling on paper and online.

1. **Practice on Paper**
   a. **Pronounce:** Read the phonetic spelling and say aloud the terms listed in the previous table, Medical Terms NOT Built from Word Parts. Refer to Table 1.3 Pronunciation Key as needed.
   b. **Spell:** Have a study partner read the terms aloud. Write the spelling of the terms on a separate sheet of paper.

2. **Practice Online** ⊕
   a. **Access** online learning resources. Go to evolve.elsevier.com > Evolve Resources > Practice Student Resources.
   b. **Pronounce:** Select Audio Glossary > Lesson 1 > Exercise H. Select a term to hear its pronunciation and repeat aloud.
   c. **Spell:** Select Activities > Lesson 1 > Spell Terms > Exercise H. Select the audio icon and type the correct spelling of the term.

❏ Check the box when complete.

 OBJECTIVE 4

Write abbreviations.

ABBREVIATIONS RELATED TO ONCOLOGY

Use the online **flashcards** to familiarize yourself with the following abbreviations.

ABBREVIATION	TERM	ABBREVIATION	TERM
Bx	biopsy	METS	metastasis, metastases
CA	cancer, carcinoma	PATH	pathology
CBC with diff	complete blood count with differential	Px	prognosis
chemo	chemotherapy	staph	staphylococcus, staphylococci
Dx	diagnosis	strep	streptococcus, streptococci
lab	laboratory	XRT	radiation therapy

Refer to Appendix B for Common Medical Abbreviations and an Error-Prone List.

EXERCISE I **Abbreviate Medical Terms**

Write the correct abbreviation next to its medical term.

1. Diseases and Disorders:

   _____ cancer, carcinoma

2. Descriptive of the Disease Process:

    a. _____   metastasis, metastases

    b. _____   diagnosis

    c. _____   prognosis

3. Surgical Procedures:

    _____   biopsy

4. Laboratory Terms:

    _____   complete blood count with differential

5. Treatments:

    a. _____   radiation therapy

    b. _____   chemotherapy

6. Specialties:

    _____   pathology

7. Related Terms:

    a. _____   laboratory

    b. _____   staphylococcus, staphylococci

    c. _____   streptococcus, streptococci

OBJECTIVE 5

Identify body structure, oncology, and laboratory terms.

Now that you have worked through the lesson, review and practice body structure, oncology, and laboratory terms. *Check your responses using the Answer Key in Appendix C.*

EXERCISE J Body Structure Terms

Write the medical term next to its definition.

1. _____   resembling fat

2. _____   pertaining to epithelium

3. _____   pertaining to internal organs

4. _____   pertaining to a (body) system (or the body as a whole)

EXERCISE K   **Oncology Terms**

Write the medical term next to its definition.

Signs and Symptoms

1. _____ localized, protective response to injury or tissue destruction characterized by redness, swelling, heat, and pain

2. _____ enlargement of an organ

Diseases and Disorders

3. _____ new growth

4. _____ tumor composed of epithelial tissue

5. _____ tumor composed of nerve tissue

6. _____ tumor of connective tissue

7. _____ tumor composed of fat tissue

8. _____ tumor composed of muscle tissue

9. _____ cancerous tumor

10. _____ invasion of pathogens in body tissue

Descriptive of Disease and Disease Processes

11. _____ identification of a disease

12. _____ prediction of possible outcome of a disease

13. _____ tending to become progressively worse, possibly resulting in death

14. _____ not malignant, nonrecurring

15. _____ lessening or absence of signs of disease

16. _____ beyond control (transfer of cells from one organ to another, as in malignant tumors); (singular)

Treatments

17. _____ treatment of cancer with radioactive substances, x-rays, and other forms of radiation

18. _____ treatment of cancer with pharmaceuticals that target all cells reproducing at a fast rate

19. _____ treatment of cancer with biological response modifiers that work with the immune system

Specialties and Professions

20. _____ physician who studies disease

21. _____ physician who studies and treats tumors

22. _____ study of tumors

23. _____ study of tissues

24. _____ study of disease

25. _____ study of cells

26. _____ study of x-rays (and other diagnostic imaging procedures)

27. _____ physician who studies and treats using x-rays (and other diagnostic imaging procedures)

Related Terms

28. _____ producing cancer

29. _____ producing disease

30. _____ bacterium that grows in a pattern resembling twisted chains and can cause infections (singular)

31. _____ bacterium that grows in a pattern resembling grapelike clusters and can cause infections (singular)

32. _____ resembling cancer

EXERCISE L **Laboratory Terms**

1. _____ removal of living tissue to be viewed under a microscope for diagnostic purposes

2. _____ series of laboratory tests performed on a blood sample that gives information regarding multiple systems, including the kidneys, liver, and lungs, and provides glucose and protein levels

3. _____ laboratory test for basic blood screening that measures various aspects of red blood cells (erythrocytes), white blood cells (leukocytes), and platelets

4. _____ laboratory test usually performed on a blood sample or cheek swab to examine DNA; can reveal changes in genes that may cause illness or disease

5. _____ sample of blood, urine, or body tissue that is taken for laboratory testing

---

 OBJECTIVE 6

Use medical language in clinical statements, the case study, and medical records.

EXERCISE M **Use Medical Terms in Clinical Statements**

Circle the medical term or abbreviation defined in the bolded phrases. Answers are listed in Appendix C. For pronunciation practice read the answers aloud.

1. **Producing disease** (Histology, Pathology, Pathogenic) bacteria may cause infection. A(n) **producing cancer** (carcinogenic, carcinoma, oncology) agent or substance may cause cancer.

2. A patient with a(n) **identification of a disease** (diagnosis, prognosis, remission) of **cancer** (chemo, CA, METS) may seek the services of a(n) **physician who studies and treats tumors** (histologist, pathologist, oncologist).

3. The **new growth** (neoplasm, myoma, epithelioma) was biopsied and sent to the laboratory for **study of cells** (pathology, cytology, histology) to determine if the tumor is **nonrecurring** (malignant, benign, inflammation) or **tending to become progressively worse** (malignant, benign, inflammation).

4. The **physician who studies disease** (oncologist, histologist, pathologist) described the tissue as **resembling fat** (lipoma, lipoid, carcinoid).

5. Mrs. Gonzalez' **study of disease** (pathology, cytology, histology) report indicated the presence of **tumor of connective tissue** (carcinoma, sarcoma, lipoma) with **beyond control** (metastasis, remission, neoplasm). She will be transferred to the **study of tumors** (histology, oncology, epithelial) unit of the hospital. The **prediction of a possible outcome of a disease** (Dx, Bx, Px) is poor.

6. A staph or strep **invasion of pathogens in body tissue** (metastasis, inflammation, infection) that moves into the bloodstream and spreads to other organs is considered a **pertaining to a body system or the body as a whole** (systemic, visceral, epithelial) infection.

EXERCISE N   **Apply Medical Terms to the Case Study**

Think back to Tova, who was introduced in the case study at the beginning of the lesson. After working through Lesson 1 on body structure and oncology, consider the medical terms that might be used to describe her experience. List two terms relevant to the case study and their meanings. ∎

Medical Term	**Definition**
1. _____	_____
2. _____	_____

EXERCISE O   **Use Medical Terms in a Document**

Tova was able to see her primary care physician, who referred her for further testing. The following medical document notes the care and treatment Tova received.

Use the definitions in numbers 1-12 to write medical terms within the following document.

1. removal of living tissue to be viewed under a microscope for diagnostic purpose

2. study of cells

3. physician who studies disease

4. identification of a disease

5. cancerous tumor

6. localized, protective response to injury or tissue destruction characterized by redness, swelling, heat, and pain

7. beyond control

8. tending to become progressively worse, possibly resulting in death

9. physician who studies and treats tumors

10. treatment of cancer using pharmaceuticals that target all cells reproducing at a fast rate

11. prediction of possible outcome of a disease

12. treatment of cancer with radioactive substances, x-rays, and other forms of radiation

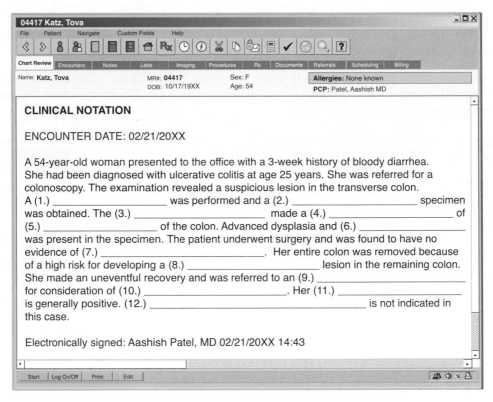

Refer to the medical record to answer the remaining questions. Mark T for true, and F for false for 13-15.

13. _____ The cancer has spread from the colon to other surrounding organs.

14. _____ Ms. Katz's prognosis is carcinoma of the colon.

15. _____ Ms. Katz was referred to a pathologist for consideration of treatment of cancer using pharmaceuticals.

16. Identify two abbreviations of medical terms used within the clinical notation.

Abbreviation _____   Term _____

Abbreviation _____   Term _____

17. Identify new medical terms in the medical record you would like to investigate. Use your medical dictionary or an online resource to look up the definition.

      Medical Term   **Definition**

1. _____   _____

2. _____   _____

EXERCISE P   **Interpret Language Used in a Medical Record**

Read the medical record and answer the questions.

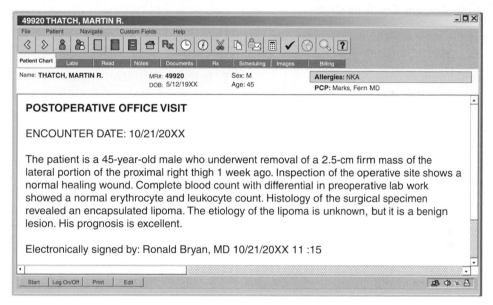

Circle the letter with the best answer for 1-3 and write your answers for 4.

1. The best description of the laboratory test included in preoperative blood work is:
   a. examines DNA to reveal changes in genes
   b. series of tests performed to assess multiple systems and provides glucose and protein levels
   c. screening of a blood sample measuring various aspects of red blood cells, white blood cells, and platelets

2. Analysis of the tissue specimen revealed an encapsulated:
   a. cancerous tumor
   b. tumor composed of fat tissue
   c. tumor composed of epithelial tissue

3. The tumor was determined to be:
   a. not malignant, not recurring
   b. beyond control (transfer of the disease beyond the tissue or organ of origin)
   c. tending to become progressively worse, possibly resulting in death

4. Identify one new medical term used in the report and research its meaning, using a medical dictionary or reliable online source.

   Term: _____

   Definition: _____

   Source: _____

OBJECTIVE 7

Recall and assess knowledge of word parts, medical terms, and abbreviations.

EXERCISE Q   **Online Review of Lesson Content**

🌐 *Recall and assess your learning from working through the lesson by completing online learning activities at evolve.elsevier.com > Evolve Resources > Student Resources.*

❑ Check the box when complete.

EXERCISE R   **Lesson Content Quiz**

Test your knowledge of the terms and abbreviations introduced in this lesson. Circle the letter for the medical term or abbreviation related to the words in italics.

1. In the medical term cytology, *logy* is the:
   a. prefix
   b. suffix
   c. combining form

2. *Neuroma*, *myoma*, and *epithelioma* are all diagnoses that indicate the presence of a:
   a. tumor
   b. growth
   c. cancer

3. The oncologist ordered *a treatment using a radioactive substance.*
   a. chemo
   b. Dx
   c. XRT

4. *Pertaining to internal organs* leishmaniasis, also called black fever, is transmitted by sand flies.
   a. visceral
   b. epithelial
   c. lipoid

5. The skin biopsy was sent to the *study of tissues* department of the medical laboratory for analysis.
   a. cytology
   b. oncology
   c. histology

6. The respiratory *invasion of pathogens in body tissue* was caused by streptococcus bacteria.
   a. inflammation
   b. infection
   c. biopsy

7. In the medical term organomegaly, the suffix *-megaly* means:
   a. control, stop
   b. enlargement
   c. resembling

8. The patient was transported to the *study of x-rays* department for her chest x-ray.
   a. radiology
   b. radiologist
   c. pathology

9. *Localized protective response to injury* was the first sign of an infection.
   a. carcinoma
   b. biopsy
   c. inflammation

10. The *physician who studies and treats using x-rays and other diagnostic procedures* interpreted the patient's CT scan of the abdomen and documented the findings.
    a. radiology
    b. radiologist
    c. oncologist

11. A *sample of blood, urine, or body tissue that is taken for laboratory testing* may aid in the diagnosis of disease.
    a. specimen
    b. biopsy
    c. chemistry panel

12. *Treatment of cancer with pharmaceuticals that target all cells reproducing at a fast rate* may be used in all stages of breast carcinoma.
    a. biological therapy
    b. chemotherapy
    c. radiation therapy

LESSON AT A GLANCE   **INTRODUCTION TO MEDICAL LANGUAGE, BODY STRUCTURE, AND ONCOLOGY WORD PARTS**

MEDICAL LANGUAGE ORIGINS
Greek and Latin word parts
acronyms
eponyms
modern language

WORD PARTS
word root
suffix
prefix
combining vowel

COMBINING FORMS
carcin/o
cyt/o
epitheli/o
hist/o
lip/o
my/o
neur/o
onc/o
organ/o
path/o
radi/o
sarc/o
system/o
viscer/o

SUFFIXES
-al
-genic
-ic
-logist
-logy
-megaly
-oid
-oma
-plasm
-stasis

PREFIXES
meta-
neo-

LESSON AT A GLANCE   **INTRODUCTION TO MEDICAL LANGUAGE, BODY STRUCTURE, AND ONCOLOGY MEDICAL TERMS AND ABBREVIATIONS**

SIGNS AND SYMPTOMS
inflammation
organomegaly

DISEASES AND DISORDERS
carcinoma (CA)
epithelioma
infection
lipoma
myoma
neoplasm
neuroma
sarcoma

DESCRIPTIVE OF DISEASE AND DISEASE PROCESSES
benign
diagnosis (Dx)
malignant
metastasis, metastases (METS)
prognosis (Px)
remission

LABORATORY TERMS
biopsy (Bx)
chemistry panel
complete blood count with differential (CBC with diff)
genetic testing
specimen

TREATMENTS
biological therapy
chemotherapy (chemo)
radiation therapy (XRT)

SPECIALTIES AND PROFESSIONS
cytology
histology
oncologist
oncology
pathologist
pathology (PATH)
radiologist
radiology

BODY STRUCTURE TERMS
epithelial
lipoid
systemic
visceral

RELATED TERMS
carcinogenic
carcinoid
pathogenic
staphylococcus, staphylococci (staph)
streptococcus, streptococci (strep)

ABBREVIATIONS

Bx	Dx	Px
CA	lab	staph
chemo	METS	strep
CBC with diff	PATH	XRT

Directional Terms, Positions, and Imaging

CASE STUDY **A'idah Khalil**

A'idah Khalil was just in a car accident, but luckily, she is awake and knows what is going on around her. The ambulance comes and the emergency team asks her where she is hurting. Her right foot hurts the most. She has pain in her upper right arm and notices some bleeding there. She also has some pain in her belly and back. The paramedics put her on a hard board, put some kind of collar around her neck, then load her into the ambulance and take her to the hospital.

■ *Consider A'idah's situation as you work through the lesson. We will return to this case study and identify medical terms used to document A'idah's experience and the care she receives.*

OBJECTIVES

1	■	Build, translate, pronounce, and spell directional terms (p. 32).
2	■	Define, pronounce, and spell medical terms used to describe anatomic planes, abdominopelvic regions, and patient positions (p. 41).
3	■	Define, pronounce, and spell diagnostic imaging terms (p. 46).
4	■	Write abbreviations (p. 49).
5	■	Identify medical terms by clinical category (p. 50).
6	■	Use medical language in clinical statements, the case study, and a medical record (p. 53).
7	■	Recall and assess knowledge of word parts, medical terms, and abbreviations (p. 57).

OBJECTIVE 1

Build, translate, pronounce, and spell directional terms.

Directional terms communicate a specific location or direction of movement and often describe:

* Locations on or within the body, organs, and anatomic structures
* Direction of x-ray beams used in radiology
* Orientation of diagnostic images
* Surgical approaches

When using directional terms, the body is assumed to be in the standard, neutral position of reference called the **anatomic position.** In this position, the body is viewed as standing erect, arms at the side, palms of the hands facing forward, and feet side by side (Figure 2.1). The directional terms are the same whether the person is standing or supine (lying face up).

Figure 2.1 Anatomic position.

CAREER FOCUS | **Professionals Who Use Directional Terms**

Professionals working in radiology frequently use directional terms, anatomic planes, and patient positions. **Radiologic technologists (RTs)**, often referred to as **rad techs** in the field, perform diagnostic imaging examinations and administer radiation therapy treatments. Types of radiologic technologists include the following:

- **Computed tomography (CT) technologists**, also called CT technicians, operate CT equipment to produce cross-sectional or "sliced" images of internal structures.
- **Magnetic resonance (MR) technologists** operate MR equipment to produce images using a strong magnetic field and radiofrequencies.
- **Radiographers** operate x-ray equipment using radiation to produce black-and-white images of bone structures and soft tissues.
- **Sonographers**, also called ultrasound technicians, operate sonography equipment to create images of internal organs using sound waves.

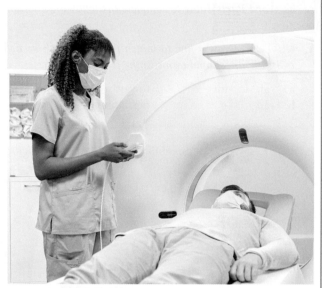
Figure 2.2 Radiologic technologist.

WORD PARTS | Use the paper or online **flashcards** to familiarize yourself with the following word parts.

COMBINING FORM (WR + CV)	DEFINITION	COMBINING FORM (WR + CV)	DEFINITION
anter/o	front	**poster/o**	back, behind
caud/o	tail (downward)	**proxim/o**	near (the point of attachment)
cephal/o	head (upward)	**radi/o**	x-rays (ionizing radiation)
dist/o	away (from the point of attachment)	**son/o**	sound
dors/o	back	**super/o**	above
infer/o	below	**tom/o**	cut, section, or slice
later/o	side	**ventr/o**	belly (front)
medi/o	middle		
SUFFIX (S)	DEFINITION	SUFFIX (S)	DEFINITION
-ad	toward	**-al, -ic, -ior**	pertaining to

For definitions of word root, suffix, prefix, and combining vowel, see Table 1.2, Using Word Parts to Build Medical Terms.

Use the **Word Parts Table** to complete the following questions. Check your responses with the Answer Key in Appendix C.

1. **MATCH:** Draw a line to match the suffix with its definition. The following suffixes will be used to build and translate directional terms in the following exercises.

   a. -al, -ic, -ior   toward
   b. -ad   pertaining to

2. **LABEL:** Write the combining forms to complete Figure 2.3.

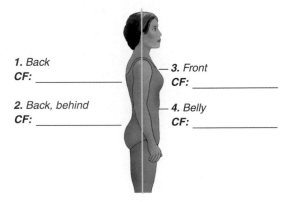

   1. *Back*
   CF: _____

   2. *Back, behind*
   CF: _____

   3. *Front*
   CF: _____

   4. *Belly*
   CF: _____

   Figure 2.3 Combining forms for *front* and *back*.

3. **TRANSLATE:** Complete the definitions of the following terms by using the meaning of word parts to fill in the blanks. Remember, the definition usually starts with the meaning of the suffix.

   a. ventr/al   _____ to the _____
   b. dors/al   pertaining _____ the _____
   c. anter/ior   _____ to the _____
   d. poster/ior   pertaining _____ the _____ (behind)

4. **READ: Ventral** (VEN-tral) and **anterior** (an-TĒR-ē-or) refer to the front of the body or anatomic structure described. The ventral cavity, located in the anterior portion of the body, is made up of the thoracic and abdominopelvic cavities. **Dorsal** (DOR-sal) and **posterior** (pos-TĒR-ē-or) refer to the back of the body or anatomic structure described. The dorsal cavity, located in the posterior portion of the body, is made up of the cranial and spinal cavities (see Figure 1.6). Anterior and posterior are also used to describe the location of anatomic structures in relation to one another. For example, the sternum is anterior to the heart.

5. LABEL: *Write word parts to complete Figure 2.4.*

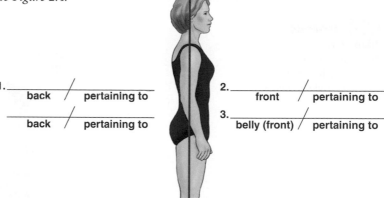

1. _____/_____
   back / pertaining to

   _____/_____
   back / pertaining to

2. _____/_____
   front / pertaining to

3. _____/_____
   belly (front) / pertaining to

Figure 2.4 Directional terms describing the front and the back.

---

6. TRANSLATE: *Complete the definitions of the following terms by using the meaning of word parts to fill in the blanks.*

   a. poster/o/anter/ior (PA)   _____ to the _____ and to the _____
   b. anter/o/poster/ior (AP)   pertaining _____ the _____ and to the _____

---

7. READ: Posteroanterior (pos-ter-ō-an-TĒR-ē-or) and **anteroposterior** (an-ter-ō-pos-TĒR-ē-or) are used to describe the direction of the x-ray beam used in radiography. PA projection for a chest radiograph is used when the heart or other anterior structures are the focus of the diagnostic study. AP projection for a chest radiograph is used when the spine is the primary focus.

---

8. LABEL: *Write word parts to complete Figure 2.5.*

X-ray machine

Path of the x-ray beams

X-ray plate

A

B

Figure 2.5 A. _____/o/_____/_____ projection
                        back   front   pertaining to

              B. _____/o/_____/_____ projection
                        front   back   pertaining to

Organs closest to the x-ray plate look the most accurate on a radiograph. In the PA projection (A), the x-ray beam moves from the back to the front of the body; in the AP projection (B), the x-ray beam moves through the front of the body to the back of the body.

9. LABEL: *Write combining forms to complete Figure 2.6.*

FYI   Head and Trunk Only
Terms built from the combining forms **cephal/o** and **caud/o** are used to describe locations in the head and trunk of the body.

1. Above
CF: _____

2. Head
CF: _____

3. Tail
CF: _____

4. Below
CF: _____

Figure 2.6 Combining forms for *above* and *below*.

---

10. TRANSLATE: *Complete the definitions of the following terms by using the meaning of word parts to fill in the blanks.*

    a. super/ior   _____ to _____

    b. infer/ior   _____ to _____

    c. anter/o/super/ior   pertaining _____ the _____ and _____

---

11. READ: When considering the head and trunk of the body, **superior** (sū-PĒR-ē-or) indicates toward the head and **inferior** (in-FĒR-ē-or) indicates toward the pelvis (these terms do not apply to the limbs). The terms can also be used to describe the position of anatomic structures in relation to one another. For example, the eyes are superior to the mouth, and conversely, the mouth is inferior to the eyes. **Anterosuperior** (an-ter-ō-sū-PĒR-ē-or) indicates direction or location toward the front and above, as might be seen in describing a surgical approach, projection angle, or location within an anatomic structure.

---

12. TRANSLATE: *Complete the definitions of the following terms by using the meaning of word parts to fill in the blanks.*

    a. cephal/ic   _____ to the _____

    b. caud/al   pertaining _____ the _____

    c. cephal/ad   _____ the _____

    d. caud/ad   _____ the _____

13. READ: **Cephalic** (se-FAL-ik) and **caudal** (KAW-dal) are used to describe locations within the head and trunk of the body and are not used to describe the limbs. *Cephalic*, literally translated as *pertaining to the head*, refers to a position above. *Caudal*, literally translated as *pertaining to the tail*, indicates a position below. It might be helpful to consider the final portion of the spine as the "tail" and the use of caudal as referring to the bottom portion of the trunk of the body. **Cephalad** (SEF-a-lad) and **caudad** (KAW-dad) indicate movement in a specific direction, as might be seen in describing a surgical approach or diagnostic projection angle. *Cephalad* indicates *toward the head* or *upward*. *Caudad* indicates *toward the tail* or *downward*.

14. LABEL: *Write word parts to complete Figure 2.7.*

> **FYI** **Terms Used Interchangeably**
> When describing anatomic structures in the head and trunk of the body, the following terms are used synonymously:
> **Anterior** and **ventral** describe the front.
> **Posterior** and **dorsal** describe the back.
> **Superior** and **cephalic** describe above.
> **Inferior** and **caudal** describe below.

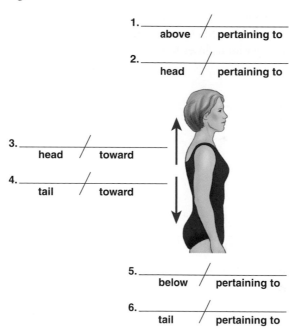

1. ___/___ above / pertaining to
2. ___/___ head / pertaining to
3. ___/___ head / toward
4. ___/___ tail / toward
5. ___/___ below / pertaining to
6. ___/___ tail / pertaining to

Figure 2.7 Directional terms describing *above* and *below*.

15. LABEL: *Write combining forms to complete Figure 2.8.*

> **FYI** **The midline** is a common reference point when describing anatomic locations. It is an imaginary line visualized in the middle of the body or anatomic structure, running from top to bottom and dividing the structure in half.

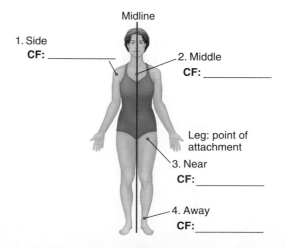

Midline
1. Side CF: ___
2. Middle CF: ___
Leg: point of attachment
3. Near CF: ___
4. Away CF: ___

Figure 2.8 Combining forms for *middle*, *side*, *near*, and *away*.

16. **BUILD:** *Write the word parts to build the following directional terms. Use the suffix –al.*

    a. pertaining to near [the point of attachment]   _____/_____

                                                       wr   s

    b. pertaining to away [from the point of attachment]   _____/_____

                                                       wr   s

---

17. **READ:** **Proximal** (PROK-si-mal) and **distal** (DIS-tal) are both used in reference to the point of attachment of the limb or anatomic structure described. When referring to a location on the arm, the shoulder is considered the point of attachment. Proximal indicates a location near the shoulder; distal indicates a position closer to the wrist (Figure 2.9).

Figure 2.9 Proximal and distal.

---

18. **BUILD:** *Write the word parts to build the following directional terms. Use the suffix -al.*

    a. pertaining to the middle   _____/_____

                                      wr   s

    b. pertaining to the side   _____/_____

                                      wr   s

---

19. **READ:** **Medial** (MĒ-dē-al) describes a location closer to the middle of the structure or the midline of the body. **Lateral** (LAT-e-ral) describes away from the middle of the structure or the midline of the body (Figure 2.10).

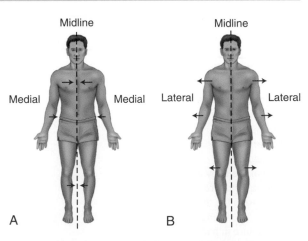

Figure 2.10 A. Medial, toward the midline. B. Lateral, toward the side.

20. LABEL: *Write word parts to complete Figure 2.11.*

Figure 2.11 Chest radiograph, left _____/_____ position.
                                          side   pertaining to

21. BUILD: *Write the word parts to build the following directional terms used to describe projection angles, surgical approaches, and specific locations within anatomic structures. Use the suffix -al.*

a. pertaining to the middle and to the side   _____/ o /_____/_____
                                                          wr   **cv**   **wr**   **s**

b. pertaining to the front and to the middle   _____/ o /_____/_____
                                                          wr   **cv**   **wr**   **s**

c. pertaining to the back and to the side   _____/ o /_____/_____
                                                          wr   **cv**   **wr**   **s**

d. pertaining to above and to the side   _____/ o /_____/_____
                                                          wr   **cv**   **wr**   **s**

e. pertaining to below and to the side   _____/ o /_____/_____
                                                          wr   **cv**   **wr**   **s**

f. pertaining to the front and to the side   _____/ o /_____/_____
                                                          wr   **cv**   **wr**   **s**

22. REVIEW OF DIRECTIONAL TERMS: The following is an alphabetical list of terms built and translated in the previous exercises.

DIRECTIONAL TERMS			
TERM	**DEFINITION**	**TERM**	**DEFINITION**
1. anterior (ant) (an-TĒR-ē-or)	pertaining to the front (Figure 2.4)	**3. anteromedial** (an-ter-ō-MĒD-ē-al)	pertaining to the front and to the middle
2. anterolateral (an-ter-ō-LAT-er-al)	pertaining to the front and to the side	**4. anteroposterior (AP)** (an-ter-ō-pos-TĒR-ē-or)	pertaining to the front and to the back (Figure 2.5, B)

Continued

DIRECTIONAL TERMS—cont'd

TERM	DEFINITION	TERM	DEFINITION
5. anterosuperior (an-ter-ō-sū-PĒR-ē-or)	pertaining to the front and above	**15. medial (med)** (MĒ-dē-al)	pertaining to the middle (Figure 2.10, A)
6. caudad (KAW-dad)	toward the tail (Figure 2.7)	**16. mediolateral** (mē-dē-ō-LAT-er-al)	pertaining to the middle and to the side
7. caudal (KAW-dal)	pertaining to the tail (Figure 2.7)	**17. posterior (post)** (pos-TĒR-ē-or)	pertaining to back, behind (Figure 2.4)
8. cephalad (SEF-a-lad)	toward the head (Figure 2.7)	**18. posteroanterior (PA)** (pos-ter-ō-an-TĒR-ē-or)	pertaining to the back and to the front (Figure 2.5, A)
9. cephalic (se-FAL-ik)	pertaining to the head (Figure 2.7)	**19. posterolateral** (pos-ter-ō-LAT-er-al)	pertaining to the back and to the side
10. distal (DIS-tal)	pertaining to away (from the point of attachment) (Figure 2.9)	**20. proximal** (PROK-si-mal)	pertaining to near (the point of attachment) (Figure 2.9)
11. dorsal (DOR-sal)	pertaining to the back (Figure 2.4)	**21. superior (sup)** (sū-PĒR-ē-or)	pertaining to above (Figure 2.7)
12. inferior (inf) (in-FĒR-ē-or)	pertaining to below (Figure 2.7)	**22. superolateral** (sū-per-ō-LAT-er-al)	pertaining to above and to the side
13. inferolateral (in-fer-ō-LAT-er-al)	pertaining to below and to the side	**23. ventral** (VEN-tral)	pertaining to the belly (Figure 2.4)
14. lateral (lat) (LAT-e-ral)	pertaining to the side (Figure 2.10, B; 2.11)		

EXERCISE B   Pronounce and Spell Directional Terms

Practice pronunciation and spelling on paper and online.

1. **Practice on Paper**
   a. **Pronounce:** Read the phonetic spelling and say aloud the terms listed in the previous table, Review of Directional Terms. Refer to Table 1.3 Pronunciation Key as needed.
   b. **Spell:** Have a study partner read the terms aloud. Write the spelling of the terms on a separate sheet of paper.

2. **Practice Online** ⊕
   a. **Access** online learning resources. Go to evolve.elsevier.com > Evolve Resources > Practice Student Resources.
   b. **Pronounce:** Select Audio Glossary > Lesson 2 > Exercise B. Select a term to hear its pronunciation and repeat aloud.
   c. **Spell:** Select Activities > Lesson 2 > Spell Terms > Exercise B. Select the audio icon and type the correct spelling of the term.

❏ Check the box when complete.

OBJECTIVE 2

Define, pronounce, and spell medical terms used to describe anatomic planes, abdominopelvic regions, and patient positions.

Anatomic Planes

Planes are imaginary flat fields used as points of reference to identify or view the location of organs and anatomic structures (Figure 2.12). The body is assumed to be in the **anatomic position** (see Figure 2.1) unless specified otherwise. References to the anatomic planes are frequently used in diagnostic imaging to describe the angle from which images are captured.

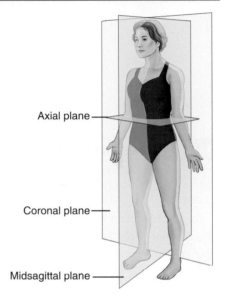

Figure 2.12 Anatomic planes.

ANATOMIC PLANES	
TERM	**DEFINITION**
1. axial plane (AK-see-uh-l) (plān)	horizontal field dividing the body into superior and inferior portions; (also called **transverse plane** and **horizontal plane**)
2. coronal plane (ko-RŌN-al) (plān)	vertical field passing through the body from side to side, dividing the body into anterior and posterior portions; (also called **frontal plane**)
3. sagittal plane (SAJ-i-tal) (plān)	vertical field running through the body from front to back, dividing the body into right and left sides.

FYI   The **midsagittal plane** is the sagittal plane at the midline of the body. A **parasagittal plane** is a plane parallel to the midsagittal plane.

Abdominopelvic Regions

To assist in communication of location, the abdomen and pelvis are divided into nine regions (Figure 2.13). Abdomino-pelvic regions are often used in the physical examination and medical history to describe signs and symptoms.

ABDOMINOPELVIC REGIONS (number of regions indicated in parentheses)	
TERM	**DEFINITION**
1. umbilical region (1) (um-BIL-i-kal) (RĒ-jun)	around the navel (umbilicus)
2. lumbar regions (2) (LUM-bar) (RĒ-junz)	to the right and left of the umbilical region, near the waist
3. epigastric region (1) (ep-i-GAS-trik) (RĒ-jun)	superior to the umbilical region
4. hypochondriac regions (2) (hī-pō-KON-drē-ak) (RĒ-junz)	to the right and left of the epigastric region
5. hypogastric region (1) (hī-pō-GAS-trik) (RĒ-jun)	inferior to the umbilical region
6. iliac regions (2) (IL-ē-ak) (RĒ-junz)	to the right and left of the hypogastric region, near the groin (also called **inguinal regions**)

Figure 2.13 Abdominopelvic regions.

TABLE 2.1	PREVENTING WRONG-SIDE ERRORS

When facing the patient, your right and left will be opposite of the patient's right and left. Confusing the patient's right and left with the provider's right and left can lead to significant errors, such as wrong-sided surgery.

Tips for preventing wrong-sided errors include:

Remember "right" and "left" pertain to the right and left of the patient's body.

Avoid saying "right" when "correct" is meant.

When a patient says the indicated side is "right" confirm the response meant "correct."

Patient Positions

Position terms are used in healthcare settings to communicate how the patient's body is placed for physical examination, diagnostic procedures, surgery, treatment, and recovery (Figure 2.17).

PATIENT POSITIONS

TERM	DEFINITION
1. lateral position (LAT-e-ral) (pe-ZISH-en)	lying on one side with knees bent (also called **side-lying position** and **lateral recumbent position**)
2. orthopnea position (or-THOP-nē-a) (pe-ZISH-en)	sitting upright in a chair or in bed supported by pillows behind the back (also called **high Fowler position**)
FYI	**Orthopnea** is built from the combining form **orth/o,** meaning *straight,* and the suffix **-pnea,** meaning *breathing.* Patients who need to sit up straight to breathe are placed in the **orthopnea** position.
3. prone position (prōn) (pe-ZISH-en)	lying on the abdomen, facing downward (head may be turned to one side)
4. semiprone position (sem-e-PRŌN) (pe-ZISH-en)	lying on one side between a lateral and prone position with the upper knee drawn up toward the chest and the lower arm drawn behind, parallel to the back
5. sitting position (SIT-ting) (pe-ZISH-en)	bed position with head of the bed elevated at an angle between 15° and 90° and with slight elevation of the knees (also called **Fowler position** and **semisitting position**)
FYI	"Right" or "left" appearing with positional terms, such as **lateral** and **semiprone**, indicates the side in contact with the supporting surface. For example, **left lateral position** means that the patient is lying on the patient's left side.

Continued

PATIENT POSITIONS—cont'd	
TERM	**DEFINITION**
6. supine position (SOO-pīn) (pe-ZISH-en)	lying on the back, facing upward
7. Trendelenburg position (tren-DEL-en-berg) (pe-ZISH-en)	lying on the back with body tilted so that the head is lower than the feet

TABLE 2.2	SITTING POSITION VARIATIONS
In general, the **sitting position** or **Fowler position** indicates the patient is sitting in bed with the head of the bed raised between 15° and 90°.	
Variations in the angle are denoted by the terms:	
High	indicating an upright position at approximately 90°
Standard	indicating an angle between 45° and 60°
Semi	indicating an angle between 30° to 45°
Low	where the head is slightly elevated between 15° to 30°

EXERCISE C   Learn Anatomic Planes, Abdominopelvic Regions, and Patient Positions

Fill in the blanks with medical terms defined using the previous tables. Check your responses with the Answer Key in Appendix C.

1. *Label Figure 2.14 by filling in the blanks.*

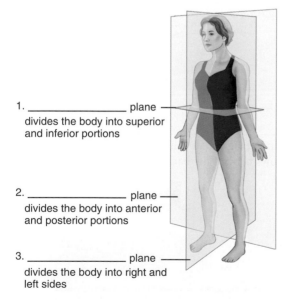

1. _____ plane
   divides the body into superior and inferior portions

2. _____ plane
   divides the body into anterior and posterior portions

3. _____ plane
   divides the body into right and left sides

Figure 2.14 Label anatomic planes.

Axial image

Coronal image   Sagittal image

Figure 2.15 MRI slices showing the view of diagnostic images taken in the axial, coronal, and sagittal planes.

2. *Label Figure 2.16 by filling in the blanks.*

5. _____ region

1. Right _____ region

6. Left _____ region

7. _____ region

2. Right _____ region

8. Left _____ region

3. Right _____ region

9. Left _____ region

4. _____ region

Figure 2.16 Label abdominopelvic regions.

3. *Label Figure 2.17 by writing the patient position pictured and defined.*

1. _____

lying on the back, facing upward

2. _____

lying on the abdomen, facing downward

3. _____

bed position with head of the bed elevated at an angle between 15° and 90° and with slight elevation of the knees

45°

4. _____

sitting upright in a chair or in bed supported by pillows behind the back

90°

5. Right _____
lying on one side with knees bent

6. Right _____
lying on one side between a lateral and prone position
with the upper knee drawn up toward the chest and
the lower arm drawn behind, parallel to the back

7. _____
lying on the back with body tilted so that the head is lower than the feet

Figure 2.17 Label patient positions.

EXERCISE D   Pronounce and Spell Anatomic Planes, Abdominopelvic Regions, and Patient Positions

1. **Practice on Paper**

    a. **Pronounce:** Read the phonetic spelling and say aloud the terms for anatomic planes, abdominopelvic regions, and patient positions. Refer to Table 1.3 Pronunciation Key as needed.

    b. **Spell:** Have a study partner read the terms aloud. Write the spelling of terms on a separate sheet of paper.

2. **Practice Online** ⊕

    a. **Access** online learning resources. Go to evolve.elsevier.com > Evolve Resources > Practice Student Resources.

    b. **Pronounce:** Select Audio Glossary > Lesson 2 > Exercise D. Select a term to hear its pronunciation and repeat aloud.

    c. **Spell:** Select Activities > Lesson 2 > Spell Terms > Exercise D. Select the audio icon and type the correct spelling of the term.

❏   Check the box when complete.

OBJECTIVE 3

Define, pronounce, and spell diagnostic imaging terms.

Diagnostic Imaging

Diagnostic imaging is an important part of the evaluation of patients with a variety of signs and symptoms. The information obtained from imaging generally reveals the presence or absence of abnormalities in the area being studied.

Radiography, or the use of x-rays, was the first form of diagnostic imaging. Because it was not fully understood when discovered by Wilhelm Conrad Roentgen in 1895, he used the name "x" rays. Today we understand that radiography produces images of internal structures using ionizing radiation emitted from an x-ray tube. An image receptor catches the radiant energy that has been transmitted through the patient. The captured energy is digitally processed to form an image called a **radiograph**, which is stored electronically and displayed on a monitor.

Since Roentgen's time, many forms of diagnostic imaging have been developed and are in use today. **Radiology** is the medical specialty dedicated to the use of imaging technology to diagnose and treat disease. Directional terms, anatomic planes, abdominopelvic regions, and patient positioning are all important aspects of diagnostic imaging. They are used to ensure that the maximum amount of information is recorded on images, while unnecessary radiation is minimized.

DIAGNOSTIC IMAGING

1. magnetic resonance imaging (MRI) (mag-NET-ik) (REZ-ō-nans) (IM-a-jing)	high-strength, computer-controlled magnetic fields produce a series of sectional images (slices) that visualize abnormalities such as swelling, infections, tumors, and herniated discs (Figure 2.19)
2. nuclear medicine (NM) (NOO-klē-er) (MED-i-sin)	imaging of internal structures by using a gamma camera to detect radiation from different parts of the body after a radioactive material (radioisotope) has been given to the patient (Figure 2.19)
3. radiography (rā-dē-OG-rah-fē)	process of recording x-rays (images of internal structures are produced using ionizing radiation) (Figure 2.18)
4. sonography (so-NOG-rah-fē)	process of recording sound (images of internal structures are produced using high-frequency sound waves); (also called **ultrasonography [US]**) (Figure 2.18)
5. tomography (to-MOG-rah-fē)	process of recording slices (images of internal structures are produced using ionizing radiation and are displayed in anatomic cross sections) (Figure 2.18)

EXERCISE E   Learn Diagnostic Imaging Terms

Use the Word Parts Table to complete the following questions. Check your responses with the Answer Key in Appendix C.

1. MATCH: *Draw a line matching the word part with its definition. The word parts will be used to build and translate diagnostic imaging terms in the following exercises.*

a. radi/o   process of recording
b. tom/o   x-rays (ionizing radiation)
c. son/o   slice(s)
d. -graphy   sound

2. TRANSLATE: *Complete the definitions of the following terms by using the meaning of word parts to fill in the blanks. Remember, the definition usually starts with the meaning of the suffix.*

a. son/o/graphy   process of_____   _____

b. radi/o/graphy   _____ of recording _____

c. tom/o/graphy   _____ of _____slices

3. LABEL: *Write combining forms and suffixes to complete Figure 2.18.*

A. Radiograph captured by   _____ / o / _____
                                     x-ray   cv   process of recording

B. Sonogram captured by   _____ / o / _____
                                     sound   cv   process of recording

C. Scan captured by computed   _____ / o / _____
                                     slices   cv   process of recording

Figure 2.18 Label diagnostic images.

4. READ: **Radiography** (rā-dē-OG-rah-fē) produces images called radiographs. Radiography, the procedure, and radiograph, the resulting image, are both also called x-ray. Diagnostic x-rays are primarily used to visualize anatomic structures, such as the lungs. Like radiography, **tomography** (to-MOG-rah-fē) uses ionizing radiation, though resulting images are called scans. Types of tomography include computed tomography (**CT**), positron emission tomography (**PET**), and single photon emission tomography (**SPECT**). **Sonography** (so-NOG-rah-fē) uses sound to generate images called sonograms. In sonography, a transducer producing sound waves is placed directly on the skin or inside a body opening. Sonography is also called ultrasonography, which is abbreviated as US.

5. IDENTIFY: *Fill in the blanks with medical terms defined using the Diagnostic Imaging term table. Check your responses with the Answer Key in Appendix C.*

a. _____ produces images of internal structures by using a gamma camera to detect radiation from different parts of the body after a radioactive material has been given to the patient and is abbreviated as _____.

b. The procedure using high-strength, computer-controlled magnetic fields to produce a series of sectional images (slices) is called _____ and abbreviated as _____ .

6. **LABEL**: *Write the diagnostic term pictured and defined in Figure 2.19.*

A. Scan produced by _____

high-strength, computer-controlled magnetic fields producing a series of sectional images (slices) that visualize abnormalities such as swelling, infections, tumors, and herniated discs

B. Scans produced by _____

imaging of internal structures by using a gamma camera to detect radiation from different parts of the body after a radioactive material has been given to the patient

Figure 2.19 Label scans.

7. **READ**: Anatomic planes are used in **magnetic resonance imaging** (mag-NET-ik) (REZ-ō-nans) (IM-a-jing), computed tomography, and sonography to identify the direction of "cuts" or "slices" used in the specific procedure and demonstrated in the resulting images. **Nuclear medicine** (NOO-klē-er) (MED-i-sin) uses small amounts of radioactive materials to create scans that provide information about the structure and function of tissues and organs studied. Many diagnostic imaging procedures, such as CT and MRI, may be combined with nuclear medicine to enhance images and to generate information about molecular activity that may indicate disease.

> **FYI** **Scans** are images resulting from diagnostic imaging procedures using sensing devices. Computer software assembles data from several different angles or sections and generates images. Images produced by **tomography, magnetic resonance imaging**, and **nuclear medicine** procedures are called scans.

EXERCISE F   **Pronounce and Spell Diagnostic Imaging Terms**

Practice pronunciation and spelling on paper and online.

1. **Practice on Paper**
   a. **Pronounce:** Read the phonetic spelling and say aloud the terms listed in the Diagnostic Imaging Terms table. Refer to Table 1.3 Pronunciation Key as needed.
   b. **Spell:** Have a study partner read the terms aloud. Write the spelling of the terms on a separate sheet of paper.

2. **Practice Online** ⊕
   a. **Access** online learning resources. Go to evolve.elsevier.com>Evolve Resources > Practice Student Resources.
   b. **Pronounce**: Select Audio Glossary > Lesson 2 > Exercise F. Select a term to hear its pronunciation and repeat aloud.
   c. **Spell:** Select Activities > Lesson 2 > Spell Terms > Exercise F. Select the audio icon and type the correct spelling of the term.

OBJECTIVE 4

Write abbreviations.

Abdominopelvic Quadrants

The abdominopelvic area also can be divided into four quadrants by using imaginary vertical and horizontal lines that intersect at the umbilicus. These divisions are used to communicate the location of pain, incisions, markings, and so forth (Figure 2.20). The four divisions are:

1. right upper quadrant (RUQ)
2. left upper quadrant (LUQ)
3. right lower quadrant (RLQ)
4. left lower quadrant (LLQ)

FYI   The **abdominopelvic quadrants** provide a more general denotation than **abdominopelvic regions**. The quadrants are often used to describe signs and symptoms.

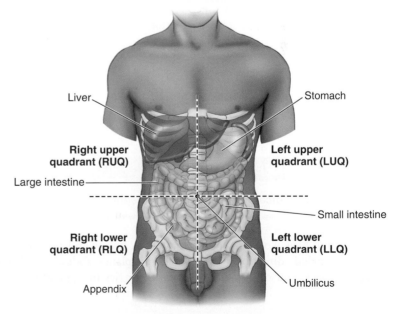

Figure 2.20 Abdominopelvic quadrants.

ABBREVIATIONS FOR ABDOMINOPELVIC QUADRANTS AND DIRECTIONAL TERMS

Use the online **flashcards** to familiarize yourself with the following abbreviations.

ABBREVIATION	TERM	ABBREVIATION	TERM
ant	anterior	NM	nuclear medicine
AP	anteroposterior	PA	posteroanterior
inf	inferior	post	posterior
lat	lateral	RLQ	right lower quadrant
LLQ	left lower quadrant	RUQ	right upper quadrant
LUQ	left upper quadrant	sup	superior
med	medial	US	ultrasonography
MRI	magnetic resonance imaging		

Refer to Appendix B for Common Medical Abbreviations and an Error-Prone List.

EXERCISE G   Abbreviate Medical Terms

Write the correct abbreviation next to its medical term.

1. Directional Terms:

a. _____ superior

b. _____ inferior

c. _____ medial

d. _____ lateral

e. _____ posteroanterior

f. _____ anteroposterior

g. _____ posterior

h. _____ anterior

2. Abdominopelvic Quadrants:

a. _____ right upper quadrant

b. _____ right lower quadrant

c. _____ left upper quadrant

d. _____ left lower quadrant

3. Diagnostic Imaging:

a. _____ ultrasonography

b. _____ nuclear medicine

c. _____ magnetic resonance imaging

OBJECTIVE 5

Identify medical terms by clinical category.

Now that you have worked through the lesson, review and practice medical terms grouped by clinical category. Categories include directional terms, anatomic planes, abdominopelvic regions, patient positions, and diagnostic imaging. Check your responses with the Answer Key in Appendix C.

EXERCISE H **Directional Terms**

Write the directional term next to its definition.

1. _____ pertaining to the head

2. _____ pertaining to above

3. _____ pertaining to above and to the side

4. _____ pertaining to the back and to the side

5. _____ pertaining to the back and to the front

6. _____ pertaining to back, behind (starts with "p")

7. _____ pertaining to the back (starts with "d")

8. _____ pertaining to the middle and to the side

9. _____ pertaining to the front and to the middle

10. _____ pertaining to the middle

11. _____ pertaining to the side

12. _____ pertaining to below and to the side

13. _____ pertaining to below

14. _____ pertaining to near (the point of attachment)

15. _____ pertaining to away (from the point of attachment)

16. _____ toward the tail

17. _____ toward the head

18. _____ pertaining to the tail

19. _____ pertaining to the belly

20. _____ pertaining to the front

21. _____ pertaining to the front and above

22. _____ pertaining to the front and to the back

23. _____ pertaining to the front and to the side

EXERCISE I **Anatomic Planes**

Write the anatomic plane next to its definition.

1. _____ plane   horizontal field dividing the body into superior and inferior portions

2. _____ plane   vertical field passing through the body from side to side, dividing the body into anterior and posterior portions

3. _____ plane   vertical field running through the body from front to back, dividing the body into right and left sides

EXERCISE J   Abdominopelvic Regions

Write the abdominopelvic region(s) next to its definition.

1. _____ region   around the navel

2. _____ region   superior to the umbilical region

3. _____ region   inferior to the umbilical region

4. _____ regions   to the right and left of the epigastric region

5. _____ regions   to the right and left of the umbilical region

6. _____ regions   to the right and left of the hypogastric region

EXERCISE K   Patient Positions

Write the patient position next to its definition.

1. _____ position   lying on the back, facing upward

2. _____ position   lying on the abdomen, facing downward

3. _____ position   sitting upright in a chair or in a bed supported by pillows behind the back

4. _____ position   lying on the back with body tilted so that the head is lower than the feet

5. _____ position   lying on one side between a lateral and prone position with the upper knee drawn up toward the chest and with the lower arm drawn behind, parallel to the back

6. _____ position   bed position with head of the bed elevated at an angle between 15° and 90° and with slight elevation of the knees (also called **Fowler position** and **semisitting position**)

7. _____ position   lying on one side with knees bent (also called **side-lying position** and **lateral recumbent position**)

EXERCISE L   **Diagnostic Imaging**

Write the diagnostic imaging procedure next to its definition.

1. _____   process of recording x-rays (images of internal structures are produced using ionizing radiation)

2. _____   process of recording slices (images of internal structures are produced using ionizing radiation and are displayed in anatomic cross sections)

3. _____   process of recording sound (images of internal structures are produced using high-frequency sound waves)

4. _____   high-strength, computer-controlled magnetic fields produce a series of sectional images (slices) that visualize abnormalities such as swelling, infections, tumors, and herniated discs

5. _____   imaging of internal structures by using a gamma camera to detect radiation from different parts of the body after a radioactive material (radioisotopes) has been given to the patient

OBJECTIVE 6

Use medical language in clinical statements, the case study, and a medical record.

EXERCISE M   **Use Medical Terms in Clinical Statements**

Read the Procedure for Palpating Arterial Pulses and answer questions 1-4.

Procedure for Palpating Arterial Pulses

Palpate arteries with the distal pads of the first two fingers. The fingertips are used because they are the most sensitive parts of the hand. Unless contraindicated, simultaneous palpation is preferred.

Temporal: Palpate over the temporal bone on each side of the head, lateral to each eyebrow.

Carotid: Palpate the anterior edge of the sternocleidomastoid muscle, just medial and inferior to the angle of the jaw. To avoid reduction of blood flow, do not palpate right and left carotid pulses simultaneously.

Radial: Palpate anterolateral side of wrist, proximal to the radio-carpal junction.

Femoral: This pulse is inferior to the medial inguinal ligament; the pulse is found midway between anterosuperior iliac spine and pubic tubercle.

Posterior tibial: This pulse is found posterior and slightly inferior to the medial malleolus of the ankle.

Dorsalis pedis: With the foot slightly dorsiflexed, lightly palpate the dorsal surface of the foot, just lateral to the first metatarsal.

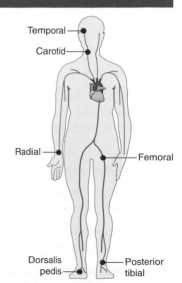

> **FYI**   **Dorsal:** When used with the foot, the directional term **dorsal** describes the upper surface of the foot opposite the sole.

Answer the following questions. For questions 2 to 4, circle the letter that correctly completes the sentence. Check answers in Appendix C.

1. Underline the directional terms used in the section titled Procedure for Palpating Arterial Pulses.

2. The temporal pulse is palpated
   a. just above the eyebrow.
   b. to the side of the eyebrow.
   c. below the eyebrow.
   d. to the middle of the eyebrow.

3. The radial pulse is palpated on the
   a. front and side of the wrist.
   b. back and side of the wrist.
   c. back and middle of the wrist.
   d. front and middle of the wrist.

4. The femoral pulse is located
   a. below the inguinal ligament.
   b. above the inguinal ligament.
   c. to the front of the inguinal ligament.
   d. medial to the inguinal ligament.

For the following questions, circle the medical term defined in the bolded phrases. Medical terms from Lesson 1 may be included. Answers are listed in Appendix C. For pronunciation practice read the answers aloud.

5. The primary care physician ordered a(n) **pertaining to the front and to the back** (AP, PA, lat) radiographic image of the chest.

6. A(n) **pertaining to the side** (lateral, medial, anterior) chest radiograph displays the anatomy in the **plane that divides the body into right and left sides** (sagittal, coronal, axial) plane.

7. An intravenous catheter was used to administer a radioisotope before the patient's **imaging of internal structures by using a gamma camera to detect radiation from different parts of the body** (nuclear medicine, magnetic resonance imaging, sonography) procedure.

8. The patient presented to her physician with pain in the right **regions to the right and left of the umbilical region** (hypochondriac, lumbar, iliac) region.

9. The electrocardiogram showed no ST changes in the **pertaining to the front** (anterior, posterior, dorsal) leads.

10. Computed tomography (CT) images can be produced from the sagittal plane, the **dividing the body into anterior and posterior portions** (coronal, axial, sagittal) plane, and the **dividing the body into superior and inferior portions** (coronal, axial, sagittal) plane.

11. The doctor's order indicated that the patient with dyspnea was to be placed in the **sitting upright supported by pillows behind the back** (supine, semiprone, orthopnea) position to facilitate breathing.

12. The patient being treated for cardiovascular shock was placed in the **lying on back with the head lower than the feet** (prone, Trendelenburg, sitting) position.

13. **Pertaining to the back** (Dorsal, Ventral, Medial) is often used to describe the back of the hand or upper surface of the foot.

14. Just before birth, the fetus shifted to a **pertaining to the head** (cephalic, caudal, anterior) presentation.

EXERCISE N **Apply Medical Terms to the Case Study**

Think back to A'idah who was introduced in the case study at the beginning of the lesson. After working through Lesson 2, consider the directional terms and abdominopelvic regions that might be used to describe the location of the pain she experienced. List three terms and their meanings. ■

Medical Term   **Definition**

1. _____   _____

2. _____   _____

3. _____   _____

EXERCISE O **Use Medical Terms in a Document**

Paramedics transported A'idah to the emergency department (ED) of the nearest hospital. The following medical record documents the encounter.

Use the definitions in 1-7 to write medical terms in the blanks on the following ED note.

1. to the right and left of the hypogastric region

2. to the right and left of the umbilical region

3. pertaining to away

4. pertaining to the middle

5. pertaining to the side

6. pertaining to near

7. process of recording slices

Refer to the medical record to answer questions 8-9.

8. In the Physical Exam section of the document, identify and define the directional term ending in **ly.** The addition of **ly** transforms the term from adjective to adverb. Adjectives describe nouns, whereas adverbs describe verbs.

   Term: _____ Definition: _____

9. Identify and define the directional term abbreviated in the Diagnostic Imaging section of the note.

   Term: _____ Definition: _____

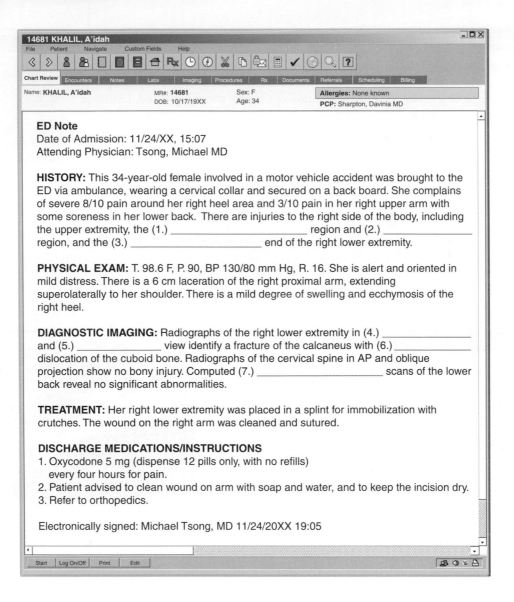

14681 KHALIL, A'idah

File   Patient   Navigate   Custom Fields   Help

Chart Review | Encounters | Notes | Labs | Imaging | Procedures | Rx | Documents | Referrals | Scheduling | Billing

Name: KHALIL, A'idah   MR#: **14681**   Sex: F   **Allergies:** None known
                              DOB: 10/17/19XX   Age: 34   PCP: Sharpton, Davinia MD

ED Note
Date of Admission: 11/24/XX, 15:07
Attending Physician: Tsong, Michael MD

HISTORY: This 34-year-old female involved in a motor vehicle accident was brought to the ED via ambulance, wearing a cervical collar and secured on a back board. She complains of severe 8/10 pain around her right heel area and 3/10 pain in her right upper arm with some soreness in her lower back. There are injuries to the right side of the body, including the upper extremity, the (1.) _____ region and (2.) _____ region, and the (3.) _____ end of the right lower extremity.

PHYSICAL EXAM: T. 98.6 F, P. 90, BP 130/80 mm Hg, R. 16. She is alert and oriented in mild distress. There is a 6 cm laceration of the right proximal arm, extending superolaterally to her shoulder. There is a mild degree of swelling and ecchymosis of the right heel.

DIAGNOSTIC IMAGING: Radiographs of the right lower extremity in (4.) _____ and (5.) _____ view identify a fracture of the calcaneus with (6.) _____ dislocation of the cuboid bone. Radiographs of the cervical spine in AP and oblique projection show no bony injury. Computed (7.) _____ scans of the lower back reveal no significant abnormalities.

TREATMENT: Her right lower extremity was placed in a splint for immobilization with crutches. The wound on the right arm was cleaned and sutured.

DISCHARGE MEDICATIONS/INSTRUCTIONS
1. Oxycodone 5 mg (dispense 12 pills only, with no refills)
   every four hours for pain.
2. Patient advised to clean wound on arm with soap and water, and to keep the incision dry.
3. Refer to orthopedics.

Electronically signed: Michael Tsong, MD 11/24/20XX 19:05

Start | Log On/Off | Print | Edit

OBJECTIVE 7

Recall and assess knowledge of word parts, medical terms, and abbreviations.

EXERCISE P **Online Review of Lesson Content**

🌐 *Recall and assess your learning from working through the lesson by completing online learning activities at evolve.elsevier.com > Evolve Resources > Student Resources.*

❏ Check the box when complete.

EXERCISE Q **Lesson Content Quiz**

Test your knowledge of the terms and abbreviations introduced in this lesson. Circle the letter for the medical term or abbreviation related to the words in italics.

1. A patient with pancreatitis presents with severe pain and tenderness in the *superior to the umbilical* region.
   a. lumbar
   b. hypogastric
   c. epigastric

2. In preparation for his physical exam, the patient transferred onto the exam table and moved into a *bed position with head of the bed elevated at an angle between 15° and 90° and with slight elevation of the knees.*
   a. sitting position
   b. semiprone position
   c. lateral position

3. The MRI scan showed images of the brain from the perspective of the *vertical field passing through the body from side to side, dividing the body into anterior and posterior portions.*
   a. axial plane
   b. coronal plane
   c. sagittal plane

4. A 74-year-old male presented with pain in the *LLQ* consistent with diverticulitis.
   a. left leg quadrant
   b. lower left quadrant
   c. left lower quadrant

5. A patient with heart failure may experience shortness of breath when *in the position of lying on the back, facing upward.*
   a. prone position
   b. supine position
   c. Trendelenburg position

6. The thyroid gland is *pertaining to above* to the sternum.
   a. anterior
   b. inferior
   c. superior

7. The computed tomography scan of the chest showed images from *the perspective of the horizontal field dividing the body into superior and inferior portions.*
   a. axial plane
   b. coronal plane
   c. sagittal plane

8. The patient presented with a mass in the *pertaining to above and to the side* portion of the left breast.
   a. anteroposterior
   b. superolateral
   c. mediolateral

9. A *pertaining to the tail* epidural steroid injection may be performed to relieve chronic low back pain.
   a. cephalic
   b. caudal
   c. dorsal

10. The gastroenterologist found a polyp in the colon *pertaining to away from the point of attachment* to the splenic flexure.
    a. proximal
    b. medial
    c. distal

11. The diagnostic imaging procedure *using high-strength, computer-controlled magnetic fields to produce a series of sectional images* is particularly effective in visualizing soft tissues, such as the brain, spinal cord, nerves, muscles, tendons, and ligaments.
    a. magnetic resonance imaging
    b. sonography
    c. radiography

12. The patient's computed *process of recording slices* scans revealed changes in both lungs with ground-glass opacities consistent with a diagnosis of COVID-19.
    a. nuclear medicine
    b. ultrasonography
    c. tomography

LESSON AT A GLANCE — DIRECTIONAL TERMS, POSITIONS, AND IMAGING WORD PARTS

COMBINING FORMS

anter/o	poster/o
caud/o	proxim/o
cephal/o	radi/o
dist/o	son/o
dors/o	super/o
infer/o	tom/o
later/o	ventr/o
medi/o	

SUFFIXES

-ad
-al
-graphy
-ic
-ior

LESSON AT A GLANCE — DIRECTIONAL TERMS, POSITIONS, AND IMAGING MEDICAL TERMS AND ABBREVIATIONS

DIRECTIONAL TERMS
anterior (ant)
anterolateral
anteromedial
anteroposterior (AP)
anterosuperior
caudad
caudal
cephalad
cephalic
distal
dorsal
inferior (inf)
inferolateral
lateral (lat)
medial (med)
mediolateral
posterior (post)
posteroanterior (PA)
posterolateral
proximal
superior (sup)
superolateral
ventral

ANATOMIC PLANES
axial plane
coronal plane
sagittal plane

ABDOMINOPELVIC REGIONS
epigastric region
hypochondriac regions
hypogastric region
iliac regions
lumbar regions
umbilical region

PATIENT POSITIONS
lateral position
orthopnea position
prone position
semiprone position
sitting position
supine position
Trendelenburg position

DIAGNOSTIC IMAGING
magnetic resonance imaging
nuclear medicine
radiography
sonography
tomography

ABDOMINOPELVIC QUADRANTS
left lower quadrant (LLQ)
left upper quadrant (LUQ)
right lower quadrant (RLQ)
right upper quadrant (RUQ)

ABBREVIATIONS

ant	LUQ	post
AP	med	RLQ
inf	MRI	RUQ
lat	NM	sup
LLQ	PA	US

Integumentary System, Colors, and Plural Endings

Amanda Sheehan

Amanda has a dark spot on her arm that worries her. She noticed it for the first time this morning as she put lotion on after her shower. It is fairly smooth and brown, but it isn't round like her other moles. When she runs her finger over it, the new spot feels more bumpy. Her other moles and freckles are flat. A few years ago she had a mole with what looked like small black bubbles removed and looked at. It turned out to be skin cancer. She had another minor skin cancer removed from her ear a year later. The specialist that Amanda saw told her to come back right away if she noticed any changes in her moles or any new spots on her skin.

■ *Consider Amanda's situation as you work through the lesson on the integumentary system. At the end of the lesson, we will return to this case study and identify related medical terms.*

OBJECTIVES

1 ■ Build, translate, pronounce, and spell medical terms built from word parts (p. 61).

2 ■ Define, pronounce, and spell medical terms NOT built from word parts (p. 72).

3 ■ Write abbreviations (p. 77).

4 ■ Distinguish plural endings from singular endings (p. 78).

5 ■ Identify medical terms by clinical category (p. 80).

6 ■ Use medical language in clinical statements, the case study, and a medical record (p. 82).

7 ■ Recall and assess knowledge of word parts, medical terms, and abbreviations (p. 85).

INTRODUCTION TO THE INTEGUMENTARY SYSTEM

Anatomic Structures of the Integumentary System	
skin (skin)	organ covering the body; made up of layers
epidermis (ep-i-DUR-mis)	outer layer of skin
dermis (DUR-mis)	inner layer of skin; also called **true skin**
hair (hār)	compressed, keratinized cells that arise from hair follicles
nails (nālz)	horny plates made from flattened epithelial cells, found on the dorsal surface of the ends of fingers and toes
sweat glands (swet) (glandz)	tiny, coiled, tubular structures that emerge through pores on the skin's surface and secrete sweat

Continued

Anatomic Structures of the Integumentary System—cont'd

sebaceous glands (se-BĀ-shas) (glandz)	special oil glands that secrete sebum (oil) into the hair follicles
appendages of the skin (a-PEN-da-jez) (of) (the) (skin)	common reference to hair, nails, sweat glands, and sebaceous glands
nerve endings (nurv) (EN-dingz)	provide sensory information, such as heat, cold, pain, and vibration

Functions of the Integumentary System

- Protects against harmful environmental elements
- Protects against fluid loss
- Produces vitamin D
- Regulates body temperature
- Excretes waste
- Provides sensory information

How the Integumentary System Works

The medical term *integumentary* originates from the Latin word *tegere*, meaning *to cover*. The integumentary system literally covers the body, providing a barrier to the external environment. The skin (also called the cutaneous membrane) is the largest organ in the human body and is made up of two layers: the epidermis and the dermis (Figure 3.2). The dermis is thicker, made of connective tissue, and contains blood vessels and nerve endings. Hair, nails, sweat glands, and sebaceous glands are referred to as the appendages of the skin. The skin and its appendages make up the integumentary system.

Colors

In addition to introducing word parts and medical terms relating to the integumentary system, this lesson includes combining forms indicating color. Medical terms built from word parts conveying color are often used to describe signs of a disease process or condition.

CAREER FOCUS   Professionals Who Work with the Integumentary System

- **Nursing assistants** provide daily care for hospital and long-term care patients, including skin care and observation of changes in the skin (Figure 3.1).

- **Medical aestheticians** perform procedures such as skin evaluation, facial massages, and hair removal. They support dermatologists and plastic surgeons with patients' preoperative and postoperative exams.

Figure 3.1 Nursing assistant providing skin care for a resident.

OBJECTIVE 1

Build, translate, pronounce, and spell medical terms built from word parts.

WORD PARTS	Presented with the Integumentary System and Colors

Use the paper or online **flashcards** to familiarize yourself with the following word parts.

COMBINING FORM (WR + CV)	DEFINITION	COMBINING FORM (WR + CV)	DEFINITION
Integumentary System		**Colors**	
acr/o	extremities	**cyan/o**	blue
cutane/o	skin	**erythr/o**	red
derm/o	skin	**leuk/o**	white
dermat/o	skin	**melan/o**	black
FYI Cutane/o is of Latin origin; **derm/o** and **dermat/o** are of Greek origin.		**xanth/o**	yellow
myc/o	fungus		
onych/o	nail		

SUFFIX (S)	DEFINITION	SUFFIX (S)	DEFINITION
-a, -e, -y	no meaning	**-lysis**	dissolution, separating
-itis	inflammation	**-ous**	pertaining to
-osis	abnormal condition		

PREFIX (P)	DEFINITION	PREFIX (P)	DEFINITION
epi-	on, upon, over	**per-**	through
hypo-	below, deficient, under	**sub-**	below, under
intra-	within	**trans-**	through, across, beyond

WORD PARTS PRESENTED IN PREVIOUS LESSONS	Used to Build Integumentary System and Color Terms

COMBINING FORM (WR + CV)	DEFINITION	COMBINING FORM (WR + CV)	DEFINITION
cyt/o	cell(s)	**path/o**	disease

SUFFIX (S)	DEFINITION	SUFFIX (S)	DEFINITION
-al, -ic	pertaining to	**-logy**	study of
-logist	one who studies and treats (specialist, physician)	**-oma**	tumor

Refer to Appendix A, Word Parts Used in *Basic Medical Language*, for alphabetical lists of word parts and their meanings.

EXERCISE A   Build and Translate Terms Built from Word Parts

*Use the **Word Parts Tables** to complete the following questions. Check your responses with the Answer Key in Appendix C.*

1. **LABEL:** *Write the combining forms for anatomic structures of the integumentary system on Figure 3.2. The combining forms will be used to build and translate medical terms in Exercise A.*

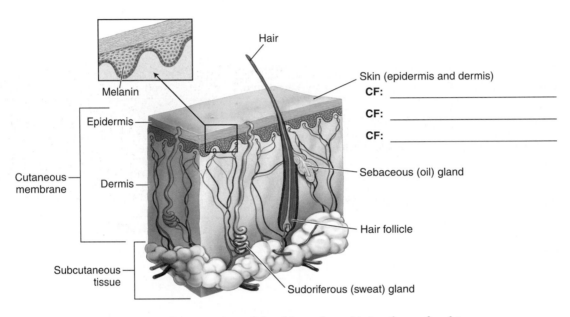

Figure 3.2 Cross section of the skin and combining forms for skin.

2. **MATCH:** *Draw a line to match the word part with its definition.*

   a. -logist   study of
   b. -logy   inflammation
   c. path/o   one who studies and treats (specialist, physician)
   d. -itis   no meaning
   e. -y   disease

3. **TRANSLATE:** *Complete the definitions of the following terms by using the meaning of word parts to fill in the blanks. Remember, the definition usually starts with the meaning of the suffix.*

   a. dermat/o/logy   _____ of the _____
   b. dermat/o/logist   physician who _____ and _____ diseases of the _____
   c. dermat/o/path/y   (any) _____ of the _____
   d. dermat/itis   _____ of the _____
   e. dermat/o/path/o/logist _____ who (microscopically) studies _____ of the skin

TABLE 3.1	USE OF COMBINING VOWELS		
TERM	**WORD PARTS**	**COMBINING VOWEL**	**EXPLANATION**
dermat/o/logy	a word root and a suffix that begins with a consonant	o	The combining vowel **o** is inserted between the word root **dermat** and the suffix **-logy** to ease pronunciation.
dermat/o/path/y	2 word roots and a suffix that is a vowel	o	To ease pronunciation of the term, the combining vowel **o** is inserted between the word roots and **dermat** and **path**. The suffix is a vowel, so there is no need to insert a combining vowel after the word root **path**.
dermat/itis	a word root and a suffix that begins with a vowel	none	The suffix **-itis** begins with a vowel, which provides the vowel sound needed for pronunciation; therefore, a combining vowel is not needed to connect the word root **dermat** and suffix **-itis**.

4. **READ: Dermatology** (der-ma-TOL-o-jē) is the medical specialty dedicated to the study of the skin, hair, nails, and mucous membranes of the eyelids, nose, and mouth. A **dermatologist** (der-ma-TOL-o-jist) diagnoses and treats pediatric and adult patients presenting with various forms of **dermatopathy** (der-ma-TOP-a-thē), including skin cancer, **dermatitis** (der-ma-TĪ-tis), and other skin conditions. A **dermatopathologist** (der-ma-tō-pat-THOL-o-jist) is trained in dermatology and pathology. A dermatopathologist works in the lab and makes diagnoses based on microscopic examination of tissue samples of skin, hair, and nails.

5. **LABEL:** *Write word parts to complete Figure 3.3.*

Figure 3.3 _____/_____ may be caused by an allergen, infection, or other disease.
                     skin   inflammation

6. **MATCH:** *Draw a line to match the word part with its definition.*

    a. epi-   below, deficient, under
    b. hypo-   within
    c. intra-   pertaining to
    d. trans-   on, upon, over
    e. -al, -ic   through, across, beyond

7. **BUILD:** *Using the combining form* **derm/o** *and the word parts reviewed in the previous exercise, build the following descriptive terms. Remember, the definition usually starts with the meaning of the suffix. Hint: Use the suffix* **-al** *for all but the last term.*

a. pertaining to the skin   _____/_____
                                       wr   s

b. pertaining to upon the skin   _____/_____/_____
                                              p   wr   s

c. pertaining to within the skin   _____/_____/_____
                                               p   wr   s

d. pertaining to through the skin   _____/_____/_____
                                                p   wr   s

e. pertaining to under the skin   _____/_____/_____
                                              p   wr   s

> **FYI**   A combining vowel is not placed between a prefix and a word root, as seen in the medical terms **trans/derm/al** and other terms built in the previous exercise.

8. **READ:** **Dermal** (DER-mal) is a general term denoting relationship to the skin, specifically the dermis. The term **epidermal** (ep-i-DER-mal) refers to the uppermost layer of skin or the epidermis. The adjectives **hypodermic** (hī-pō-DER-mik), **intradermal** (in-tra-DER-mal), and **transdermal** (trans-DER-mel) are used to describe administration of medications. Injections may be given with a syringe and hypodermic needle, which penetrates the skin. An intradermal injection places a small amount of liquid within the dermis. Transdermal administration, using a patch, cream, or ointment, slowly introduces medication as it absorbs through the skin.

9. **LABEL:** *Write word parts to complete Figure 3.4.*

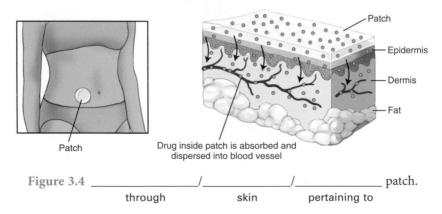

Patch

Drug inside patch is absorbed and dispersed into blood vessel

Patch

Epidermis

Dermis

Fat

Figure 3.4 _____/_____/_____ patch.
                  through   skin   pertaining to

10. **MATCH:** *Draw a line to match the word part with its definition.*

a. per-   below, under
b. -ous   pertaining to
c. sub-   through

11. TRANSLATE: *Use the meaning of word parts to complete the definitions of the following terms built from the combining form **cutane/o**, meaning skin. Remember, the definition usually starts with the meaning of the suffix.*

   a. cutane/ous   _____ to the _____

   b. sub/cutane/ous   pertaining to _____ the _____

   c. per/cutane/ous   _____ to _____ the skin

TABLE 3.2	TERMS WITH THE SAME DEFINITION, BUT USED DIFFERENTLY	
TERMS	**SAME MEANING**	**DIFFERENT USAGE**
percutaneous, transdermal	through the skin	**Percutaneous** describes surgical procedures performed through the skin. **Transdermal** describes a route of administration introducing medicine into the bloodstream by absorption through the skin.
hypodermic, subcutaneous	under the skin	**Hypodermic** describes the needle and syringe used to inject substances into the body. **Subcutaneous** describes the injection itself. For example, a hypodermic needle is used to administer a subcutaneous injection.

12. READ: The **cutaneous** (kū-TĀ-nē-us) membrane refers to the epidermis and the dermis. **Subcutaneous** (sub-kū-TĀ-nē-us) tissue lies beneath the dermis and contains fat, connective tissue, larger blood vessels and nerves. A subcutaneous injection delivers fluid to the tissue below the dermis. **Percutaneous** (per-kū-TĀ-nē-us) is used to describe procedures performed through the skin of the patient by the physician, such as a percutaneous endoscopic gastrostomy (PEG) and percutaneous coronary intervention (PCI).

13. LABEL: *Write word parts to complete Figure 3.5.*

FYI
MEMORY TIP
Hypodermic explains
how.
Subcutaneous **s**hows
where.

Figure 3.5 Insertion of a _____/_____/_____ needle into the
                              under   skin   pertaining to

_____/_____/_____ tissue.
    under   skin   pertaining to

14. LABEL: *Write the combining form for nail to complete Figure 3.6.*

Lunula   Nail   **CF:** _____

Figure 3.6 Cross section of the finger with nail and the combining form for nail.

---

15. MATCH: *Draw a line to match the word part with its definition.*

   a. -osis   separation
   b. -lysis   abnormal condition
   c. myc/o   fungus

---

16. BUILD: *Using the combining form* **onych/o**, *write the word parts to build terms related to the nail.*

   a. abnormal condition of the nail   _____ / _____
                                                   wr   **s**

   b. abnormal condition of fungus in the nail   _____ / _o_ / _____ / _____
       Hint: The combining form for nail appears first.   **wr**   **cv**   **wr**   **s**

   c. separation of the nail   _____ / _o_ / _____
                                           wr   **cv**   **s**

---

17. READ: **Onychosis** (on-i-KŌ-sis) describes any disease or disorder of the nail. **Onychomycosis** (on-i-kō-mī-KŌ-sis), the most common nail disorder, encompasses all fungal infections of the toenails and fingernails. **Onycholysis** (on-ē-KOL-i-sis) is another common disorder that may be caused by psoriasis, fungal infections, or traumatic injury.

---

18. LABEL: *Write word parts to complete Figure 3.7.*

Figure 3.7 Examples of _____ / o / _____ / _____ .
                                 nail   fungus   abnormal condition

19. REVIEW OF INTEGUMENTARY SYSTEM TERMS BUILT FROM WORD PARTS: The following is an alphabetical list of terms built and translated in the previous exercises.

MEDICAL TERMS BUILT FROM WORD PARTS

TERM	DEFINITION	TERM	DEFINITION
1. **cutaneous** (kū-TĀ-nē-us)	pertaining to the skin	9. **hypodermic (hypo)** (hī-pō-DER-mik)	pertaining to under the skin (Figure 3.5)
2. **dermal** (DER-mal)	pertaining to the skin	10. **intradermal (ID)** (in-tra-DER-mal)	pertaining to within the skin
3. **dermatitis** (der-ma-TĪ-tis)	inflammation of the skin (Figure 3.3)	11. **onychomycosis** (on-i-kō-mī-KŌ-sis)	abnormal condition of fungus in the nail (Figure 3.7)
4. **dermatologist** (der-ma-TOL-o-jist)	physician who studies and treats diseases of the skin	12. **onychosis** (on-i-KŌ-sis)	abnormal condition of the nail
5. **dermatology (DERM)** (der-ma-TOL-o-jē)	study of the skin	13. **onycholysis** (on-ē-KOL-i-sis)	separation of the nail
6. **dermatopathologist** (der-ma-tō-pat-THOL-o-jist)	physician who (microscopically) studies diseases of the skin	14. **percutaneous** (per-kū-TĀ-nē-us)	pertaining to through the skin
7. **dermatopathy** (der-ma-TOP-a-thē)	(any) disease of the skin	15. **subcutaneous (subcut)** (sub-kū-TĀ-nē-us)	pertaining to under the skin (Figure 3.5)
8. **epidermal** (ep-i-DER-mal)	pertaining to upon the skin	16. **transdermal (TD)** (trans-DER mel)	pertaining to through the skin (Figure 3.4)

EXERCISE B   Pronounce and Spell Terms Built from Word Parts

Practice pronunciation and spelling on paper and online.

1. **Practice on Paper**
    a. **Pronounce:** Read the phonetic spelling and say aloud the terms listed in the previous table, Review of Terms Built from Word Parts. Refer to Table 1.3 Pronunciation Key as needed.
    b. **Spell:** Have a study partner read the terms aloud. Write the spelling of the terms on a separate sheet of paper.

2. **Practice Online** 🌐
    a. **Access** online learning resources. Go to evolve.elsevier.com > Evolve Resources > Practice Student Resources.
    b. **Pronounce:** Select Audio Glossary > Lesson 3 > Exercise B. Select a term to hear its pronunciation and repeat aloud.
    c. **Spell:** Select Activities > Lesson 3 > Spell Terms > Exercise B. Select the audio icon and type the correct spelling of the term.

❏   Check the box when complete.

EXERCISE C	Build and Translate MORE Terms Built from Word Parts

*Use the **Word Parts Tables** near the beginning of the lesson to complete the following questions. Check your responses with the Answer Key in Appendix C.*

1. **LABEL:** *Write the combining forms for colors in Figure 3.8. The combining forms will be used to build and translate medical terms in Exercise C.*

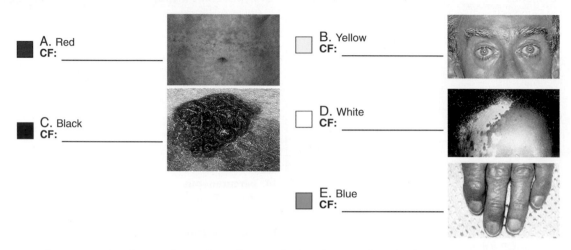

A. Red
CF: _____

B. Yellow
CF: _____

C. Black
CF: _____

D. White
CF: _____

E. Blue
CF: _____

Figure 3.8 Combining forms for color matched with examples of color as seen in the skin.

2. **MATCH:** *Draw a line to match the word part with its definition.*

   a. derm/o   skin
   b. -a   no meaning

3. **TRANSLATE:** *Use the meaning of word parts to complete the definitions of terms built from the combining form **derm/o**.*

   a. leuk/o/derm/a   _____   _____
   b. melan/o/derm/a   _____   _____
   c. erythr/o/derm/a   _____   _____
   d. xanth/o/derm/a   _____   _____

4. **READ:** **Leukoderma** (lū-kō-DER-ma) describes white patches of skin resulting from a disease process or reaction to a chemical substance. In leukoderma, there is an abnormal lack of pigmentation in the skin. Conversely, **melanoderma** (mel-a-nō-DER-ma) describes an abnormal increase in pigmentation, resulting in darkening of the skin. **Xanthoderma** (zan-thō-DER-ma) is a general term describing any yellow discoloration of the skin, such as seen in jaundice. **Erythroderma** (e-rith-rō-DER-ma) indicates abnormal redness of large areas of the skin. Inflammatory skin disease and adverse drug reactions may cause erythroderma, though in some cases no cause is identified (idiopathic erythroderma). If peeling of skin accompanies erythroderma, it may also be called exfoliative dermatitis.

5. LABEL: *Write word parts to complete Figure 3.9.*

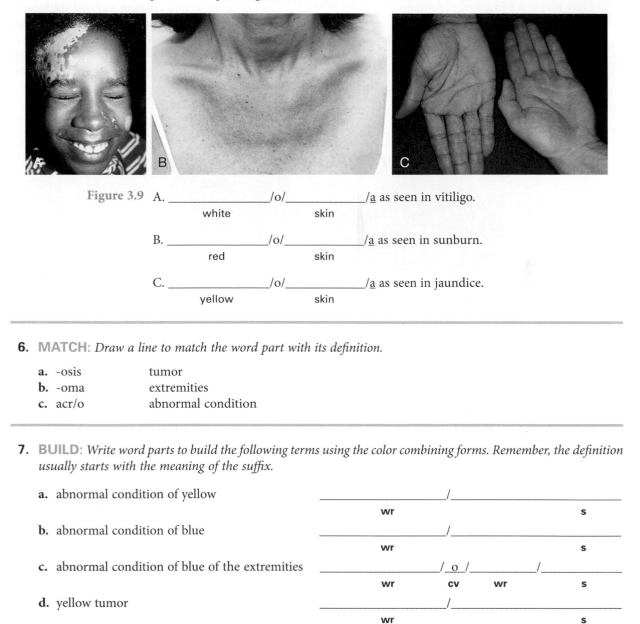

Figure 3.9   A. _____/o/_____/a as seen in vitiligo.
                        white   skin

             B. _____/o/_____/a as seen in sunburn.
                         red   skin

             C. _____/o/_____/a as seen in jaundice.
                        yellow   skin

---

6. MATCH: *Draw a line to match the word part with its definition.*

   a. -osis   tumor
   b. -oma   extremities
   c. acr/o   abnormal condition

---

7. BUILD: *Write word parts to build the following terms using the color combining forms. Remember, the definition usually starts with the meaning of the suffix.*

   a. abnormal condition of yellow   _____/_____
                                                        wr   s

   b. abnormal condition of blue   _____/_____
                                                        wr   s

   c. abnormal condition of blue of the extremities   _____/_o_/_____/_____
                                                                  wr   cv   wr   s

   d. yellow tumor   _____/_____
                                                        wr   s

   e. black tumor   _____/_____
                                                        wr   s

8. **READ: Melanoma** (mel-a-NŌ-ma) is a malignant tumor that occurs primarily on the skin. **Xanthoma** (zan-THŌ-ma) is a benign tumor usually occurring in the subcutaneous tissue and creating a raised skin lesion yellowish in color. **Cyanosis** (sī-a-NŌ-sis) describes a bluish discoloration of the skin or mucous membranes caused by an inadequate supply of oxygen in the blood. **Acrocyanosis** (ak-rō-sī-a-NŌ-sis) refers to an abnormal bluish discoloration of the skin limited to the extremities, usually the hands and feet, which may be caused by narrowing of the arteries in distal portions of the arms and legs. **Xanthosis** (zan-THŌ-sis) is an abnormal condition of yellowing, sometimes associated with cancer.

9. **LABEL:** *Write word parts to complete Figure 3.10.*

Figure 3.10   A._____/_____.
                           black   tumor
                B._____/_____ of the nail beds.
                           blue   abnormal condition

10. **MATCH:** *Draw a line to match the word part with its definition.*

   a. cyt/o   no meaning
   b. -e   cell(s)

11. **TRANSLATE:** *Using the meaning of word parts, complete the definitions of the following terms referring to types of blood cells.*

   a. leuk/o/cyt/e   _____ (blood) _____
   b. erythr/o/cyt/e   _____ (blood) _____

> **FYI**   The final **e** in **erythr/o/cyt/e** and **leuk/o/cyt/e** is a noun suffix that has no meaning and does not alter the meaning of the medical term.

12. **READ: Erythrocyte** (e-RITH-rō-sīt) and **leukocyte** (LŪ-kō-sīt) refer to cells contained in the blood. They are often referred to as red blood cells **(RBC)** and white blood cells **(WBC),** although the word root for blood does not appear in the definition of each medical term. Erythrocytes carry oxygen and carbon dioxide. Leukocytes help fight infection.

13. LABEL: *Write word parts to complete Figure 3.11.*

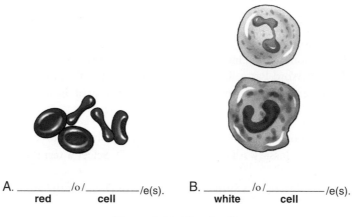

A. _____/o/_____/e(s).   B. _____/o/_____/e(s).
     red   cell   white   cell

Figure 3.11 Blood cells.

14. **REVIEW OF MORE INTEGUMENTARY SYSTEM TERMS BUILT FROM WORD PARTS:** The following is an alphabetical list of terms built and translated in the previous exercises.

MEDICAL TERMS BUILT FROM WORD PARTS

TERM	DEFINITION	TERM	DEFINITION
1. acrocyanosis (ak-rō-sī-a-NŌ-sis)	abnormal condition of blue of the extremities	**7. melanoderma** (mel-a-nō-DER-ma)	black skin
2. cyanosis (sī-a-NŌ-sis)	abnormal condition of blue (Figure 3.10, *B*)	**8. melanoma** (mel-a-NŌ-ma)	black tumor (malignant, primarily of the skin) (Figure 3.10, *A*)
3. erythrocyte (e-RITH-rō-sīt)	red (blood) cell (Figure 3.11, *A*)	**9. xanthoderma** (zan-thō-DER-ma)	yellow skin (Figure 3.9, *C*)
4. erythroderma (e-rith-rō-DER-ma)	red skin (Figure 3.9, *B*)	**10. xanthoma** (zan-THŌ-ma)	yellow tumor (benign, primarily in the skin)
5. leukocyte (LŪ-kō-sīt)	white (blood) cell (Figure 3.11, *B*)	**11. xanthosis** (zan-THŌ-sis)	abnormal condition of yellow
6. leukoderma (lū-kō-DER-ma)	white skin (Figure 3.9, *A*)		

FYI Additional combining forms describing color are **chlor/o**, meaning green, and **glauc/o** and **poli/o**, both meaning gray. **Chrom/o** is the combining form for color. See your medical dictionary or a reliable online resource for more information on how they are used.

EXERCISE D **Pronounce and Spell MORE Terms Built from Word Parts**

Practice pronunciation and spelling on paper and online.

1. **Practice on Paper**
   a. **Pronounce**: Read the phonetic spelling and say aloud the terms listed in the previous table, Review of MORE Terms Built from Word Parts. Refer to Table 1.3 Pronunciation Key as needed.
   b. **Spell**: Have a study partner read the terms aloud. Write the spelling of the terms on a separate sheet of paper.

2. **Practice Online** 🌐
   a. **Access** online learning resources. Go to evolve.elsevier.com > Evolve Resources > Practice Student Resources.
   b. **Pronounce:** Select Audio Glossary > Lesson 3 > Exercise D. Select a term to hear its pronunciation and repeat aloud.
   c. **Spell:** Select Activities > Lesson 3 > Spell Terms > Exercise D. Select the audio icon and type the correct spelling of the term.

❑ Check the box when complete.

 OBJECTIVE 2

Define, pronounce, and spell medical terms NOT built from word parts.

The terms listed below may contain word parts, but are difficult to translate literally.

MEDICAL TERMS NOT BUILT FROM WORD PARTS

TERM	DEFINITION
1. **abscess** (AB-ses)	localized collection of pus accompanied by swelling and inflammation; abscesses can occur in tissues, organs (e.g., skin abscess), and contained spaces (e.g., abdominal abscess)
2. **basal cell carcinoma (BCC)** (BĀ-sal) (sel) (kar-si-NŌ-ma)	malignant epithelial tumor arising from the bottom layer of the epidermis called the basal layer; it seldom metastasizes, but invades local tissue and often recurs in the same location
3. **cellulitis** (sel-ū-LĪ-tis)	inflammation of the skin and subcutaneous tissue caused by infection; characterized by redness, pain, heat, and swelling
4. **eczema** (EK-ze-ma)	noninfectious, inflammatory skin disease characterized by redness, blisters, scabs, and itching
5. **edema** (e-DĒ-ma)	puffy swelling of tissue from the accumulation of fluid
6. **erythema** (er-i-THĒ-ma)	redness
7. **herpes** (HER-pēz)	inflammatory skin disease caused by one of a number of viruses; the rash appears as small blisters in clusters
8. **impetigo** (im-pe-TĪ-gō)	superficial skin infection characterized by red lesions that progress to blisters and then honey-colored crusts; most commonly caused by either staphylococcus or streptococcus bacteria
9. **jaundice** (JAWN-dis)	condition characterized by a yellow tinge to the skin, mucous membranes, and sclera (whites of the eyes)

Continued

MEDICAL TERMS **NOT** BUILT FROM WORD PARTS—cont'd

TERM	DEFINITION
10. laceration (lac) (las-er-Ā-shun)	torn, ragged-edged wound
11. lesion (LĒ-zhun)	any visible change in tissue resulting from injury or disease
12. methicillin-resistant *Staphylococcus aureus* **(MRSA)** (meth-i-SIL-in) (rē-ZIS-tent) (staf-uh-lō-KOK-us)(OR-ē-us)	strain of common bacteria that has developed resistance to methicillin and other antibiotics. It can produce skin and soft tissue infections, and sometimes bloodstream infections and pneumonia, which can be fatal if not treated.
13. nevus (pl. nevi) (NĒ-vus), (NĒ-vī)	malformation of the skin, usually brown, black, or flesh colored (also called a **mole** or a **birthmark**)
14. pallor (PAL-or)	paleness
15. pressure injury (PRESH-ur) (IN-ju-rē)	damage of the skin and the subcutaneous tissue caused by prolonged pressure, often occurring in bedridden patients (also called **pressure ulcer** and **bedsore**; formerly called decubitus ulcer)
16. squamous cell carcinoma (SCC) (SQWĀ-mus) (sel) (kar-si-NO-ma)	malignant growth developing from scalelike epithelial tissue of the surface layer of the epidermis; it invades local tissue and may metastasize. While most commonly appearing on the skin, SCC can occur in other parts of the body including mouth, lips, and genitals.

EXERCISE E Label

Write the medical terms pictured and defined using the previous table of Medical Terms NOT Built from Word Parts. Check your work with the Answer Key in Appendix C.

1. _____

malignant epithelial tumor arising from the bottom layer of the epidermis called the basal layer

2. _____

malignant growth developing from scalelike epithelial tissue of the surface layer of the epidermis

3. _____

damage of the skin and the subcutaneous tissue caused by prolonged pressure

4. _____

inflammation of the skin and subcutaneous tissue caused by infection; characterized by redness, pain, heat, and swelling

5. _____

inflammatory skin disease caused by one of a number of viruses

6. _____

malformation of the skin, usually brown, black, or flesh colored

7. _____

bacterial skin infection characterized by red lesions that progress to blisters and then honey-colored crusts

8. _____

torn, ragged-edged wound

9. _____

puffy swelling of tissue from the accumulation of fluid

10. _____

noninfectious, inflammatory skin disease characterized by redness, blisters, scabs, and itching

---

EXERCISE F   **Match**

Match the terms in the first column with their correct definitions in the second column. Check your responses with the Answer Key in Appendix C.

_____ **1.** lesion

_____ **2.** pallor

_____ **3.** abscess

_____ **4.** erythema

_____ **5.** jaundice

_____ **6.** methicillin-resistant *Staphylococcus aureus*

a. redness

b. any visible change in tissue resulting from injury or disease

c. strain of common bacteria that has developed resistance to methicillin and other antibiotics

d. localized collection of pus accompanied by swelling and inflammation

e. characterized by a yellow tinge to the skin, mucous membranes, and sclera

f. paleness

EXERCISE G   **Learn Medical Terms NOT Built from Word Parts**

*Fill in the blanks with medical terms defined in **bold** using the Medical Terms NOT Built from Word Parts table. Check your responses with the Answer Key in Appendix C.*

1. **Any visible change in tissue resulting from injury or disease** _____ is a broad term that includes sores, wounds, ulcers, and tumors.

2. **Damage of the skin and the subcutaneous tissue caused by prolonged pressure** _____ (*plural form*) often occur in bedridden patients.

3. A boil is a(n) **localized collection of pus** _____ involving the hair follicle and subcutaneous tissue.

4. Torn, ragged-edged wounds _____(s) may be caused by sharp objects cutting the skin and may result in pain and bleeding.

5. Puffy swelling of tissue from the accumulation of fluid _____ of the ankles and feet often makes it difficult to wear shoes.

6. The dermatologist performed a biopsy of the patient's **malformation of the skin** _____, which recently showed changes in shape and color.

7. Unlike **malignant tumor arising from the bottom layer of the epidermis** _____ _____, a **malignant growth developing from scalelike epithelial tissue** _____ _____ has the potential to metastasize.

8. Many types of **inflammatory skin disease caused by one of a number of viruses** _____ exist. *Herpes simplex*, for example, causes fever blisters; *herpes zoster*, also called shingles, is characterized by painful skin eruptions that follow nerves inflamed by the virus.

9. **Superficial skin infection characterized by red lesions which progress to blisters and then honey-colored crusts** _____ is highly contagious and most commonly occurs in infants and young children.

10. Strep and staph may also cause a more serious infection called **inflammation of the skin and subcutaneous tissue** _____. This bacterial skin infection, which can spread rapidly, is characterized by **redness** _____, pain, heat, and swelling.

11. **Paleness** _____, an abnormal loss of color in skin and mucous membranes, can be widespread or localized and is caused by a reduction in blood flow.

12. **Yellow tinge to the skin, mucous membranes, and sclera** _____ occurs in adults and infants and results from an excess of bilirubin, a yellow-colored pigment of erythrocytes. Infant jaundice is common and usually resolves without treatment. Adult jaundice may indicate a more serious disease process affecting liver function.

13. **Strain of common bacteria that has developed resistance to methicillin and other antibiotics** _____ is quite common in hospitals and long-term care facilities but is increasingly emerging as an important infection in the general population.

14. **Noninfectious, inflammatory skin disease characterized by redness, blisters, scabs, and itching** _____ is commonly seen in people who have allergies and asthma.

EXERCISE H   Pronounce and Spell Medical Terms NOT Built from Word Parts

Practice pronunciation and spelling with the textbook and online.

1. **Practice on Paper**
   a. **Pronounce:** Read the phonetic spelling and say aloud the terms listed in the previous table, Medical Terms NOT Built from Word Parts. Refer to Table 1.3 Pronunciation Key as needed.
   b. **Spell:** Have a study partner read the terms aloud. Write the spelling of the terms on a separate sheet of paper.

2. **Practice Online** 🌐
   a. **Access** online learning resources. Go to evolve.elsevier.com > Evolve Resources > Practice Student Resources.
   b. **Pronounce:** Select Audio Glossary > Lesson 3 > Exercise H. Select a term to hear its pronunciation and repeat aloud.
   c. **Spell:** Select Activities > Lesson 3 > Spell Terms > Exercise H. Select the audio icon and type the correct spelling of the term.

❑ Check the box when complete.

OBJECTIVE 3

Write abbreviations.

ABBREVIATIONS RELATED TO THE INTEGUMENTARY SYSTEM

Use the online **flashcards** to familiarize yourself with the following abbreviations.

ABBREVIATION	TERM	ABBREVIATION	TERM
BCC	basal cell carcinoma	RBC	erythrocyte
DERM	dermatology	SCC	squamous cell carcinoma
hypo	hypodermic	TD	transdermal
ID	intradermal	subcut	subcutaneous
lac	laceration	WBC	leukocyte
MRSA	methicillin-resistant *Staphylococcus aureus*		

EXERCISE I   Abbreviate Medical Terms

Write the correct abbreviation next to its medical term. Check your responses with the Answer Key in Appendix C.

1. Diseases and Disorders:

   a. _____   laceration

   b. _____   squamous cell carcinoma

   c. _____   basal cell carcinoma

2. Related Terms:

a. _____   dermatology

b. _____   hypodermic

c. _____   methicillin-resistant *Staphylococcus aureus*

d. _____   leukocyte

e. _____   erythrocyte

f. _____   transdermal

g. _____   intradermal

h. _____   subcutaneous

 OBJECTIVE 4

Distinguish plural endings from singular endings.

In the English language, plurals are formed by simply adding an **s** or **es** to the end of a word. For example, hand becomes plural by adding an **s** to form hands. Likewise, box becomes plural by adding **es** to become boxes. In the language of medicine, many terms have Latin or Greek suffixes, and forming plurals for these terms is not quite as easy. Listed below are singular and plural endings used in medical language.

TABLE 3.3   SINGULAR AND PLURAL ENDINGS

LATIN ENDINGS		GREEK ENDINGS	
SINGULAR	PLURAL	SINGULAR	PLURAL
-a	-ae	-ma	-mata
-ax	-aces	-nx	-nges
-ex	-ices	-on	-a
-is	-es	-sis	-ses
-ix	-ices		
-um	-a		
-us	-i		

EXERCISE J **Learn Plural Endings**

Using the Singular and Plural Endings box, convert the following terms from singular form to plural form and identify the plural ending. Check your answers with the answer key in Appendix C.

SINGULAR TERM	ENDING	PLURAL TERM	ENDING
Example: vertebra	*-a*	vertebrae	*-ae*
1. thorax	-ax	_____	_____
2. appendix	-ix	_____	_____
3. cervix	-ix	_____	_____
4. diagnosis	-sis	_____	_____
5. prognosis	-sis	_____	_____
6. metastasis	-sis	_____	_____
7. pelvis	-is	_____	_____
8. testis	-is	_____	_____
9. bronchus	-us	_____	_____
10. nevus	-us	_____	_____
11. streptococcus	-us	_____	_____
12. fungus	-us	_____	_____
13. bacterium	-um	_____	_____
14. ovum	-um	_____	_____
15. sarcoma	-ma	_____	_____
16. fibroma	-ma	_____	_____
17. pharynx	-nx	_____	_____
18. larynx	-nx	_____	_____
19. apex	-ex	_____	_____
20. cortex	-ex	_____	_____
21. ganglion	-on	_____	_____
22. spermatozoon	-on	_____	_____
23. pleura	-a	_____	_____
24. sclera	-a	_____	_____
25. bursa	-a	_____	_____

OBJECTIVE 5

Identify medical terms by clinical category.

Now that you have worked through the integumentary system lesson, review and practice medical terms grouped by clinical category. Categories include signs and symptoms, diseases and disorders, surgical procedures, specialties and professions, and other terms related to the integumentary system. Check your responses with the Answer Key in Appendix C.

EXERCISE K   **Signs and Symptoms**

Write the medical terms for signs and symptoms next to their definitions.

1. _____   puffy swelling of tissue from the accumulation of fluid

2. _____   any visible change in tissue resulting from injury or disease

3. _____   paleness

4. _____   condition characterized by a yellow tinge to the skin, mucous membranes, and whites of the eyes

5. _____   redness

6. _____   abnormal condition of blue of the extremities

7. _____   abnormal condition of blue

8. _____   black skin

9. _____   white skin

10. _____   yellow skin

11. _____   red skin

12. _____   abnormal condition of yellow

EXERCISE L   **Diseases and Disorders**

Write the medical terms for diseases and disorders next to their definitions.

1. _____   localized collection of pus accompanied by swelling and inflammation

2. _____   inflammation of the skin and subcutaneous tissue caused by infection, characterized by redness, pain, heat, and swelling

3. _____   damage of the skin and the subcutaneous tissue caused by prolonged pressure

4. _____   torn, ragged-edged wound

5. _____   abnormal condition of the nail

6. _____   (any) disease of the skin

7. _____   inflammation of the skin

8. _____ noninfectious, inflammatory skin disease characterized by redness, blisters, scabs, and itching

9. _____ abnormal condition of fungus in the nail

10. _____ superficial skin infection characterized by red lesions that progress to blisters and then honey-colored crusts

11. _____ inflammatory skin disease caused by one of a number of viruses; the rash appears as small blisters in clusters

12. _____ yellow tumor (benign, primarily in the skin)

13. _____ black tumor (primarily of the skin)

14. _____ malignant growth developing from scalelike epithelial tissue of the surface layer of the epidermis

15. _____ malignant epithelial tumor arising from the bottom layer of the epidermis called the basal layer

16. _____ strain of common bacteria that has developed resistance to methicillin and other antibiotics

17. _____ separation of the nail

18. _____ malformation of the skin, usually brown, black, or flesh colored (also called a mole or birthmark)

EXERCISE M   Specialties and Professions

Write the medical terms for specialties and professions next to their definitions.

1. _____ study of the skin

2. _____ physician who studies and treats diseases of the skin

3. _____ physician who (microscopically) studies diseases of the skin

---

EXERCISE N   Medical Terms Related to the Integumentary System and Colors

Write the medical terms related to the integumentary system and color next to their definitions.

1. _____ red (blood) cell

2. _____ white (blood) cell

3. a._____ pertaining to the skin

   b._____

4. _____ pertaining to upon the skin

5. _____ pertaining to within the skin

6. a._____ pertaining to under the skin

   b._____

7. a._____ pertaining to through the skin

   b._____

OBJECTIVE 6

Use medical language in clinical statements, the case study, and a medical record.

Check your responses for the following exercises with the Answer Key in Appendix C.

EXERCISE O Use Medical Terms in Clinical Statements

Circle the medical term defined in the bolded phrases. Medical terms from previous lessons are included. For pronunciation practice read the answers aloud.

1. As the patient became more immobile, she was at increased risk of developing a(n) **damage of the skin and the subcutaneous tissue caused by prolonged pressure** (abscess, laceration, pressure injury). The nursing assistant took preventative measures, including changing the patient's position, keeping her skin dry, and looking for **redness** (erythema, jaundice, pallor).

2. The 2-year-old patient who presented with several pimplelike **visible change in tissue resulting from injury or disease** (lesions, lacerations, pressure ulcers) accompanied by erythema was diagnosed with **superficial skin infection characterized by red lesions that progress to blisters and then honey-colored crusts** (herpes, impetigo, jaundice).

3. After clearing out a weedy patch in his front yard, Mr. Pisaniello noticed **red skin** (melanoderma, leukoderma, erythroderma) on his forearm that itched quite a bit. He sought treatment from a **physician who studies and treats diseases of the skin** (dermatopathy, dermatologist, dermatopathologist). He was diagnosed as having contact **inflammation of the skin** (dermatitis, erythroderma, dermatopathy) thought to be caused by poison ivy.

4. Fungal infections can occur in various areas of the body, including the skin, hair, and nails. **Abnormal condition of fungus in the nail(s)** (onychomycosis, onychosis, onycholysis) occurs more frequently in toenails and may lead to discoloration, thickening, crumbling, and/or splitting of the nail.

5. The skin test for tuberculosis is administered by a(n) **within the skin** (hypodermic, intradermal, percutaneous) injection.

6. The hospice patient had **black tumor** (melanoma, melanoderma, xanthoma), a form of skin cancer, with **beyond control** (benign, malignant, metastasis) to the brain. To relieve her pain, the nurse used a **pertaining to under the skin** (percutaneous, transdermal, hypodermic) needle to administer morphine into the **pertaining to under the skin** (intradermal, epidermal, subcutaneous) tissue.

7. The most common form of skin cancer is **malignant epithelial tumor arising from the bottom layer of the epidermis** (basal cell carcinoma, squamous cell carcinoma, melanoma), and it most often occurs on sun-exposed skin. **Malignant growth developing from scalelike epithelial tissue of the surface layer of the epidermis** (basal cell carcinoma, squamous cell carcinoma, melanoma) is also a common form of skin cancer. BCC and SCC are both linked to long-term sun exposure and are likely to occur on the head, neck, and backs of the hands.

8. **Strain of common bacteria that has developed resistance to many antibiotics** (SCC, BCC, MRSA) is common in hospitals, but is also occurring more frequently in the general population. First symptoms often include **inflammation of the skin and subcutaneous tissue characterized by redness, heat, pain, and swelling** (edema, dermatitis, cellulitis) and a(n) **localized collection of pus accompanied by swelling and inflammation** (abscess, laceration, lesion).

9. Plural and Singular Endings: For the following statements, circle the correct form of term in the parentheses.

    a. The patient had (metastasis, metastases) from the primary site of cancer of the breast to her lymph glands and bone.

    b. Several pulmonary (embolus, emboli) were identified on the CT scan.

    c. An (ova, ovum) is a female egg cell.

    d. Two (testis, testes) are enclosed in the scrotum.

    e. The patient had two small (lipoma, lipomata) removed from his upper back.

EXERCISE P **Apply Medical Terms to the Case Study**

Think back to Amanda, who was introduced in the case study at the beginning of the lesson. After working through Lesson 3 on the integumentary system, consider the medical terms that might be used to describe her experience. List three terms relevant to the case study and their meanings. ■

Medical Term	**Definition**
1. _____	_____
2. _____	_____
3. _____	_____

EXERCISE Q **Use Medical Terms in a Document**

Amanda was able to see her dermatologist, who surgically removed the lesion for examination. The following medical record documents the biopsy results.

Use the definitions in numbers 1-10 to write medical terms within the following document.

1. study of disease

2. black tumor (primarily skin cancer)

3. malignant epithelial tumor arising from the bottom layer of the epidermis called the basal layer

4. malformation of the skin, usually brown, black, or flesh colored

5. removal of living tissue to be viewed under a microscope for diagnostic purposes

6. pertaining to near the point of attachment

7. pertaining to upon the skin

8. pertaining to the front

9. not malignant, not recurring

10. physician who (microscopically) studies diseases of the skin

```
┌──────────────────────────────────────────────────────────────────────────────┐
│ 49785 Sheehan, Amanda                                                 _ □ ✕   │
│  File    Patient    Navigate    Custom Fields    Help                          │
│  ‹  ›  👤 👥 ▯ ▤ ▤ ⌂ Rx ◷ ⓘ ✂ ▯ ▦ ▦ ✓ ◔ ◌ ?                                   │
│ ┌────────┬──────────┬───────┬──────┬─────────┬──────────┬────┬───────────┬─────────┬──────────┬────────┐ │
│ │Chart Review│Encounters│ Notes │ Labs │ Imaging │Procedures│ Rx │ Documents │Referrals│Scheduling│ Billing│ │
│ └────────┴──────────┴───────┴──────┴─────────┴──────────┴────┴───────────┴─────────┴──────────┴────────┘ │
│ Name: Sheehan, Amanda       MR#: 49785        Sex: F      ┌──────────────────────────────┐│
│                             DOB: 6/15/19XX    Age: 29     │ Allergies: None              ││
│                                                           │ PCP: Papas, Aenea MD         ││
│                                                           └──────────────────────────────┘│
```

(1.) _____ REPORT
DATE/TIME COLL: Jun 12 20XX, 12:00

DATE RECEIVED: Jun 12 20XX, 16:00

DATE REPORTED: Jun 15 20XX

REPORT STATUS: FINAL REPORT

HISTORY: Previous incidence of (2.) _____ and
(3.) _____, no metastases

PRE-OP DIAGNOSIS: Melanoma vs. compound (4.) _____

PROCEDURE: Tissue (5.) _____

SPECIMEN: Skin biopsy, anterior, (6.) _____ right arm

GROSS DESCRIPTION: One container is received. Specimen in formalin labeled with the
patient's name is a shave biopsy of gray-white hair-bearing skin measuring 0.4 × 0.3 cm in
surface dimension and averaging 0.1 cm in thickness. The (7.) _____ surface
contains a symmetric, smooth, ordered, pigmented lesion measuring 0.3 cm in greatest
diameter. The specimen is bisected and totally submitted.

MICROSCOPIC EXAMINATION: A microscopic examination has been performed.

DIAGNOSIS: Lesion, (8.) _____, proximal right arm;
(9.) _____compound nevus.

Electronically signed: J. Alvarez, MD, (10.) _____,
6/15/20XX 10:48

```
│  Start │ Log On/Off │ Print │ Edit │                            🖨 ◌ ◌ 🔒 │
└──────────────────────────────────────────────────────────────────────────────┘
```

Refer to the medical record as needed to answer questions 11-13.

11. The skin biopsy was obtained from:
   a. near the shoulder on the back of the right arm
   b. near the shoulder on the front of the right arm
   c. near the wrist on the back of the right arm
   d. near the wrist on the front of the right arm

12. Identify singular and plural forms of medical terms used in the pathology report. Write "P" for plural and "S" for singular next to the terms. Refer to Table 3.3 Singular and Plural Endings.

   a. melanoma _____   **e.** metastasis _____
   b. melanomata _____   **f.** metastases _____
   c. nevi _____   **g.** biopsy _____
   d. nevus _____   **h.** biopsies _____

13. Using a medical dictionary or a reliable online source, write the meanings of the following terms used in the pathology report:

   a. compound _____

   b. pigmented _____

   c. bisected _____

   d. microscopic _____

OBJECTIVE 7

Recall and assess knowledge of word parts, medical terms, and abbreviations.

EXERCISE R **Online Review of Lesson Content**

🌐 *Recall and assess your learning from working through the lesson by completing online learning activities at evolve.elsevier.com > Evolve Resources > Student Resources.*

❑ Check the box when complete.

EXERCISE S **Lesson Content Quiz**

Test your knowledge of the terms and abbreviations introduced in this lesson. Circle the letter for the medical term or abbreviation related to the words in italics.

1. Vitiligo is a progressive skin condition that is a form of *white skin.*
   a. melanoderma
   b. leukoderma
   c. erythroderma

2. A *physician who (microscopically) studies diseases of the skin* may examine deep samples of tissue to evaluate skin cancer.
   a. dermatologist
   b. pathologist
   c. dermatopathologist

3. A *malignant epithelial tumor arising from the bottom layer of the epidermis called the basal layer* may occur on the tip of the nose, the ears, or other sun-exposed areas.
   a. BCC
   b. SCC
   c. RBC

4. *Yellow skin* refers to any yellowish discoloration of the skin, while jaundice is an indicator of disease, and is usually caused by obstruction in the gastrointestinal system.
   a. xanthoma
   b. xanthosis
   c. xanthoderma

5. A *malformation of the skin, usually brown, black, or flesh colored* that changes significantly should be examined by a physician to rule out melanoma.
   a. nevus
   b. laceration
   c. abscess

6. *Inflammation of the skin and subcutaneous tissue caused by infection* can become very serious and should be treated immediately with antibiotics and supportive measures.
   a. dermatitis
   b. cellulitis
   c. cyanosis

7. A tuberculosis (TB) skin test, is a(n) *pertaining to within the skin* injection that must be interpreted 48-72 hours later.
   a. hypodermic
   b. transdermal
   c. intradermal

8. *Abnormal condition of fungus in the nail* is often caused by *T. rubrum* and may be preceded by "athlete's foot," a fungal dermatopathy.
   a. onychomycosis
   b. onycholysis
   c. onychosis

9. Pallor may sometimes be caused by anemia, which is a(n) *red (blood) cell* deficiency.
   a. leukocyte
   b. erythrocyte
   c. cyanosis

10. *Inflammatory skin disease caused by one of a number of viruses; the rash appears as small blisters in clusters* is one of many infections that affect that skin.
    a. impetigo
    b. herpes
    c. acrocyanosis

11. *Superficial skin infection characterized by pustules and caused by either staphylococci or streptococci* is common in young children.
    a. impetigo
    b. measles
    c. herpes

12. Compression of the lateral femoral *pertaining to the skin* nerve results in sensations of aching, burning, stabbing, and/or numbness in the thigh area.
    a. epidermal
    b. cutaneous
    c. intradermal

13. The *localized collection of pus* was incised and drained.
    a. nevus
    b. abscess
    c. laceration

14. A culture swab of the wound revealed *invasion of body tissue by methicillin-resistant Staphylococcus aureus*.
    a. MRSA infection
    b. herpes
    c. cellulitis

LESSON AT A GLANCE   INTEGUMENTARY SYSTEM, COLORS, AND PLURAL ENDINGS WORD PARTS

COMBINING FORMS	SUFFIXES	PREFIXES	SINGULAR ENDINGS	PLURAL ENDINGS
Integumentary System	-a, -e, -y	epi-	-a	-ae
acr/o	-itis	hypo-	-ax	-aces
cutane/o	-lysis	intra-	-ex	-ices
derm/o	-osis	per-	-is	-es
dermat/o	-ous	sub-	-ix	-ices
myc/o		trans-	-ma	-mata
onych/o			-nx	-nges
			-on	-a
Colors			-sis	-ses
cyan/o			-um	-a
erythr/o			-us	-i
leuk/o				
melan/o				
xanth/o				

SIGNS AND SYMPTOMS
acrocyanosis
cyanosis
edema
erythema
erythroderma
jaundice
lesion
leukoderma
melanoderma
pallor
xanthoderma
xanthosis

DISEASES AND DISORDERS
abscess
basal cell carcinoma (BCC)
cellulitis
dermatitis
dermatopathy

eczema
herpes
impetigo
laceration (lac)
melanoma
methicillin-resistant *Staphylococcus aureus* (MRSA)
nevus
onycholysis
onychomycosis
onychosis
pressure injury
squamous cell carcinoma (SCC)
xanthoma

SPECIALTIES AND PROFESSIONS
dermatologist
dermatology (DERM)
dermatopathologist

RELATED TERMS
cutaneous
dermal
epidermal
erythrocyte (RBC)
hypodermic (hypo)
intradermal (ID)
leukocyte (WBC)
percutaneous
subcutaneous (subcut)
transdermal (TD)

ABBREVIATIONS

BCC	RBC
DERM	SCC
hypo	TD
ID	subcut
lac	WBC
MRSA	

Respiratory System

CASE STUDY
 Roberta Pawlaski

Roberta is experiencing difficulty breathing. She notices it gets worse when she tries to do chores around the house. This has been going on for about four days. She also has a cough and a runny nose. Today when she woke up, she noticed that her throat was very sore. She also thinks that she might have a fever because she feels hot all over. She tried taking some over-the-counter cough medicine, but this didn't seem to help. She notices when she coughs that a thick yellow mucus comes out. She hasn't had a cough like this since before she quit smoking about 10 years ago. She remembers that her grandson who stays with her after school has missed school because of a cold. She decides to call her doctor's office for advice.

■ *Consider Roberta's situation as you work through the lesson on the respiratory system. At the end of the lesson, we will return to this case study and identify medical terms used to document Roberta's experience and the care she receives.*

OBJECTIVES

1	■ Build, translate, pronounce, and spell medical terms built from word parts (p. 90).
2	■ Define, pronounce, and spell medical terms NOT built from word parts (p. 108).
3	■ Write abbreviations (p. 114).
4	■ Identify medical terms by clinical category (p. 116).
5	■ Use medical language in clinical statements, the case study, and a medical record (p. 119).
6	■ Recall and assess knowledge of word parts, medical terms, and abbreviations (p. 123).

INTRODUCTION TO THE RESPIRATORY SYSTEM

Anatomic Structures of the Respiratory System	
alveoli (s. alveolus) (al-VĒ-ō-lī), (al-VĒ-o-lus)	air sacs at the smallest subdivision of the bronchial tree; oxygen and carbon dioxide are exchanged through the alveolar walls and the capillaries that surround them
bronchus (pl. bronchi) (BRONG-kus), (BRONG-kī)	one of two branches from the trachea that conducts air into the lungs, where it divides and subdivides. The branchings resemble a tree; therefore, they are referred to as a **bronchial tree**.
larynx (LAR-inks)	location of vocal cords; air enters from the pharynx; (also called **voice box**)
lungs (lungs)	two spongelike organs in the thoracic cavity. The right lung has three lobes, and the left lung has two lobes.
nose (nōz)	lined with mucous membranes and fine hairs; acts as a filter to moisten and warm air

Continued

Anatomic Structures of the Respiratory System—cont'd

pharynx (FAR-inks)	serves as food and air passageway; air enters from the nasal cavities and/or mouth and passes through the pharynx to the larynx. Food enters the pharynx from the mouth and passes into the esophagus; (also called **throat**)
sinuses (SĪ-nus-es)	air cavities within the cranial bones; membrane lining the air cavities produces mucus, which drains into the nasal passages; (also called **paranasal sinuses**)
thorax (THOR-aks)	chest; the part of the body between the neck and the diaphragm encased by the ribs. The **thoracic cavity** is the hollow space between the neck and diaphragm.
trachea (TRĀ-kē-a)	passageway for air from the larynx to the bronchi; (also called **windpipe**)

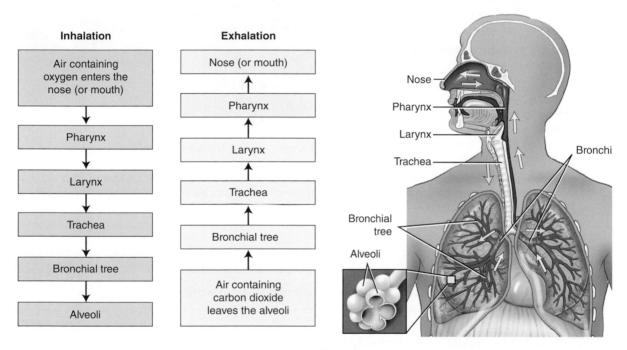

Figure 4.1 Flow of air.

Functions of the Respiratory System

- Moves air in and out of lungs
- Provides for intake of oxygen and release of carbon dioxide
- Provides air flow for speech
- Enables sense of smell

How the Respiratory System Works

The respiratory system is divided into two parts: the upper respiratory tract and the lower respiratory tract. **The upper respiratory tract** includes the nose, pharynx, and larynx. **The lower respiratory tract** includes the trachea, bronchi, and lungs. The thoracic cavity, or chest cavity, encases the lower respiratory tract. The function of the respiratory system is the exchange of oxygen (O_2) and carbon dioxide (CO_2) between the atmosphere and the body's cells. The process is called respiration or breathing. **Inhalation** occurs as air passes through the **nose** or mouth into the **pharynx, larynx,** and **trachea** before entering the **lungs** through the **bronchi.** There, oxygen passes from the sacs in the lungs, called **alveoli,** to the blood in tiny vessels called **capillaries. Exhalation** occurs as carbon dioxide passes back from the capillaries to the alveoli and is expelled through the respiratory tract (see Figure 4.1).

CAREER FOCUS   Professionals Who Work with the Respiratory System

- **Respiratory therapists (RTs)** treat, evaluate, and maintain function of the heart and lungs. RTs are highly skilled and perform pulmonary function tests; provide treatments, such as oxygen therapy and intermittent positive pressure breathing (IPPB); draw blood for an arterial blood gas (ABG) to monitor carbon dioxide and oxygen in the blood; and assist with ventilation of seriously ill patients.

- **Respiratory therapy technicians** provide respiratory care under the supervision of respiratory therapists and physicians.

- **Sleep technologists**, also called **registered polysomnographic technologists (RPSGTs)**, perform polysomnography and other tests to diagnose and monitor sleep disorders. RPSGTs work under the guidance of a physician.

Figure 4.2 Respiratory therapist assisting a patient.

- **Sleep technicians**, also called **certified polysomnographic technicians (CPSGTs)**, prepare sleep testing equipment, gather patient information, and provide explanations of procedures. CPSGTs work under the guidance of sleep technologists or respiratory therapists.

 OBJECTIVE 1

Build, translate, pronounce, and spell medical terms built from word parts.

WORD PARTS   Presented with the Respiratory System

Use paper or online **flashcards** to familiarize yourself with the following word parts.

COMBINING FORM (WR + CV)	DEFINITION	COMBINING FORM (WR + CV)	DEFINITION
bronch/o	bronchus (*s.*), bronchi (*pl.*)	**pneumon/o**	lung, air
capn/o	carbon dioxide	**pulmon/o**	lung
laryng/o	larynx (voice box)	**rhin/o**	nose
muc/o	mucus	**sinus/o**	sinus (*s.*), sinuses (*pl.*)
nas/o	nose	**somn/o**	sleep
ox/i	oxygen	**spir/o**	breathe, breathing
pharyng/o	pharynx (throat)	**thorac/o**	chest, chest cavity
pneum/o	lung, air	**trache/o**	trachea (windpipe)

Continued

WORD PARTS	Presented with the Respiratory System—cont'd		
SUFFIX (S)	**DEFINITION**	**SUFFIX (S)**	**DEFINITION**
-ary, -eal	pertaining to	**-rrhea**	flow, discharge
-centesis	surgical puncture to remove fluid (with a sterile needle)	**-scope**	instrument used for visual examination
-ectomy	surgical removal, excision	**-scopic**	pertaining to visual examination
-gram	record, radiographic image	**-scopy**	visual examination
-ia	diseased state, condition of	**-stomy**	creation of an artificial opening
-meter	instrument used to measure	**-thorax**	chest, chest cavity
-pnea	breathing	**-tomy**	cut into, incision
-rrhagia	excessive bleeding		
PREFIX (P)	**DEFINITION**	**PREFIX (P)**	**DEFINITION**
a-, an-	absence of, without	**hyper-**	above, excessive
dys-	difficult, painful, abnormal	**poly-**	many, much
endo-	within		

WORD PARTS PRESENTED IN PREVIOUS LESSONS	Used to Build Terms for the Respiratory System		
SUFFIX (S)	**DEFINITION**	**SUFFIX (S)**	**DEFINITION**
-al, -ous	pertaining to	**-logist**	one who studies and treats (specialist, physician)
-graphy	process of recording, radiographic imaging	**-logy**	study of
-itis	inflammation		
PREFIX (P)	**DEFINITION**		
hypo-	below, deficient, under		

Refer to Appendix A, Word Parts Used in *Basic Medical Language*, for alphabetical lists of word parts and their meanings.

EXERCISE A **Build and Translate Terms Built from Word Parts**

Use the **Word Parts Tables** to complete the following questions. Check your responses with the Answer Key in Appendix C.

1. MATCH: *Draw a line to match the suffix with its definition.*

   a. -rrhea   inflammation
   b. -rrhagia   excessive bleeding
   c. -itis   flow, discharge

> **FYI** -rrhagia and -rrhea are two of four **rrh** suffixes you will learn in medical terminology. Note the **h** in **rrh**. The **h** is often missing in misspelled words.

2. LABEL: *Write the combining forms for anatomic structures of the respiratory system on Figure 4.3. These anatomic combining forms will be used to build and translate medical terms in Exercise A.*

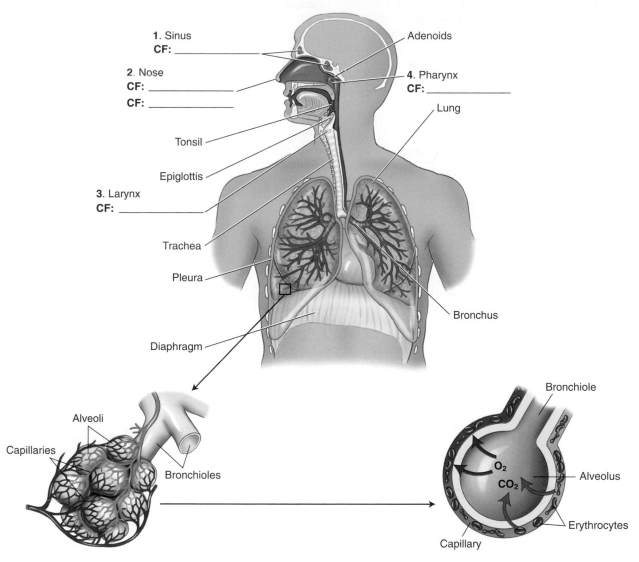

Figure 4.3 The respiratory system and combining forms for sinus, nose, larynx, and pharynx.

3. **BUILD:** *Using the combining form* **rhin/o** *and the suffixes reviewed in the previous exercise, build the following terms describing conditions related to the nose and nasal membranes:*

   a. inflammation of the nose (nasal membranes)   _____/_____
                                                              wr   s

   b. discharge from the nose   _____/_o_/_____
                                                              wr   cv   s

   c. excessive bleeding from the nose   _____/_o_/_____
                                                              wr   cv   s

4. **READ:** **Rhinorrhagia** (rī-nō-RĀ-ja), also called **epistaxis**, refers to a nosebleed. **Rhinorrhea** (rī-nō-RĒ-a), the medical term for "runny nose," describes discharge from the nose as seen in the common cold and in **rhinitis** (rī-NĪ-tis), a symptom of allergies.

5. **MATCH:** *Draw a line to match the combining form or suffix with its definition.*

   a. -tomy   mucus
   b. -al, -ous   inflammation
   c. muc/o   pertaining to
   d. -itis   cut into, incision

> **FYI**   **Incision** refers to the surgical cutting of skin and deeper anatomic structures as necessary to perform procedures.

6. **TRANSLATE:** *Complete the definitions of the following terms by using the meaning of word parts to fill in the blanks. Remember, the definition usually starts with the meaning of the suffix.*

   a. nas/al   _____ to the _____
   b. muc/ous   _____ to _____
   c. sinus/itis   _____ of the _____ (membranes)
   d. sinus/o/tomy   (cut into or)_____ of a _____

7. **READ:** Paranasal sinuses are hollow spaces located near the **nasal** (NĀ-zal) cavity and drain into it. The paranasal sinuses produce mucus, a slimy fluid that lubricates and protects the **mucous** (MŪ-kus) membranes. **Sinusitis** (sī-nū-SĪ-tis), which presents with nasal congestion, headache, and fever, often extends into the nasal passageways. A **sinusotomy** (sī-nū-SOT-o-mē) may be performed to relieve symptoms in more severe cases. An otolaryngologist, often referred to as an ENT, is a specialist trained to treat problems of the ear, nose, and throat. ENTs also perform surgeries of the head and neck, including sinusotomy.

> **FYI**   **Mucus** and **mucous** are pronounced the same. **Mucus** is a noun, the substance, whereas **mucous** is an adjective describing a noun, as in mucous membrane.

8. LABEL: *Write word parts to complete Figure 4.4.*

A   B

Inflammation

Normal

Mucus-filled
sinuses

Figure 4.4 A) Normal sinuses. B) _____/_____.
                                        sinus   inflammation

9. MATCH: *Draw a line to match the suffix with its definition.*

a. -itis	pertaining to	
b. -eal	inflammation	
c. -ectomy	visual examination	
d. -scope	surgical removal, excision	
e. -scopy	instrument used for visual examination	

> **FYI** **Excision** refers
> to the surgical removal
> of all or part of an
> anatomic structure or
> diseased tissue, such
> as a tumor.

10. BUILD: *Write word parts to build terms describing inflammation. (Hint: Use **nas/o** for the combining form meaning nose.)*

a. inflammation of the pharynx (throat)   _____/_____
                                                        wr   s

b. inflammation of the nose (nasal membranes) and   _____/ o /_____/_____
    pharynx (throat)   wr   cv   wr   s

c. inflammation of the larynx (voice box)   _____/_____
                                                        wr   s

11. READ: **Pharyngitis** (far-in-JĪ-tis) is the medical term for sore throat. The larynx, commonly referred to as the voice box, contains the vocal cords. Frequently caused by a virus, **laryngitis** (lar-in-JĪ-tis) may be characterized by hoarseness or loss of voice.

12. BUILD: *Write word parts to build descriptive terms using the suffix –eal, meaning **pertaining to.***

a. pertaining to the pharynx (throat)   _____/_____
                                                        wr   s

b. pertaining to the larynx (voice box)   _____/_____
                                                     wr   s

FYI   The suffixes **-ic, -al, -ous, -ary,** and **-eal** all mean **pertaining to.** As you practice and use the medical terms, you will become more familiar with which suffix is used.

13. TRANSLATE: *Complete the definitions of the following terms built from the combining form **laryng/o**, meaning larynx. Use the meaning of word parts to fill in the blanks. Remember, the definition usually starts with the meaning of the suffix.*

    a. laryng/o/scope   _____ used for _____ examination of the larynx

    b. laryng/o/scopy   visual _____ of the _____

    c. laryng/ectomy   _____ (or surgical removal) of the _____

14. READ: A **laryngoscope** (lar-RING-gō-skōp) is used to perform **laryngoscopy** (lar-in-GOS-ko-pē). Treatment of **laryngeal** (lar-IN-jē-al) cancer may include a **laryngectomy** (lar-in-JEK-to-mē).

FYI   Manuel Garcia, a Spanish singing teacher, invented the modern **laryngoscope** in 1854. The first successful **laryngectomy** was performed in 1873 by the famous Viennese surgeon Christian Albert Theodor Billroth.

15. MATCH: *Draw a line to match the prefix or suffix with its definition.*

    a. a-, an-   breathing

    b. dys-   absence of, without

    c. hyper-   difficult, painful, abnormal

    d. hypo-   below, deficient, under

    e. -pnea   above, excessive

FYI   **Tips for Use of Word Parts**
- The prefix **a-** is used when the following word root begins with a consonant. **An-** is used when the following word root begins with a vowel.
- For translating the meaning of respiratory system terms, use "excessive" for the definition of **hyper-** and use "deficient" for the definition of **hypo-**.
- The suffix **–pnea** is used with a prefix only. The word root **pne** means breathing and is embedded in the suffix **-pnea**.

16. TRANSLATE: *Complete the definitions of the following terms by using the meaning of word parts to fill in the blanks. Remember, the definition usually starts with the meaning of the suffix. Terms built using the suffix **-pnea**:*

    a. a/pnea   _____ of _____

    b. dys/pnea _____ breathing

    c. hypo/pnea deficient _____

    d. hyper/pnea _____ breathing

17. READ: Apnea (AP-nē-a) refers to absence of spontaneous respiration. **Dyspnea** (DISP-nē-a), a symptom, describes shortness of breath or any other breathing difficulty outside of a person's normal experience. **Hypopnea** (hī-POP-nē-a) and **hyperpnea** (hī-perp-NĒ-a) describe airflow in terms of rate and quantity. Hypopnea represents a deficient or decreased rate and depth of breathing. Hyperpnea represents an excessive or increased rate and depth of breathing. The medical terms apnea and hypopnea are key findings in obstructive sleep apnea.

18. MATCH: *Draw a line to match the combining form, prefix, or suffix with its definition.*

a.	-ia	above, excessive
b.	-meter	instrument used to measure
c.	hyper-	condition of
d.	hypo-	below, deficient, under
e.	capn/o	oxygen
f.	ox/i	breathing
g.	spir/o	carbon dioxide

19. BUILD: *Write word parts to build terms describing excessive or deficient amounts of oxygen and carbon dioxide in the body:*

a. condition of excessive oxygen (in the tissues)

_____ / _____ / _____
    p   wr   s

b. condition of excessive carbon dioxide (in the blood)

_____ / _____ / _____
    p   wr   s

c. condition of deficient carbon dioxide (in the blood)

_____ / _____ / _____
    p   wr   s

d. condition of deficient oxygen (in the tissues)

_____ / _____ / _____
    p   wr   s

> **FYI**   The **o** from **hypo** has been dropped in the medical term **hypoxia**. The final vowel of a prefix may be dropped when the word to which it is added begins with a vowel.

20. READ: Condition of deficient oxygen in the tissues, or **hypoxia** (hī-POK-sē-a), may be caused by the inability of erythrocytes to transport oxygen to the tissues or from being at high altitude. Condition of excessive oxygen, **hyperoxia** (hī-per-OK-sē-a), usually results from an increase in the concentration of oxygen given to a patient. Condition of excessive carbon dioxide, or **hypercapnia** (hī-per-KAP-nē-a), can result from disorders such as emphysema or chronic obstructive pulmonary disease, whereas condition of deficient carbon dioxide, or **hypocapnia** (hī-pō-KAP-nē-a), usually results from hyperventilation, which is ventilation of the lungs beyond normal body needs.

21. TRANSLATE: *Complete the definitions of the following terms by using the meaning of word parts to fill in the blanks. Remember, the definition usually starts with the meaning of the suffix. Terms built using the suffix -**meter**:*

   a. capn/o/meter _____ used to measure _____ _____

   b. ox/i/meter   instrument used to _____ _____

   c. spir/o/meter _____ used to measure _____ (or lung volumes)

22. READ: A **capnometer** (kap-NOM-e-ter) measures carbon dioxide concentration in exhaled air. A pulse **oximeter** (ok-SIM-e-ter) is placed on a fingertip and measures the oxygen level in the blood. A **spirometer** (spī-ROM-e-ter) measures the amount of air that can be inhaled and exhaled.

23. LABEL: *Write word parts to complete Figure 4.5.*

A   B   C

Figure 4.5   A) Pulse _____/i/_____.
                               oxygen   instrument used to measure
                  B) _____/o/_____.
                       carbon dioxide   instrument used to measure
                  C) _____/o/_____.
                       breathing   instrument used to measure

24. REVIEW OF RESPIRATORY SYSTEM TERMS BUILT FROM WORD PARTS: The following is an alphabetical list of terms built and translated in the previous exercises.

MEDICAL TERMS BUILT FROM WORD PARTS

TERM	DEFINITION	TERM	DEFINITION
1. apnea (AP-nē-a)	absence of breathing	**3. dyspnea** (DISP-nē-a)	difficult breathing
2. capnometer (kap-NOM-e-ter)	instrument used to measure carbon dioxide (Figure 4.5, *B*)	**4. hypercapnia** (hī-per-KAP-nē-a)	condition of excessive carbon dioxide

Continued

MEDICAL TERMS BUILT FROM WORD PARTS—cont'd

TERM	DEFINITION	TERM	DEFINITION
5. hyperoxia (hī-per-OK-sē-a)	condition of excessive oxygen	16. nasal (NĀ-zal)	pertaining to the nose
6. hyperpnea (hī-perp-NĒ-a)	excessive breathing	17. nasopharyngitis (nā-zō-far-in-JĪ-tis)	inflammation of the nose and pharynx
7. hypocapnia (hī-pō-KAP-nē-a)	condition of deficient carbon dioxide	18. oximeter (ok-SIM-e-ter)	instrument used to measure oxygen (Figure 4.5, A)
8. hypopnea (hī-POP-nē-a)	deficient breathing	19. pharyngeal (fa-RIN-jē-al)	pertaining to the pharynx
9. hypoxia (hī-POK-sē-a)	condition of deficient oxygen	20. pharyngitis (far-in-JĪ-tis)	inflammation of the pharynx
10. laryngeal (lar-IN-jē-al)	pertaining to the larynx	21. rhinitis (rī-NĪ-tis)	inflammation of the nose (nasal membranes)
11. laryngectomy (lar-in-JEK-to-mē)	excision of the larynx	22. rhinorrhagia (rī-nō-RĀ-ja)	excessive bleeding from the nose (also called epistaxis)
12. laryngitis (lar-in-JĪ-tis)	inflammation of the larynx	23. rhinorrhea (rī-nō-RĒ-a)	discharge from the nose
13. laryngoscope (lar-RING-gō-skōp)	instrument used for visual examination of the larynx (Figure 4.7)	24. sinusitis (sī-nū-SĪ-tis)	inflammation of the sinus (membranes) (Figure 4.4, B)
14. laryngoscopy (lar-in-GOS-ko-pē)	visual examination of the larynx	25. sinusotomy (sī-nū-SOT-o-mē)	incision of a sinus
15. mucous (MŪ-kus)	pertaining to mucus	26. spirometer (spī-ROM-e-ter)	instrument used to measure breathing (lung volume) (Figure 4.5, C)

EXERCISE B   Pronounce and Spell Terms Built from Word Parts

Practice pronunciation and spelling on paper and online.

1. **Practice on Paper**
   a. **Pronounce:** Read the phonetic spelling and say aloud the terms listed in the previous table, Review of Terms Built from Word Parts. Refer to Table 1.3 Pronunciation Key as needed.
   b. **Spell:** Have a study partner read the terms aloud. Write the spelling of the terms on a separate sheet of paper.

2. **Practice Online** 🌐
   a. **Access** online learning resources. Go to evolve.elsevier.com > Evolve Resources > Practice Student Resources.
   b. **Pronounce:** Select Audio Glossary > Lesson 4 > Exercise B. Select a term to hear its pronunciation and repeat aloud.
   c. **Spell:** Select Activities > Lesson 4 > Spell Terms > Exercise B. Select the audio icon and type the correct spelling of the term.

❑ Check the box when complete.

EXERCISE C   **Build and Translate MORE Medical Terms Built from Word Parts**

1. LABEL: *Write the word parts for anatomic structures of the respiratory system on Figure 4.6. These anatomic combining forms and suffix will be used to build and translate medical terms in Exercise C.*

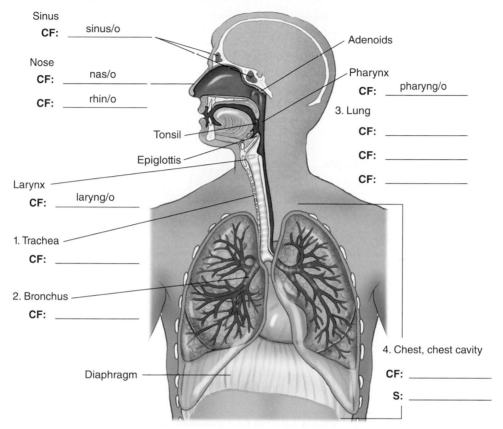

Sinus
CF: ____sinus/o____

Nose
CF: ____nas/o____
CF: ____rhin/o____

Tonsil

Epiglottis

Larynx
CF: ____laryng/o____

1. Trachea
CF: _____

2. Bronchus
CF: _____

Diaphragm

Adenoids

Pharynx
CF: ____pharyng/o____

3. Lung
CF: _____
CF: _____
CF: _____

4. Chest, chest cavity
CF: _____
S: _____

Figure 4.6 The respiratory system and word parts for trachea, bronchus, lung, and chest cavity.

2. MATCH: *Draw a line to match the prefix or suffix with its definition.*

    a. -stomy   instrument used for visual examination
    b. -tomy   creation of an artificial opening
    c. endo-   pertaining to
    d. -al   within
    e. -scope   cut into, incision

3. TRANSLATE: *Complete the definitions of terms built from the combining form **trache/o** by using the meaning of word parts to fill in the blanks. Remember, the definition usually starts with the meaning of the suffix.*

    a. trache/o/tomy   (cut into or) _____ of the _____

    b. trache/o/stomy   creation of an _____ _____ into the _____

    c. endo/trache/al   _____ to _____ the _____

4. READ: An **endotracheal** (en-dō-TRĀ-kē-al) tube, or **ET** tube, is inserted through the mouth or nose into the trachea to maintain an open airway, the passageway for the movement of the air to and from the lungs. This tube remains in place for a limited amount of time, such as during a surgical procedure. A **laryngoscope** (lar-RING-gō-skōp) is used to place the tube. Insertion of the tube is called endotracheal intubation.

5. LABEL: *Write word parts to complete Figure 4.7.*

Figure 4.7 The nurse anesthetist inserts a(n) _____/_____/_____ tube with a
within   trachea   pertaining to

_____/o/_____ to guide the tube into place.
larynx   instrument used for visual examination

6. READ: A **tracheotomy** (trā-kē-OT-o-mē) establishes an open airway when normal breathing is obstructed. An emergency tracheotomy may be performed, for instance, when a person's upper airway is blocked. If the opening needs to be maintained, a tube is inserted, creating a **tracheostomy** (trā-kē-OS-to-mē). A tracheostomy may be temporary, as for prolonged mechanical ventilation to support breathing, or it may be permanent, as in airway reconstruction after a **laryngectomy** (lar-in-JEK-to-mē) to treat **laryngeal** (lar-IN-jē-al) cancer.

FYI   The terms **tracheotomy** and **tracheostomy** are used interchangeably, though tracheotomy names the procedure entailing an incision into the trachea and tracheostomy names the resulting opening.

7. LABEL: *Write word parts to complete Figure 4.8.*

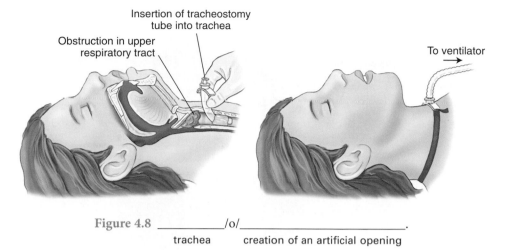

Insertion of tracheostomy
tube into trachea

Obstruction in upper
respiratory tract

To ventilator

Figure 4.8 _____ /o/ _____ .
              trachea   creation of an artificial opening

---

8. MATCH: *Draw a line to match the suffix with its definition.*

a. -scope   instrument used for visual examination
b. -scopy   inflammation
c. -itis   visual examination

---

9. BUILD: *Write word parts to build the following terms using the combining form **bronch/o**, meaning bronchi.*

a. inflammation of the bronchi   _____ / _____
                                                                         wr   s

b. instrument used for visual examination of the bronchi   _____ / o / _____
                                                                         wr   cv   s

c. visual examination of the bronchi   _____ / o / _____
                                                                         wr   cv   s

> **FYI** The medical term **bronchus** is singular; the plural form, **bronchi**, refers to the multiple branches within the lung. See Lesson 3 for plural endings.

---

10. READ: **Bronchoscopy** (bron-KOS-ko-pē) is performed by using a **bronchoscope** (BRON-kō-skōp) inserted through the nostril or mouth and passed through the pharynx, larynx, and trachea into the bronchus.

11. LABEL: *Write word parts to complete Figure 4.9.*

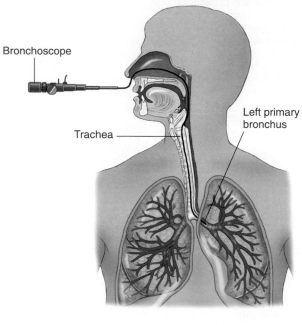

Figure 4.9 _____/o/_____.
　　　　　　　　bronchi　　　　visual examination

---

12. MATCH: *Draw a line to match the suffix with its definition.*

a. -ia　　　　　　pertaining to
b. -ectomy　　　　study of
c. -ary　　　　　　one who studies and treats (specialist, physician)
d. -logy　　　　　diseased state, condition of
e. -logist　　　　surgical removal, excision

---

13. TRANSLATE: *Complete the definitions of the following terms by using the meaning of word parts to fill in the blanks. Remember, the definition usually starts with the meaning of the suffix. Terms built from the combining form **pulmon/o**, meaning lung:*

a. pulmon/ary　　　　_____ to the _____

b. pulmon/o/logy　　　_____ of the _____

c. pulmon/o/logist　　physician who _____ and _____ diseases of the lung

14. **READ:** The medical term **pulmonary** (PUL-mō-nar-ē), an adjective, describes anatomic location, as in pulmonary artery, or the location of a disease, as in pulmonary tuberculosis. **Pulmonology** (pul-mon-OL-o-jē), a subspecialty of internal medicine, focuses on treating diseases and disorders of the lungs and bronchial tubes. The pulmonology department of a hospital provides evaluation, diagnosis, and treatment of patients with conditions affecting the lungs. **Pulmonologists** (pul-mon-OL-o-jists) may be involved with the care of hospitalized patients who are critically ill. They also care for lung transplant candidates and patients with pulmonary diseases, including severe asthma, pneumonia, emphysema, chronic obstructive pulmonary disease (COPD), cystic fibrosis (CF), and tuberculosis (TB).

15. **BUILD:** *Write word parts to build terms using the combining form **pneumon/o**, meaning lung, air.*

    a. diseased state of the lungs   _____ / _____
                                                                wr   s

    b. diseased state of the bronchi and lungs   _____ / o / _____ / _____
                                                       wr   cv   wr   s

    c. excision of a lung   _____ / _____
                                                      wr   s

16. **READ:** **Pneumonia** (nū-MŌ-nē-a) describes a diseased state of the lung and refers to an infection of the lung or, more specifically, the alveoli (air sacs within the lungs). **Bronchopneumonia** (bron-kō-nū-MŌ-nē-a) refers to an infection of the bronchi and the lung. **Pneumonectomy** (nū-mō-NEK-to-mē), excision of the whole lung, is most commonly performed to treat lung cancer.

17. **MATCH:** *Draw a line to match the combining form or suffix with its definition.*

    a. -tomy   chest, chest cavity
    b. -centesis   lung, air
    c. -thorax, thorac/o   cut into, incision
    d. pneum/o   surgical puncture to remove fluid (with a sterile needle)

> **FYI**   While pneumon/o and pneum/o can both be used to mean lung or air, when building and translating terms presented in this text, use **pneum/o** to mean **air** and **pneumon/o** to mean **lung**.

18. **BUILD:** *Write word parts to build terms using the suffix –**thorax** and the combining form **thorac/o**, meaning chest, chest cavity.*

    a. air in the chest cavity   _____ / o / _____
                                                            wr   cv   s

    b. incision into the chest cavity   _____ / o / _____
                                                             wr   cv   s

    c. surgical puncture to remove fluid from the chest cavity   thora/ _____
                                                               wr   s

> **FYI**   The combining vowel "o" and the "c" in **thorac/o** are dropped in the term **thoracentesis**.

19. **LABEL:** *Write word parts to complete Figure 4.10.*

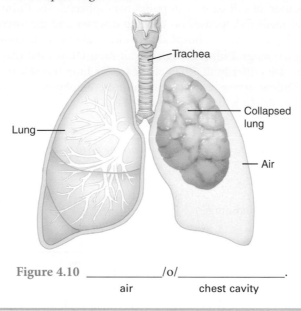

Trachea

Collapsed
lung

Air

Lung

Figure 4.10 _____/o/_____.

air   chest cavity

---

20. **READ: Pneumothorax** (nū-mō-THOR-aks), directly translated as "air in the chest cavity," specifically refers to air in the pleural space between the membrane covering the lung and the membrane lining the thoracic cavity. Pneumothorax may lead to the collapse of a lung and is often the result of an open chest wound. **Thoracotomy** (tho-ra-KOT-o-mē) is a surgical procedure performed to examine, treat, or excise organs contained in the chest cavity. Procedures involving -**centesis** are performed for therapeutic and diagnostic purposes, facilitating the body's healing processes by removing excess fluid from a body cavity and by obtaining a fluid sample for laboratory analysis, respectively. **Thoracentesis** (thor-a-sen-TĒ-sis) is performed to remove fluid from the chest cavity.

---

21. **LABEL:** *Write word parts to complete Figure 4.11.*

Ribs

Parietal
pleura

Visceral
pleura

Lung

Pleural
effusion

Area for needle insertion

Figure 4.11 A _____/_____ is used for both diagnosis and treatment.

chest cavity   surgical puncture to remove fluid

22. MATCH: *Draw a line to match the combining form, prefix or suffix with its definition.*

 a. thorac/o   instrument used for visual examination
 b. endo-   visual examination
 c. -scope   chest, chest cavity
 d. -scopy   within
 e. -scopic   pertaining to
 f. -ic   pertaining to visual examination

> **FYI**   Medical terms ending with the suffix **-scope** and **-scopy** are nouns. Medical terms ending with the suffix **-scopic** are adjectives. For example:
> endoscope = noun, the instrument
> endoscopy = noun, the procedure
> endoscopic = adjective, describes the procedure

23. TRANSLATE: *Complete the definitions of the following terms by using the meaning of word parts to fill in the blanks. Remember, the definition usually starts with the meaning of the suffix. Terms built using the prefix* ***endo-:***

 a. endo/scope   _____ used for _____ examination _____
                    (a hollow organ or body cavity)

 b. endo/scopic   _____ to visual examination _____ (a hollow organ or
                    body cavity)

 c. endo/scopy   visual _____ within (a hollow organ or body cavity)

> **FYI**   The medical terms **endo/scope**, **endo/scopic**, and **endo/scopy** appear to be made up of a prefix and a suffix. The word root **scop**, meaning "to view," is embedded in the suffixes **-scope**, **-scopic**, and **-scopy.**

24. READ: Endoscopy (en-DOS-ko-pē), the visual examination within a hollow organ or body cavity, is per-formed using an **endoscope** (EN-dō-skōp). **Endoscopic** (en-dō-SKOP-ik) surgery is used for diagnosis and treatment. A small incision is made to accommodate a specialized endoscope fitted with a video camera. Other small incisions are made to hold the surgical instruments. The surgeon uses images displayed on a monitor to perform the surgery. Endoscopic surgery, which causes less pain and reduces recovery time, has replaced many large incision surgeries.

25. BUILD: *Write word parts to build terms using the combining form* ***thorac/o,*** *meaning chest, chest cavity.*

 a. pertaining to the chest   _____/_____
                                                                  wr   s

 b. visual examination of the chest cavity   _____/_o_/_____
                                                                  wr   cv   s

 c. instrument used for visual examination of the chest cavity _____/_o_/_____
                                                                  wr   cv   s

 d. pertaining to visual examination of the chest cavity   _____/_o_/_____
                                                                  wr   cv   s

26. READ: **Thoracoscopy** (thor-a-KOS-ko-pē) is a type of **endoscopy** (en-DOS-ko-pē). **Thoracoscopic** (thor-a-kō-SKOP-ik) surgery, which employs the use of a **thoracoscope** (tho-RAK-ō-skōp), may be performed to obtain a biopsy, remove a portion of the lung, treat cysts, or treat plural effusions. A **thoracic** (thō-RAS-ik) surgeon performs the procedure.

> **FYI**   **Thoracic surgeons** and **pulmonologists** both specialize in treating disorders of the lower respiratory system; however, pulmonologists do not perform surgery.

27. LABEL: *Write word parts to complete Figure 4.12.*

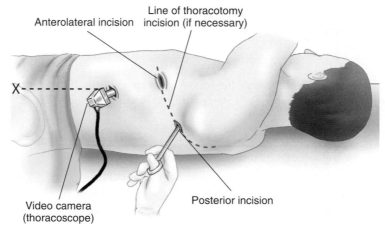

Anterolateral incision   Line of thoracotomy incision (if necessary)

X

Video camera (thoracoscope)

Posterior incision

Figure 4.12 _____/o/_____ surgery.
chest cavity   pertaining to visual examination

28. MATCH: *Draw a line to match the word part with its definition.*

a. -graphy	sleep
b. -gram	many
c. poly-	process of recording
d. somn/o	record

29. TRANSLATE: *Complete the definitions of the following terms by using the meaning of word parts to fill in the blanks. Remember, the definition usually starts with the meaning of the suffix.*

a. poly/somn/o/graphy   process of _____ many _____(tests)
b. poly/somn/o/gram   _____ of _____ sleep (tests)

30. READ: Polysomnography (pol-ē-som-NOG-rah-fē), abbreviated as **PSG**, is used to diagnose and evaluate sleep disorders, including sleep-related respiratory disorders. A battery of tests is performed during sleep to monitor oxygen levels, heart rate, eye movements, brain waves, and other measures. The resulting **polysomnogram** (pol-ē-SOM-nō-gram) documents information gathered from the various tests.

31. LABEL: *Write word parts to complete Figure 4.13.*

Figure 4.13 A. _____/_____/o/_____
                        many   sleep (tests)   process of recording

              B. _____/_____/o/_____
                        many   sleep (tests)   record

32. REVIEW OF MORE RESPIRATORY SYSTEM TERMS BUILT FROM WORD PARTS: The following is an alphabetical list of terms built and translated in the previous exercises.

MEDICAL TERMS BUILT FROM WORD PARTS

TERM	DEFINITION	TERM	DEFINITION
1. bronchitis (bron-KĪ-tis)	inflammation of the bronchi	**6. endoscopic** (en-dō-SKOP-ik)	pertaining to visual examination within (a hollow organ or cavity)
2. bronchopneumonia (bron-kō-nū-MŌ-nē-a)	diseased state of the bronchi and lungs	**7. endoscopy** (en-DOS-ko-pē)	visual examination within (a hollow organ or cavity)
3. bronchoscope (BRON-kō-skōp)	instrument used for visual examination of the bronchi	**8. endotracheal (ET)** (en-dō-TRĀ-kē-al)	pertaining to within the trachea
4. bronchoscopy (bron-KOS-ko-pē)	visual examination of the bronchi (Figure 4.9)	**9. pneumonectomy** (nū-mō-NEK-to-mē)	excision of a lung
5. endoscope (EN-dō-skōp)	instrument used for visual examination within (a hollow organ or cavity)	**10. pneumonia** (nū-MŌ-nē-a)	diseased state of the lungs

Continued

MEDICAL TERMS BUILT FROM WORD PARTS—cont'd

TERM	DEFINITION	TERM	DEFINITION
11. **pneumothorax** (nū-mō-THOR-aks)	air in the chest cavity (Figure 4.10)	18. **thoracic** (thō-RAS-ik)	pertaining to the chest
12. **polysomnography (PSG)** (pol-ē-som-NOG-rah-fē)	process of recording many (tests) during sleep; (also called **sleep study**)	19. **thoracoscope** (tho-RAK-ō-skōp)	instrument used for visual examination of the chest cavity
13. **polysomnogram** (pol-ē-SOM-nō-gram)	record of many sleep tests	20. **thoracoscopic** (thor-a-kō-SKOP-ik)	pertaining to visual examination of the chest cavity (Figure 4.12)
14. **pulmonary** (PUL-mō-nar-ē)	pertaining to the lung	21. **thoracoscopy** (tho-a-KOS-ko-pē)	visual examination of the chest cavity
15. **pulmonologist** (pul-mon-OL-o-jist)	physician who studies and treats diseases of the lung	22. **thoracotomy** (tho-ra-KOT-o-mē)	incision into the chest cavity
16. **pulmonology** (pul-mon-OL-o-jē)	study of the lung	23. **tracheostomy** (trā-kē-OS-to-mē)	creation of an artificial opening into the trachea (Figure 4.8)
17. **thoracentesis** (thor-a-sen-TĒ-sis)	surgical puncture to remove fluid from the chest cavity (Figure 4.11)	24. **tracheotomy** (trā-kē-OT-o-mē)	incision into the trachea

EXERCISE D   Pronounce and Spell MORE Terms Built from Word Parts

Practice pronunciation and spelling on paper and online.

1. **Practice on Paper**
   a. **Pronounce**: Read the phonetic spelling and say aloud the terms listed in the previous table, Review of MORE Terms Built from Word Parts. Refer to Table 1.3 Pronunciation Key as needed.
   b. **Spell**: Have a study partner read the terms aloud. Write the spelling of the terms on a separate sheet of paper.

2. **Practice Online** 🌐
   a. **Access** online learning resources. Go to evolve.elsevier.com > Evolve Resources > Practice Student Resources.
   b. **Pronounce**: Select Audio Glossary > Lesson 4 > Exercise D. Select a term to hear its pronunciation and repeat aloud.
   c. **Spell**: Select Activities > Lesson 4 > Spell Terms > Exercise D. Select the audio icon and type the correct spelling of the term.

❑ Check the box when complete.

OBJECTIVE 2

Define, pronounce, and spell medical terms NOT built from word parts.

The terms listed below may contain word parts, but are difficult to translate literally.

MEDICAL TERMS NOT BUILT FROM WORD PARTS

TERM	DEFINITION
1. **asthma** (AZ-ma)	respiratory disease characterized by coughing, wheezing, and shortness of breath; caused by constriction and inflammation of airways that is reversible between attacks
2. **chronic obstructive pulmonary disease (COPD)** (KRON-ik) (ob-STRUK-tive) (PUL-mō-nar-ē) (di ZĒZ)	progressive lung disease blocking air flow, which makes breathing difficult. Chronic bronchitis and emphysema are two main components of COPD. Most COPD is a result of cigarette smoking.
3. **computed tomography (CT)** (kom-PU-ted) (tō-MOG-re-fē)	diagnostic imaging test producing scans composed from sectional radiographic images, which can be taken in any of the anatomic planes for a multidimensional view of internal structures. Chest computed tomography is often performed to follow up on abnormalities identified on previous chest radiographs. (Figure 4.14, *B*)
4. **coronavirus disease (COVID-19)** (kō-RŌ-na-vī-rus) (di-ZĒZ)	respiratory illness caused by a newly discovered virus with symptoms that include fever, cough, fatigue, difficulty breathing, and digestive upset; the disease course can range from mild to severe with the possibility of acute respiratory distress syndrome and multisystem organ failure

FYI Several strains of **coronavirus** exist, including those that cause severe acute respiratory syndrome (SARS), Middle East respiratory syndrome (MERS), and coronavirus disease (COVID-19).

TERM	DEFINITION
5. **culture and sensitivity (C&S)** (KUL-cher) (sen-si-TIV-i-tē)	laboratory test performed on a collected sample to determine the presence of pathogenic bacteria or fungi and to identify the most effective antimicrobial treatment. The test may be performed on sputum, throat cultures, blood, urine, and other fluids. Sputum culture and sensitivity tests are frequently used in the diagnosis of lower respiratory tract infections such as bronchitis and pneumonia.
6. **emphysema** (em-fi-SĒ-ma)	loss of elasticity of the alveoli results in distension, causing stretching of the lung. As a result, the body does not receive enough oxygen. (component of COPD)
7. **influenza (flu)** (in-flū-EN-za)	highly contagious and often severe viral infection of the respiratory tract

FYI **Influenza pandemic** is the sudden outbreak of a flu that becomes widespread, affecting a region, a continent, or the world. Examples are H1N1 swine flu and H5N1 avian flu.

TERM	DEFINITION
8. **obstructive sleep apnea (OSA)** (ob-STRUK-tiv) (slēp) (AP-nē-a)	repetitive pharyngeal collapse during sleep, which leads to short absences of breathing (apnea); can produce daytime drowsiness and elevated blood pressure
9. **radiograph** (RĀ-dē-ō-graf)	image created by ionizing radiation; chest radiographs are frequently performed to diagnose respiratory conditions; (also called an **x-ray**) (Figure 4.14, *A*)
10. **sputum** (SPŪ-tum)	mucous secretion from the lungs, bronchi, and trachea expelled through the mouth
11. **tuberculosis (TB)** (tū-ber-kū-LŌ-sis)	infectious bacterial disease, most commonly spread by inhalation of small particles and usually affecting the lungs (may spread to other organs)
12. **upper respiratory infection (URI)** (UP-er) (RES-pi-ra-tor-ē) (in-FEK-shun)	infection of the nasal cavity, pharynx, or larynx, usually caused by a virus; (commonly called a **cold**) (Figure 4.15)

FYI   **Diagnostic imaging**
is a general term referring to procedures that generate images of internal structures, including radiography (also called x-ray), computed tomography (CT), magnetic resonance (MR), nuclear medicine (NM), and sonography (also called ultrasonography, abbreviated as US) .

Figure 4.14 Diagnostic imaging. **A,** Radiographic table and chest radiograph (x-ray). **B,** CT scanner and scan of the chest.

EXERCISE E   Match

Match the terms in the first column with their correct descriptions in the second column.

_____ **1.** asthma

_____ **2.** tuberculosis

_____ **3.** sputum

_____ **4.** influenza

_____ **5.** coronavirus disease

_____ **6.** chronic obstructive pulmonary disease

a. highly contagious and often severe viral infection of the respiratory tract

b. respiratory illness caused by a newly discovered virus, which ranges from mild to severe with the possibility of acute respiratory distress syndrome and multisystem organ failure

c. chronic bronchitis and emphysema are two main components of this progressive lung disease

d. infectious bacterial disease, most commonly spread by inhalation of small particles and usually affecting the lungs (may spread to other organs)

e. caused by constriction and inflammation of airways that is reversible between attacks

f. mucous secretion from the lungs, bronchi, and trachea expelled through the mouth

EXERCISE F   Label

Write the medical terms pictured and defined using the previous table of Medical Terms NOT Built from Word Parts.
Check your work with the Answer Key in Appendix C.

1. _____

diagnostic imaging test producing scans composed from sectional radiographic images, which can be taken in any of the anatomic planes for a multidimensional view of internal structures

2. _____

image created by ionizing radiation

3. _____

repetitive pharyngeal collapse during sleep, which leads to short absences of breathing; the lack of activity of the pharyngeal muscle structure allows the airway to close

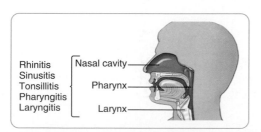

4. _____

loss of elasticity of the alveoli results in distension, causing stretching of the lung

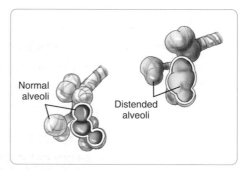

5. _____

infection of the nasal cavity, pharynx, or larynx, usually caused by a virus and commonly called a cold

6. _____

laboratory test performed on a collected sample to determine the presence of pathogenic bacteria or fungi and to identify the most effective antimicrobial treatment

---

| **EXERCISE G** | **Learn Medical Terms NOT Built from Word Parts** |

Fill in the blanks with medical terms defined in bold and abbreviations using the Medical Terms NOT Built from Word Parts table. Check your responses with the Answer Key in Appendix C.

1. COPD is the abbreviation for the medical term _____.

A person with COPD has dyspnea, especially with physical activity. Emptying the lungs, or exhalation, is particularly difficult; a visible hyperinflation of the chest may be observed. A chest _____, or **image created by ionizing radiation,** abbreviated as CXR, may be used to monitor COPD.

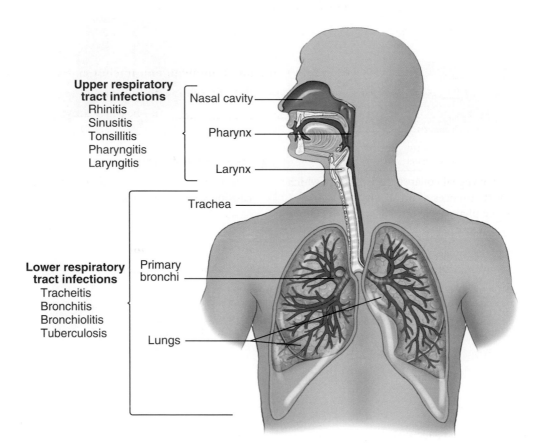

Figure 4.15 Upper and lower respiratory tract infections.

2. A person diagnosed with _____ has a **respiratory disease characterized by cough, wheezing and shortness of breath**. Allergens, toxins, or exercise cause recurring spasms of the smooth muscles of the bronchial airways, resulting in dyspnea, especially with inhalation.

> **FYI** **SOB** is the abbreviation for "shortness of breath."

3. **An infection of the nasal cavity, pharynx, or larynx** is known as a(n) _____ _____. A patient may have signs and symptoms of a **URI** from a **highly contagious and often severe viral infection** known as _____.

4. A patient with a pulmonary **infectious bacterial disease usually affecting the lungs and which may spread to other organs,** or _____, may be asked to cough to bring up _____, **mucous secretion from the lungs, bronchi, and trachea expelled through the mouth. A laboratory test performed on a collected sample to determine the presence of pathogenic bacteria or fungi,** or _____, may be performed to assess the effectiveness of medication to treat TB.

5. Prolonged cigarette smoking is the most common cause of the **loss of elasticity of the alveoli resulting in distension and causing stretching of the lung** or _____. There is no cure for this disease.

6. Chest _____, a **diagnostic imaging test producing scans composed from sectional radiographic images taken in any of the anatomic planes for a multidimensional view of internal structures,** offers a more detailed image than a chest radiograph. Chest CT scans may be ordered to diagnose unexplained respiratory symptoms such as dyspnea and coughing.

> **FYI** **Computed tomography** is also used to visualize other anatomic structures, such as the abdomen and brain.

7. **Repetitive pharyngeal collapse during sleep, leading to short absences of breathing,** or _____ _____, abbreviated as _____, is associated with increased risk for elevated blood pressure, cardiovascular disease, diabetes, and stroke. Nocturnal polysomnography as performed by a sleep technologist is frequently used in the diagnosis of this disorder. Continuous positive airway pressure, abbreviated as CPAP, is a common therapy used in treating OSA and involves the use of a machine to provide mild air pressure to keep airways open.

8. There are multiple variants of SARS-CoV-2, the virus causing _____ or a potentially life-threatening **respiratory illness with symptoms including fever, cough, fatigue, difficulty breathing, and digestive upset.**

EXERCISE H | Pronounce and Spell Medical Terms NOT Built from Word Parts

Practice pronunciation and spelling on paper and online.

1. **Practice on Paper**
   a. **Pronounce:** Read the phonetic spelling and say aloud the terms listed in the previous table of Medical Terms NOT Built from Word Parts. Refer to Table 1.3 Pronunciation Key as needed.
   b. **Spell:** Have a study partner read the terms aloud. Write the spelling of the terms on a separate sheet of paper.

2. **Practice Online** ⊕
   a. **Access** online learning resources. Go to evolve.elsevier.com > Evolve Resources > Practice Student Resources.
   b. **Pronounce:** Select Audio Glossary > Lesson 4 > Exercise H. Select a term to hear its pronunciation and repeat aloud.
   c. **Spell:** Select Activities > Lesson 4 > Spell Terms > Exercise H. Select the audio icon and type the correct spelling of the term.

❏ Check the box when complete.

OBJECTIVE 3

Write abbreviations.

Medical Record Abbreviations

Documentation of a patient's medical history and health care received is stored in medical records. Medical records are the who, what, when, where, and how of patient care. A common format used to record information is the **SOAP note**. SOAP is an acronym formed from the first letters of the note's section titles, including subjective, objective, assessment, and plan (Table 4.1). In documentation of a visit with a primary care provider, the objective section will include the patient's **vital signs (VS)**, including **temperature (T)**, **blood pressure (BP)**, **pulse (P)** rate, and **respiration (R)** rate.

TABLE 4.1	SOAP NOTE FORMAT	
Section	**Abbreviation**	**Description**
Subjective	S	Patient's words describing their health and problems experienced
Objective	O	Physical exam findings and diagnostic test results
Assessment	A	Provider's interpretation of the patient's condition
Plan	P	Therapeutic treatment, further diagnostic procedures, patient education, follow-up

ABBREVIATIONS RELATED TO THE RESPIRATORY SYSTEM

Use the online **flashcards** to familiarize yourself with the following abbreviations.

ABBREVIATION	TERM	ABBREVIATION	TERM
ABG	arterial blood gas	P	pulse
BP	blood pressure	PFTs	pulmonary function tests
CO_2	carbon dioxide	PSG	polysomnography
COPD	chronic obstructive pulmonary disease	R	respiration
COVID-19	coronavirus disease	RT	respiratory therapist
CPAP	continuous positive airway pressure	SOAP	subjective, objective, assessment, plan (note format)
C&S	culture and sensitivity	SOB	shortness of breath
CT	computed tomography	T	temperature
CXR	chest radiograph (chest x-ray)	TB	tuberculosis
ET	endotracheal	URI	upper respiratory infection
flu	influenza	VS	vital signs
O_2	oxygen	V/Q scan	lung ventilation/perfusion scan
OSA	obstructive sleep apnea		

EXERCISE I   Abbreviate Medical Terms

Write the correct abbreviation next to its medical term. Check your responses with the Answer Key in Appendix C.

1. Signs and Symptoms:

_____ shortness of breath

2. Diseases and Disorders:

a. _____ tuberculosis

b. _____ chronic obstructive pulmonary disease

c. _____ influenza

d. _____ upper respiratory infection

e. _____ obstructive sleep apnea

f. _____ coronavirus disease

3. Diagnostic Tests and Equipment:

a. _____ culture and sensitivity

b. _____ computed tomography

c. _____ chest radiograph (chest x-ray)

d. _____ lung ventilation/perfusion scan

e. _____ polysomnography

f. _____ pulmonary function tests

g. _____ arterial blood gas

4. Professions:

_____ respiratory therapist

5. Medical Record Abbreviations:

   a. _____ vital signs

   b. _____ temperature

   c. _____ pulse

   d. _____ respiration

   e. _____ blood pressure

   f. _____ subjective, objective, assessment, plan (note format)

6. Related Terms:

   a. _____ continuous positive airway pressure

   b. _____ carbon dioxide

   c. _____ endotracheal

   d. _____ oxygen

OBJECTIVE 4

Identify medical terms by clinical category.

Now that you have worked through the respiratory system lesson, review and practice medical terms grouped by clinical category. Categories include signs and symptoms, diseases and disorders, diagnostic tests and equipment, surgical procedures, specialties and professions, and other terms related to the respiratory system.

EXERCISE J Signs and Symptoms

Write the medical terms for signs and symptoms next to their definitions.

1. _____ absence of breathing
2. _____ difficult breathing
3. _____ excessive breathing
4. _____ deficient breathing
5. _____ condition of excessive oxygen
6. _____ condition of deficient oxygen
7. _____ condition of deficient carbon dioxide
8. _____ condition of excessive carbon dioxide
9. _____ discharge from the nose
10. _____ excessive bleeding from the nose (also called epistaxis)

EXERCISE K Diseases and Disorders

Write the medical terms for diseases and disorders next to their definitions.

1. _____ inflammation of the sinus (membranes)

2. _____ inflammation of the larynx

3. _____ inflammation of the pharynx

4. _____ inflammation of the nose and pharynx

5. _____ infection of the nasal cavity, pharynx, or larynx

6. _____ inflammation of the nose (nasal membranes)

7. _____ highly contagious and often severe viral infection of the respiratory tract

8. _____ infectious bacterial disease most commonly spread by inhalation of small particles and usually affecting the lungs (may spread to other organs)

9. _____ air in the chest cavity

10. _____ diseased state of the lungs

11. _____ diseased state of the bronchi and lungs

12. _____ inflammation of the bronchi

13. _____ loss of elasticity of the alveoli results in distension, causing stretching of the lung

14. _____ progressive lung disease blocking airflow, which makes breathing difficult. Chronic bronchitis and emphysema are two main components.

15. _____ repetitive pharyngeal collapse during sleep, which leads to short absences of breathing; can produce daytime drowsiness and elevated blood pressure

16. _____ respiratory disease characterized by coughing, wheezing, and shortness of breath; caused by constriction and inflammation of airways that is reversible between attacks

17. _____ respiratory infection caused by a newly discovered virus with symptoms that include fever, cough, fatigue, difficulty breathing, and digestive upset; the disease course can range from mild to severe with the possibility of acute respiratory distress syndrome and multisystem organ failure

EXERCISE L   Diagnostic Tests and Equipment

Write the medical terms for diagnostic tests and equipment next to their definitions.

1. _____ instrument used to measure carbon dioxide

2. _____ instrument used to measure oxygen

3. _____ instrument used to measure breathing (lung volume)

4. _____ pertaining to visual examination within (a hollow organ or cavity)

5. _____ visual examination of the chest cavity

6. _____ visual examination of the larynx

7. _____ visual examination of the bronchi

8. _____ instrument used for visual examination within (a hollow organ or cavity)

9. _____ instrument used for visual examination of the larynx

10. _____ instrument used for visual examination of the bronchi

11. _____ instrument used for visual examination of the chest cavity

12. _____ visual examination within (a hollow organ or cavity)

13. _____ pertaining to visual examination of the chest cavity

14. _____ image created by ionizing radiation

15. _____ diagnostic imaging test producing scans composed from sectional
    _____ radiographic images, which can be taken in any of the anatomic
    planes for a multidimensional view of internal structures

16. _____ laboratory test performed on a collected sample to determine
    _____ the presence of pathogenic bacteria or fungi and to identify the
    most effective antimicrobial treatment

17. _____ process of recording many sleep (tests)

18. _____ record of many sleep (tests)

EXERCISE M   Surgical Procedures

Write the medical terms for surgical procedures next to their definitions.

1. _____ surgical puncture to remove fluid from the chest cavity

2. _____ incision into the chest cavity

3. _____ incision of a sinus

4. _____ incision into the trachea

5. _____ creation of an artificial opening into the trachea

6. _____ excision of the larynx

7. _____ excision of a lung

EXERCISE N **Specialties and Professions**

Write the medical terms for specialties and professions next to their definitions.

1. _____ study of the lung

2. _____ physician who studies and treats diseases of the lung

EXERCISE O **Medical Terms Related to the Respiratory System**

Write the medical terms related to the respiratory system next to their definitions.

1. _____ pertaining to the chest

2. _____ pertaining to the lung

3. _____ pertaining to the nose

4. _____ pertaining to the larynx

5. _____ pertaining to the pharynx

6. _____ pertaining to within the trachea

7. _____ pertaining to mucus

8. _____ mucous secretion from the lungs, bronchi, and trachea expelled through the mouth

OBJECTIVE 5

Use medical language in clinical statements, the case study, and a medical record.

EXERCISE P **Use Medical Terms in Clinical Statements**

Circle the medical terms and abbreviations defined in the bolded phrases. Medical terms from previous lessons are included. Answers are listed in Appendix C. For pronunciation practice, read the answers aloud.

1. Mrs. Tsunde was experiencing **deficient breathing** (hyperpnea, hypopnea, hypercapnia) and, at times, had periods of **absence of breathing** (apnea, dyspnea, hyperoxia). As a result, she was observed as having **abnormal condition of blue of the extremities** (apnea, asthma, acrocyanosis).

2. The physician performed a **visual examination of the bronchus** (bronchoscopy, bronchoscope) to assist in diagnosing a **cancerous tumor** (neoplasm, carcinoma, abscess) in Mrs. Rabin. No **beyond control** (benign, metastasis, malignant) was noted. Treatment included a **surgical puncture to remove fluid from the chest cavity** (thoracoscopy, thoracotomy, thoracentesis) followed by a partial **excision of the lung** (pneumonectomy, pneumothorax, laryngectomy).

3. Sudden sharp chest pain and **difficult breathing** (apnea, dyspnea, asthma) are signs of **air in the chest cavity** (influenza, pneumothorax, tuberculosis). Treatment includes a(n) **incision into the chest cavity** (tracheostomy, thoracentesis, thoracotomy) and insertion of a chest tube to remove the air.

4. Inflammation of the sinus (membranes) (Sinusitis, Sinusotomy, Nasopharyngitis) is caused by bacteria, viruses, or fungi. It often occurs after an upper respiratory infection or may follow an acute allergic **inflammation of the nose (nasal membranes)** (rhinorrhagia, rhinorrhea, rhinitis). Symptoms include **discharge from the nose** (rhinorrhagia, rhinorrhea, rhinitis), malaise, pain, and mucopurulent drainage. **Pertaining to visual examination within** (Endoscope, Endoscopic, Endoscopy) surgery, drugs, and heat therapy may be used as treatment.

5. A chest **image created by ionizing radiation** (bronchoscopy, spriometer, radiograph) is used to assist in the diagnosis and monitoring of **an infectious bacterial disease usually affecting the lungs and which may spread to other organs** (tuberculosis, emphysema, influenza), **diseased state of the lung** (pneumothorax, bronchopneumonia, pneumonia), **progressive lung disease that blocks airflow** (COPD, OSA, TB), and other **pertaining to the lung** (pulmonary, laryngeal, pharyngeal) diseases.

6. An **instrument used to measure oxygen** (oximeter, capnometer, spirometer) is used to perform pulse oximetry, which measures the amount of oxygen in the blood. Oximetry, chest **image created by ionizing radiation** (radiograph, polysomnogram, computed tomography), and chest **scans composed from sectional radiographic images** (radiograph, polysomnogram, computed tomography) are often used to diagnose lung disorders such **as loss of elasticity of the alveoli results in distension causing stretching of the lung** (asthma, emphysema, URI). **Condition of excessive carbon dioxide** (Hypercapnia, Hyperoxia, Hyperpnea) can occur with severe emphysema.

7. **Arterial blood gas** (ABG, BP, PFTs) is a laboratory test performed on a blood sample to measure pH and the amount of **oxygen** (CO_2, O_2, R) and **carbon dioxide** (CO_2, O_2, R) in the blood. The test is commonly ordered when respiratory symptoms, such as dyspnea or **shortness of breath** (COPD, TB, SOB), worsen.

8. A **lung ventilation/perfusion scan** (PFTs, V/Q scan, C&S) is a form of diagnostic imaging often performed to identify a blood clot in the lungs, which may result from a **pertaining to the lung** (thoracic, endotracheal, pulmonary) embolus.

9. The sleep technologist compiled results of the **process of recording many sleep (tests)** (polysomnography, polysomnogram, PFTs) and forwarded the resulting **record of many sleep (tests)** (polysomnography, polysomnogram, PFTs) to the **physician who studies and treats diseases of the lung** (pulmonology, pulmonologist, respiratory therapist).

10. The patient was diagnosed with **repetitive pharyngeal collapse during sleep, which leads to short absences of breathing** (URI, COPD, OSA). **Continuous positive airway pressure** (CXR, PFTs, CPAP) therapy, involving the use of a mask worn while sleeping to administer a steady stream of air, was prescribed.

EXERCISE Q   **Apply Medical Terms to the Case Study**

Think back to Roberta, who was introduced in the case study at the beginning of the lesson. After working through Lesson 4 on the respiratory system, consider the medical terms that might be used to describe her experience. List three terms relevant to the case study and their meanings. ■

    Medical Term   **Definition**

1. _____   _____

2. _____   _____

3. _____   _____

EXERCISE R Use Medical Terms in a Document

Roberta was seen at her doctor's office later that afternoon. Her vital signs were taken, and she was examined by the nurse practitioner. Roberta's office visit, test results, and course of care were documented in the following medical record.

Use the definitions in numbers 1-9 to write medical terms within the document on the next page.

1. difficult breathing

2. mucous secretion from the lungs, bronchi, and trachea expelled through the mouth

3. discharge from the nose

4. pertaining to the nose

5. puffy swelling of tissue from the accumulation of fluid

6. abnormal condition of blue

7. image created by ionizing radiation (plural)

8. diseased state of the lungs

9. infection of the nasal cavity, pharynx, or larynx

Refer to the medical record to answer questions 10-14.

10. Write out the vital signs measurements as noted in the Objective section of the report.
    Temperature: _____
    Pulse: _____
    Respiration: _____
    Blood Pressure: _____

11. The term **mucoid**, used in the medical record to describe the sputum observed, is built from word parts. Use your knowledge of word parts to define the term.
    muc/o means _____
    -oid means _____
    Remember, most definitions begin with the suffix.
    muc/oid means _____

12. List two medical terms in the report related to diagnostic tests or equipment:
    _____
    _____

13. PA is the abbreviation for _____, which indicates the x-ray beam for the chest radiograph was projected from the _____ to the _____.

14. Identify two new medical terms in the medical record you would like to investigate. Use your medical dictionary or a reliable online resource to look up the definition.

    Medical Term   **Definition**

1. _____   _____

2. _____   _____

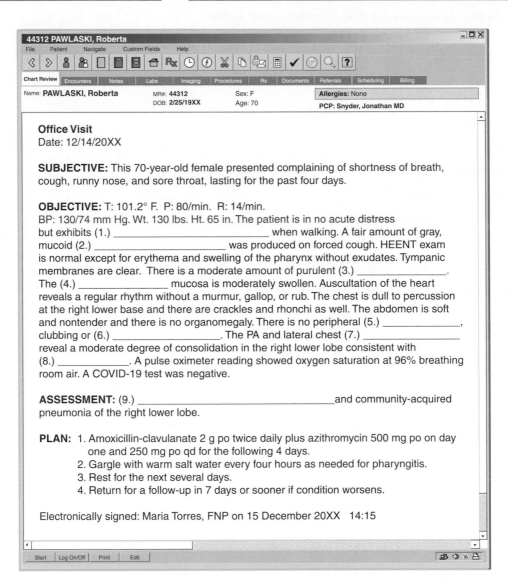

44312 PAWLASKI, Roberta

File   Patient   Navigate   Custom Fields   Help

Chart Review | Encounters | Notes | Labs | Imaging | Procedures | Rx | Documents | Referrals | Scheduling | Billing

Name: **PAWLASKI, Roberta**   MR#: **44312**   Sex: F   **Allergies:** None
DOB: **2/25/19XX**   Age: 70   PCP: Snyder, Jonathan MD

Office Visit
Date: 12/14/20XX

SUBJECTIVE: This 70-year-old female presented complaining of shortness of breath, cough, runny nose, and sore throat, lasting for the past four days.

OBJECTIVE: T: 101.2° F. P: 80/min. R: 14/min.
BP: 130/74 mm Hg. Wt. 130 lbs. Ht. 65 in. The patient is in no acute distress but exhibits (1.) _____ when walking. A fair amount of gray, mucoid (2.) _____ was produced on forced cough. HEENT exam is normal except for erythema and swelling of the pharynx without exudates. Tympanic membranes are clear. There is a moderate amount of purulent (3.) _____.
The (4.) _____ mucosa is moderately swollen. Auscultation of the heart reveals a regular rhythm without a murmur, gallop, or rub. The chest is dull to percussion at the right lower base and there are crackles and rhonchi as well. The abdomen is soft and nontender and there is no organomegaly. There is no peripheral (5.) _____, clubbing or (6.) _____. The PA and lateral chest (7.) _____ reveal a moderate degree of consolidation in the right lower lobe consistent with (8.) _____. A pulse oximeter reading showed oxygen saturation at 96% breathing room air. A COVID-19 test was negative.

ASSESSMENT: (9.) _____and community-acquired pneumonia of the right lower lobe.

PLAN: 1. Amoxicillin-clavulanate 2 g po twice daily plus azithromycin 500 mg po on day one and 250 mg po qd for the following 4 days.
2. Gargle with warm salt water every four hours as needed for pharyngitis.
3. Rest for the next several days.
4. Return for a follow-up in 7 days or sooner if condition worsens.

Electronically signed: Maria Torres, FNP on 15 December 20XX 14:15

Start | Log On/Off | Print | Edit

EXERCISE S **Use Medical Language in Online Electronic Health Records**

Select the correct medical terms to complete three medical records in one patient's electronic file.

Access online resources at evolve.elsevier.com > Evolve Resources > Practice Student Resources > Activities > Lesson 4 > Electronic Health Records

Topic: COPD
Record 1: Progress Note
Record 2: Radiology Report
Record 3: Pulmonary Function Department Note

❏ Check the box when complete.

OBJECTIVE 6

Recall and assess knowledge of word parts, medical terms, and abbreviations.

EXERCISE T **Online Review of Lesson Content**

Recall and assess your learning from working through the lesson by completing online learning activities at evolve. elsevier.com > Evolve Resources > Student Resources.

❏ Check the box when complete.

EXERCISE U **Lesson Content Quiz**

Test your knowledge of the terms and abbreviations introduced in this lesson. Circle the letter for the medical term or abbreviation related to the words in italics.

1. After weeks of experiencing a hoarse voice, the patient underwent a *visual examination of the larynx* performed by an otolaryngologist to determine the cause.
   a. laryngoscope
   b. laryngoscopy
   c. laryngectomy

2. The breathing disorder involving the *absence of spontaneous respiration* is called:
   a. apnea
   b. hypopnea
   c. dyspnea

3. Following a car accident, the occupant experienced chest pain and dyspnea. CXR demonstrated *air in the chest cavity* or:
   a. pneumothorax
   b. thoracentesis
   c. pneumonia

4. A polysomnography test was ordered to rule out *repetitive pharyngeal collapse during sleep* or:
   a. OSA
   b. SOB
   c. C&S

5. During evaluation of the patient presenting with dyspnea, *the condition of excessive carbon dioxide* was discovered.
   a. hyperoxia
   b. hypercapnia
   c. hypoxia

6. After undergoing many diagnostic tests, the patient received the diagnosis of a *progressive lung disease blocking air flow, which makes breathing difficult.*
   a. obstructive sleep apnea
   b. upper respiratory infection
   c. chronic obstructive pulmonary disease

7. To assist with long-term mechanical ventilation of the comatose patient, a *creation of an artificial opening into the trachea* was performed.
   a. thoracotomy
   b. tracheostomy
   c. laryngectomy

8. To rule out tuberculosis in a patient who had been coughing up blood, the pulmonologist ordered a TB *laboratory test performed on a collected sample to determine the presence of pathogenic bacteria or fungi and to identify the most effective antimicrobial treatment.*
   a. culture and sensitivity
   b. computed tomography
   c. bronchoscopy

9. A *physician who treats diseases of the lung* was consulted to treat the patient diagnosed with COPD.
   a. respiratory therapist
   b. pulmonology
   c. pulmonologist

10. A chest *diagnostic imaging test producing scans composed from sectional radiographic images, which can be taken in any of the anatomic planes for a multidimensional view of internal structures* was ordered to monitor growth of a small cell carcinoma in the right lung.
    a. CT
    b. CXR
    c. C&S

11. A patient came to the emergency department of the hospital with *excessive bleeding from the nose.*
    a. rhinitis
    b. rhinorrhagia
    c. rhinorrhea

12. The patient had a sore throat. Her physician referred to the condition as *inflammation of the throat.*
    a. rhinitis
    b. laryngitis
    c. pharyngitis

13. The RT taught the patient recovering from pneumonia how to use an incentive *instrument used to measure breathing* to reduce fluid build up in her lungs.
    a. oximeter
    b. thoracoscope
    c. spirometer

14. The ICU intubation team carefully followed infection control protocol as they readied the patient with COVID-19 for the insertion of a(n) *pertaining to within the trachea* tube.
    a. endotracheal
    b. laryngeal
    c. pharyngeal

LESSON AT A GLANCE   RESPIRATORY SYSTEM WORD PARTS

COMBINING FORMS		SUFFIXES		PREFIXES
bronch/o	pneumon/o	-ary	-rrhagia	a-, an-
capn/o	pulmon/o	-centesis	-rrhea	dys-
laryng/o	rhin/o	-eal	-scope	endo-
muc/o	sinus/o	-ectomy	-scopic	hyper-
nas/o	somn/o	-gram	-scopy	poly-
ox/i	spir/o	-ia	-stomy	
pharyng/o	thorac/o	-meter	-thorax	
pneum/o	trache/o	-pnea	-tomy	

LESSON AT A GLANCE RESPIRATORY SYSTEM MEDICAL TERMS AND ABBREVIATIONS

SIGNS AND SYMPTOMS
apnea
dyspnea
hypercapnia
hyperoxia
hyperpnea
hypocapnia
hypopnea
hypoxia
rhinorrhagia
rhinorrhea

DISEASES AND DISORDERS
asthma
bronchitis
bronchopneumonia
chronic obstructive pulmonary disease
  (COPD)
coronavirus disease (COVID-19)
emphysema
influenza (flu)
laryngitis
nasopharyngitis
obstructive sleep apnea (OSA)
pharyngitis
pneumonia
pneumothorax
rhinitis
sinusitis
tuberculosis (TB)
upper respiratory infection (URI)

DIAGNOSTIC TESTS
AND EQUIPMENT
bronchoscope
bronchoscopy
capnometer
computed tomography (CT)
culture and sensitivity (C&S)
endoscope
endoscopic
endoscopy
laryngoscope
laryngoscopy
oximeter
polysomnogram
polysomnography (PSG)
radiograph
spirometer
thoracoscope
thoracoscopic
thoracoscopy

SURGICAL PROCEDURES
laryngectomy
pneumonectomy
sinusotomy
thoracentesis
thoracotomy
tracheostomy
tracheotomy

SPECIALTIES AND PROFESSIONS
pulmonologist
pulmonology

RELATED TERMS
endotracheal (ET)
laryngeal
mucous
nasal
pharyngeal
pulmonary
sputum
thoracic

ABBREVIATIONS

ABG	ET	T
BP	flu	SOAP
CO_2	O_2	SOB
COPD	OSA	TB
COVID-19	P	URI
C&S	PFTs	VS
CPAP	PSG	V/Q scan
CT	R	
CXR	RT	

5

Urinary System

Tyrone Parker

Tyrone Parker was feeling fine until about 3 days ago. He was at his job at a warehouse when he noticed pain in his back, but only on the left side. At first he thought maybe he pulled something when he was moving inventory. He took some over-the-counter pain medicine, but this didn't really seem to help. In the past when he had back pain it got better after a night of sleep. When he woke up the next morning, the pain was worse, and it had spread into the lower part of his belly and his groin, still on the left side. He also noticed blood when he urinated. He was worried that he might have an infection.

■ *Consider Tyrone's situation as you work through the lesson on the urinary system. At the end of the lesson, we will return to this case study and identify medical terms used to document Tyrone's experience and the care he receives.*

OBJECTIVES

1 ■ Build, translate, pronounce, and spell medical terms built from word parts (p. 128).

2 ■ Define, pronounce, and spell medical terms NOT built from word parts (p. 144).

3 ■ Write abbreviations (p. 148).

4 ■ Identify medical terms by clinical category (p. 149).

5 ■ Use medical language in clinical statements, the case study, and a medical record (p. 151).

6 ■ Recall and assess knowledge of word parts, medical terms, and abbreviations (p. 156).

INTRODUCTION TO THE URINARY SYSTEM

Anatomic Structures of the Urinary System	
kidneys (KID-nēz)	two bean-shaped organs in the lumbar region that filter the blood to remove waste products and produce urine
renal pelvis (RĒ-nal) (PEL-vis)	funnel-shaped reservoir in each kidney that collects urine and passes it to the ureter
ureters (Ū-re-ters)	two slender tubes that carry urine from the kidney to the bladder
urethra (ū-RĒ-thra)	narrow tube that carries urine from the bladder to the outside of the body
urinary bladder (Ū-ri-nar-ē) (BLAD-er)	muscular, hollow organ that temporarily holds urine

Continued

Anatomic Structures of the Urinary System—cont'd	
urinary meatus (Ū-ri-nar-ē) (mē-Ā-tus)	opening through which urine passes to the outside of the body
urinary tract (Ū-ri-nar-ē) (trakt)	organs and ducts responsible for the elimination of urine
urine (Ū-rin)	pale yellow liquid waste product made up of 95% water

Functions of the Urinary System

- Removes waste material from the body
- Regulates fluid volume
- Maintains electrolyte concentration in body fluid
- Assists in blood pressure regulation

How the Urinary System Works

The **kidneys,** fist-sized organs shaped like kidney beans, filter the blood and remove water, salt, amino acids, electrolytes, and other minerals (see Figure 5.1). After filtration, a portion of these materials is reabsorbed into the bloodstream, maintaining optimal levels of each. The remaining amounts are combined with uric acid, ammonia, and other substances to form **urine.** Urine collects in the **renal pelvis,** a funnel-shaped reservoir in each kidney, where it drains into the **ureter,** a tube extending from the kidney. The ureter carries urine to the **urinary bladder,** where it is temporarily stored. Urine is emptied from the bladder and eliminated from the body through the **urethra.** The **urinary meatus** is the opening through which urine passes out of the body.

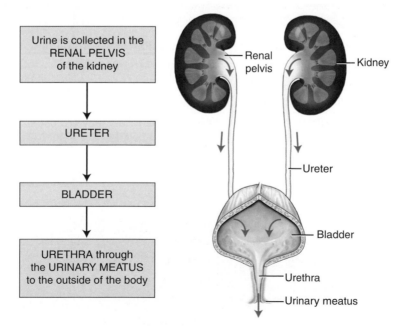

Figure 5.1 Flow of urine.

CAREER FOCUS | Professionals Who Work with the Urinary System

- **Medical/surgical nurses** care for patients who are ill or who have had surgery, implement providers' instructions, and provide pain management. They also watch for signs of infection, a risk in patients who are catheterized.

- **Nephrology nurses** play a primary role in health maintenance for those living with kidney disease through patient education and routine assessments. In patients with renal failure, they perform dialysis, a procedure in which the body's liquid wastes are removed with special machinery. Nephrology nurses also manage intravenous lines, change dressings, and administer medications.

- **Dialysis patient care technicians (PCTs)** work under the supervision of nephrology nurses and provide direct care for patients undergoing dialysis treatments (Figure 5.2). They operate the machines and monitor the fluid removal rate of the patients while using sterile techniques to make sure the risk of infection is very low.

- **Urology technicians** work in laboratories, hospitals, and clinics, assisting urologists with the diagnosis and treatment of urinary disorders. Their duties include reviewing patient records, explaining procedures, setting up equipment, and assisting with diagnostic testing. Urology technicians might also take ultrasound images of the bladder and perform catheterizations.

Figure 5.2 A dialysis patient care technician monitoring treatment.

OBJECTIVE 1

Build, translate, pronounce, and spell medical terms built from word parts.

WORD PARTS | Presented with the Urinary System

Use the paper or online **flashcards** to familiarize yourself with the following word parts.

COMBINING FORM (WR + CV)	DEFINITION	COMBINING FORM (WR + CV)	DEFINITION
cyst/o	bladder, sac	olig/o	scanty, few
hem/o, hemat/o	blood	pyel/o	renal pelvis
hydr/o	water	py/o	pus
lith/o	stone(s), calculus (pl. calculi)	ur/o	urination, urine, urinary tract
meat/o	meatus (opening)	ureter/o	ureter
nephr/o, ren/o	kidney	urethr/o	urethra
noct/i	night (Note: The combining vowel is i.)		

SUFFIX (S)	DEFINITION	SUFFIX (S)	DEFINITION
-emia	in the blood	-plasty	surgical repair
-iasis	condition	-tripsy	surgical crushing

WORD PARTS PRESENTED IN PREVIOUS LESSONS		Used to Build Urinary System Terms	
SUFFIX (S)	**DEFINITION**	**SUFFIX (S)**	**DEFINITION**
-al	pertaining to	-logist	one who studies and treats (specialist, physician)
-ectomy	surgical removal, excision		
-gram	record, radiographic image	-logy	study of
-graphy	process of recording, radiographic imaging	-osis	abnormal condition
		-scopic	pertaining to visual examination
-ia	diseased state, condition of	-scopy	visual examination
-itis	inflammation	-stomy	creation of an artificial opening
		-tomy	cut into, incision
PREFIX (P)	**DEFINITION**	**PREFIX (P)**	**DEFINITION**
a-, an-	absence of, without	dys-	difficult, painful, abnormal

Refer to Appendix A, Word Parts Used in *Basic Medical Language*, for alphabetical lists of word parts and their meanings.

EXERCISE A   **Build and Translate Medical Terms Built from Word Parts**

*Use the **Word Parts Tables** to complete the following questions. Check your responses with the Answer Key in Appendix C at the back of the book.*

1. LABEL: *Write the combining forms for anatomic structures of the urinary system on Figure 5.3. These anatomic combining forms will be used to build and translate medical terms in Exercise A.*

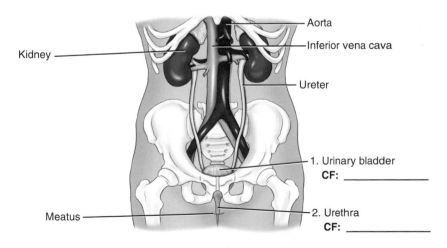

Aorta

Inferior vena cava

Kidney

Ureter

1. Urinary bladder
   CF: _____

2. Urethra
   CF: _____

Meatus

Figure 5.3 The urinary system with combining forms for bladder and urethra.

2. MATCH: *Draw a line to match the word part with its definition.*

a. -gram   inflammation
b. -graphy   stone(s), calculus (*pl.* calculi)
c. -itis   condition
d. -iasis   process of recording, radiographic imaging
e. lith/o   record, radiographic image

3. BUILD: *Using the combining form **cyst/o** and the suffixes reviewed in the previous exercise, build the following terms describing conditions related to the urinary bladder. Remember, the definition usually starts with the meaning of the suffix.*

a. inflammation of the bladder

_____/_____
          wr   s

b. radiographic imaging of the bladder

_____/ o /_____
        wr   cv   s

c. radiographic image of the bladder

_____/ o /_____
        wr   cv   s

d. condition of stone(s) in the bladder

_____/ o /_____/_____
      wr   cv   wr   s

4. READ: **Cystitis** (sis-TĬ-tis) is an inflammation of the urinary bladder. **Cystography** (sis-TOG-ra-fē) may identify this inflammation by taking a radiographic image of the bladder. A **cystogram** (SIS-tō-gram) can show whether there are stones present in the bladder. **Cystolithiasis** (sis-tō-lith-Ī-a-sis) is also referred to as bladder stones.

> **FYI**   **Bladder** is a derivative of the Anglo-Saxon **blaeddre**, meaning a **blister** or **windbag**.

5. LABEL: *Write word parts to complete Figure 5.4.*

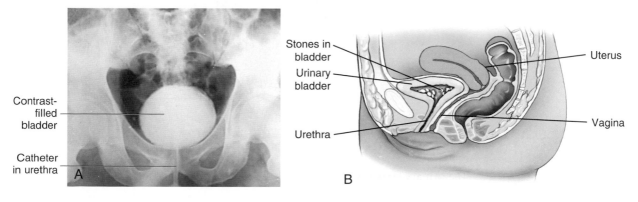

Figure 5.4 **A.** _____/o/_____.
                         bladder   radiographic image

            B. _____/o/_____/_____.
                         bladder   stone(s)   condition

6. MATCH: *Draw a line to match the word part with its definition.*

a. -stomy   stone(s), calculus (*pl.* calculi)
b. -scope   cut into, incision
c. -scopy   instrument used for visual examination
d. -tomy   surgical repair
e. -plasty   creation of an artificial opening
f. lith/o   visual examination

---

7. TRANSLATE: *Complete the definitions of the following terms by filling in the blanks for procedures related to the bladder (**cyst/o**). Remember, the definition usually starts with the meaning of the suffix.*

a. cyst/o/stomy _____ of an _____ _____ into the _____

b. cyst/o/scope _____ used for _____ _____ of the _____

c. cyst/o/scopy _____ _____ of the _____

d. cyst/o/lith/o/tomy _____ into the _____ to remove stone(s)

---

8. READ: A **cystoscope** (SIS-tō-skōp) is used to examine the inside of the bladder to look for abnormalities such as infection or cancer. **Cystoscopy** (sis-TOS-ko-pē) can also be used to treat abnormalities, such as removal of a small tumor using a tool passed through the scope. **Cystolithotomy** (sis-tō-li-THOT-o-mē) uses an incision low on the belly to access the bladder to remove large stones. A **cystostomy** (sis-TOS-to-mē) creates an artificial opening into the bladder, which allows a tube to be inserted for drainage of urine.

---

9. BUILD: *Write word parts to build terms related to the urethra, using the combining form **urethr/o**.*

a. instrument used for visual examination of the urethra   _____ / o / _____
                                                              wr   cv   s

b. inflammation of the urethra and bladder   _____ / o / _____ / _____
                                               wr   cv   wr   s

c. radiographic imaging of the bladder and urethra   _____ / o / _____ / o / _____
                                                       wr   cv   wr   cv   s

d. surgical repair of the urethra   _____ / o / _____
                                      wr   cv   s

---

10. READ: **Urethroplasty** (ū-RĒ-thrō-plas-tē) is surgical repair of the urethra and may be necessary to treat severe injury or birth defects. A **urethroscope** (ū-RĒ-thrō-skōp) may be used to diagnose narrowing of the urethra. **Urethrocystitis** (ū-rē-thrō-sis-TĪ-tis) is inflammation of the urethra and bladder and may be diagnosed by **cystourethrography** (sis-tō-ū-rē-THROG-ro-fē).

11. LABEL: *Write word parts to complete Figure 5.5.*

Urinary
bladder

Urethra

Figure 5.5 Image generated by _____/o/_____/o/_____.

bladder   urethra   radiographic imaging

---

12. MATCH: *Draw a line to match the word part with its definition.*

a. ur/o   pus
b. hem/o, hemat/o   diseased state, condition of
c. py/o   urine, urination, urinary tract
d. dys-   blood
e. -ia   difficult, painful, abnormal (*Tip: defined as "difficult or painful" when used with the combining form* **ur/o** *in the next exercise*)

---

13. TRANSLATE: *Complete the definitions of the following terms built from the combining form* **ur/o**.

a. hemat/ur/ia   _____ of blood in the _____

b. py/ur/ia   condition of _____ in the _____

c. dys/ur/ia   _____ of difficult or _____ urination

---

14. READ: Signs of a bladder infection can include difficult or painful urination, or **dysuria** (dis-Ū-rē-a), as well as blood in the urine, or **hematuria** (hem-a-TU-rē-a). **Pyuria** (pī-Ū-rē-a), a term meaning condition of pus in the urine, can cause urine to appear cloudy and is another sign of infection.

---

15. MATCH: *Draw a line to match the word part with its definition.*

    a. a-, an-   urine, urination, urinary tract
    b. noct/i   in the blood
    c. olig/o   absence of, without
    d. -emia   night
    e. ur/o   few, scanty

16. BUILD: *Write word parts to describe conditions describing urine.*

    a. condition of absence of urine

                                     p   wr   s

    b. condition of night urination

                                   wr   wr   s

    c. condition of scanty urine (amount)

                                   wr   wr   s

    d. urine in the blood

                                   wr   s

FYI Sometimes literal translation brings one close to the meaning of the word but does not account for every word in the definition used in the practice of medicine. For example, **anuria** (an-Ū-rē-a) literally means condition of absence of urine. For learning purposes, that will be the meaning used in this text. In practice, the term means failure of the kidneys to produce urine.

---

17. READ: Nocturia (nok-TŪ-rē-a) describes having to get up multiple times during the night to urinate. It may be caused by partial blockage of the urinary tract, as with an enlarged prostate gland. **Oliguria** (ol-i-GŪ-rē-a) refers to the scanty production of urine, which can be due to dehydration, blockage, infections, and many other serious causes. **Uremia** (ū-RĒ-mē-a) is a toxic condition resulting from a high level of urea and other waste products in the blood; these would normally be eliminated by the kidneys.

FYI For learning purposes, we have allowed the definition of **uremia** to be urine in the blood because urea is present in urine. The term **hematuria** means blood in the urine. Hematuria is a sign, whereas uremia is a serious disorder. Use your medical dictionary or an online source to learn more about these common terms.

18. LABEL: *Write the combining forms for anatomic structures of the urinary system on Figure 5.6. These anatomic combining forms will be used to build and translate medical terms in following exercises.*

1. Kidney
CF: _____
CF: _____

2. Renal pelvis
CF: _____

Figure 5.6 Kidney and renal pelvis with combining forms.

19. MATCH: *Draw a line to match the word part with its definition.*

   a. lith/o   condition
   b. -tripsy   surgical crushing
   c. -iasis   stone(s), calculus (*pl.* calculi)

20. TRANSLATE: *Complete the definitions of the following terms built from the combining form **lith/o**, meaning stone(s) or calculus. Use the meaning of word parts to fill in the blanks.*

   a. lith/o/tripsy   _____ _____ of stone(s)

   b. nephr/o/lith/iasis   condition of _____(s) in the _____

   c. pyel/o/lith/o/tomy   incision into the _____ _____ to remove _____(s)

> **FYI**   **Pyelos** is the Greek word for **tub-shaped vessel**, which describes the renal pelvis' shape.

21. READ: **Nephrolithiasis** (nef-rō-lith-Ī-a-sis) is the medical term for kidney stones, a common disorder. **Litho-tripsy** (LITH-ō-trip-sē) is a noninvasive procedure that uses shock waves to "crush" or break the stones into smaller pieces that can be passed through the urinary system. If stones are trapped in the renal pelvis, a minor surgery requiring a small incision in the back called **pyelolithotomy** (pī-el-ō-lith-OT-o-mē) can be used to remove the stones.

22. LABEL: *Write word parts to complete Figure 5.7*

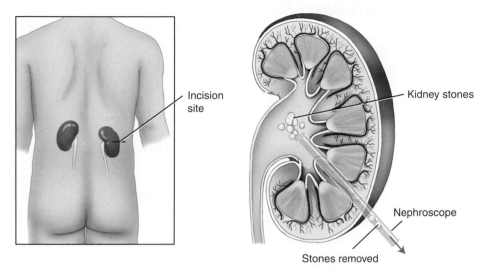

Incision
site

Kidney stones

Nephroscope

Stones removed

Figure 5.7 Percutaneous _____/o/_____/o/_____
renal pelvis   stone(s)   incision

uses a small incision into the back to remove medium or larger-size kidney stones. A nephroscope is passed into the kidney through the incision; the urologist then removes the stone(s) through the nephroscope.

23. REVIEW OF URINARY SYSTEM TERMS BUILT FROM WORD PARTS: *The following is an alphabetical list of terms built and translated in the previous exercises.*

MEDICAL TERMS BUILT FROM WORD PARTS

TERM	DEFINITION	TERM	DEFINITION
1. anuria (an-Ū-rē-a)	condition of absence of urine	**7. cystoscope** (SIS-tō-skōp)	instrument used for visual examination of the bladder
2. cystitis (sis-TĪ-tis)	inflammation of the bladder	**8. cystoscopy** (sis-TOS-ko-pē)	visual examination of the bladder
3. cystogram (SIS-tō-gram)	radiographic image of the bladder (Figure 5.4, *A*)	**9. cystostomy** (sis-TOS-to-mē)	creation of an artificial opening into the bladder
4. cystography (sis-TOG-ra-fē)	radiographic imaging of the bladder	**10. cystourethrography** (sis-tō-ū-rē-THROG-ro-fē)	radiographic imaging of the bladder and urethra (Figure 5.5)
5. cystolithiasis (sis-tō-lith-Ī-a-sis)	condition of stone(s) in the bladder (Figure 5.4, *B*)	**11. dysuria** (dis-Ū-rē-a)	condition of difficult or painful urination
6. cystolithotomy (sis-tō-li-THOT-o-mē)	incision into the bladder to remove stone(s)	**12. hematuria** (hem-a-TU-rē-a)	condition of blood in the urine

Continued

MEDICAL TERMS BUILT FROM WORD PARTS—cont'd

TERM	DEFINITION	TERM	DEFINITION
13. **lithotripsy** (LITH-ō-trip-sē)	surgical crushing of stone(s)	18. **pyuria** (pī-Ū-rē-a)	condition of pus in the urine
14. **nephrolithiasis** (nef-rō-lith-Ī-a-sis)	condition of stone(s) in the kidney	19. **uremia** (ū-RĒ-mē-a)	urine in the blood
15. **nocturia** (nok-TŪ-rē-a)	condition of night urination	20. **urethrocystitis** (ū-rē-thrō-sis-TĪ-tis)	inflammation of the urethra and bladder
16. **oliguria** (ol-i-GŪ-rē-a)	condition of scanty urine (amount)	21. **urethroplasty** (ū-RĒ-thrō-plas-tē)	surgical repair of the urethra
17. **pyelolithotomy** (pī-el-ō-lith-OT-o-mē)	incision into the renal pelvis to remove stone(s) (Figure 5.7)	22. **urethroscope** (ū-RĒ-thrō-skōp)	instrument used for visual examination of the urethra

EXERCISE B   Pronounce and Spell Terms Built from Word Parts

Practice pronunciation and spelling on paper and online.

1. **Practice on Paper**
   a. **Pronounce**: Read the phonetic spelling and say aloud the terms listed in the previous table, Review of Terms Built from Word Parts.
   b. **Spell**: Have a study partner read the terms aloud. Write the spelling of the terms on a separate sheet of paper.

2. **Practice Online** 🌐
   a. **Access** online learning resources. Go to evolve.elsevier.com > Evolve Resources > Practice Student Resources.
   b. **Pronounce**: Select Audio Glossary > Lesson 5 > Exercise B. Select a term to hear its pronunciation and repeat aloud.
   c. **Spell**: Select Activities > Lesson 5 > Spell Terms > Exercise B. Select the audio icon and type the correct spelling of the term.

❏ Check the box when complete.

EXERCISE C **Build and Translate MORE Medical Terms Built from Word Parts**

*Use the **Word Parts Tables** to complete the following questions. Check your responses with the Answer Key in Appendix C.*

1. LABEL: *Write the combining forms for anatomic structures of the urinary system on Figure 5.8. These anatomic combining forms will be used to build and translate medical terms in Exercise C.*

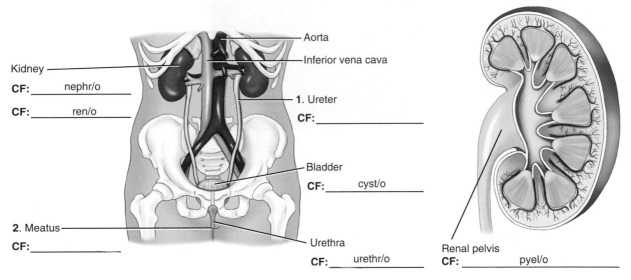

Figure 5.8 The urinary system with combining forms for ureter and meatus.

2. MATCH: *Draw a line to match the word part with its definition.*

    a. -itis   water
    b. -osis   inflammation
    c. -al   abnormal condition
    d. hydr/o   pertaining to

3. TRANSLATE: *Complete the definitions of the following terms by using the meaning of the word parts to fill in the blanks. Remember, the definition usually starts with the meaning of the suffix. Terms built from combining forms **ren/o** and **nephr/o**, meaning kidney:*

    a. nephr/itis   _____ of the _____

    b. ren/al   _____ to the _____

    c. hydr/o/nephr/osis   _____ _____ of _____ in the kidney

    d. pyel/o/nephr/itis   _____ of the _____ _____ and kidney

4. READ: Nephritis (ne-FRĪ-tis) refers to inflammation of the kidneys and is frequently caused by infections and medications. Acute **pyelonephritis** (pī-e-lō-ne-FRĪ-tis) is a bacterial infection that causes swelling and enlargement of the kidneys, while chronic **pyelonephritis** can result in scarring and loss of function.

5. LABEL: *Write word parts to complete Figure 5.9.*

Figure 5.9 **A.** Acute _____/o/_____/_____.
renal pelvis   kidney   inflammation

B. Normal-sized kidney with some scarring.

6. READ: Hydronephrosis (hī-drō-ne-FRŌ-sis), literally translated as abnormal condition of water in the kidney, is actually a buildup of urine in the kidney caused by blockage somewhere in the urinary tract, such as a stone in the ureter. This causes distension (swelling) of the renal pelvis.

7. LABEL: *Write word parts to complete Figure 5.10.*

Figure 5.10 _____/o/_____/_____.
water   kidney   abnormal condition

8. **MATCH:** *Draw a line to match the combining form or suffix with its definition.*

a. pyel/o   creation of an artificial opening
b. -ectomy   cut into, incision
c. -stomy   surgical removal, excision
d. -tomy   renal pelvis

9. **BUILD:** *Using the combining form **nephr/o** and the suffixes reviewed in the previous exercise, build the following terms describing procedures related to the kidney. Remember, the definition usually starts with the meaning of the suffix.*

a. excision of the kidney

_____/_____
                      wr   s

b. creation of an artificial opening into the kidney

_____/_o_/_____
                      wr   cv   s

c. incision into the kidney

_____/_o_/_____
                      wr   cv   s

10. **READ:** A **nephrectomy** (ne-FREK-to-mē) may be performed to treat kidney cancer. A **nephrostomy** (ne-FROS-to-mē) creates an artificial opening into the kidney to relieve hydronephrosis caused by blockage, such as when a stone gets stuck in a ureter. A **nephrotomy** (ne-FROT-o-mē) might be necessary to remove a very large kidney stone.

11. **LABEL:** *Write word parts to complete Figure 5.11.*

Figure 5.11 _____/o/_____.
                kidney   creation of an artificial opening

12. **MATCH:** *Draw a line to match the word part with its definition.*

a. -itis   surgical repair
b. -tomy   stone(s), calculus (*pl.* calculi)
c. -iasis   inflammation
d. -plasty   cut into, incision
e. lith/o   condition

13. TRANSLATE: *Complete the definitions of the following terms by using the meaning of the word parts to fill in the blanks. Terms built from the combining form **ureter/o**, meaning ureter:*

a. ureter/o/lith/iasis _____ of stone(s) in the _____

b. ureter/o/pyel/o/nephr/itis _____ of the ureter, _____ _____, and kidney

c. ureter/o/lith/o/tomy _____ into the _____ to remove _____(s)

---

14. READ: Ureterolithiasis (ū-rē-ter-ō-lith-Ī-a-sis) occurs when a stone is stuck in a ureter. The urine flow can become blocked. If bacteria are present, the area above the blockage can become infected. This is known as **ureteropyelonephritis** (ū-rē-ter-ō-pī-e-lō-ne-FRĪ-tis). A **ureterolithotomy** (ū-rē-ter-ō-lith-OT-o-mē) is generally only done if other, less invasive measures fail.

---

15. BUILD: *Using the combining form **ureter/o**, build the following terms describing procedures related to the ureter.*

a. excision of the ureter

_____/_____
           wr   s

b. surgical repair of the ureter

_____/_o_/_____
           wr   cv   s

---

16. READ: Ureterectomy (ū-rē-ter-EK-to-mē) is generally performed for cancers involving one or both ureters. **Ureteroplasty** (ū-RĒ-ter-ō-plas-tē) may be necessary if the ureter is blocked due to stones, infections, or cancer.

---

17. LABEL: *Write word parts to complete Figure 5.12.*

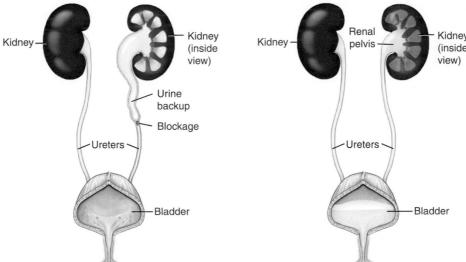

Figure 5.12 **A.** Left ureter is blocked, causing urine to back up in the kidney.

B. After _____/o/_____, the ureter is open and urine flows freely to the bladder.
          ureter   surgical repair

18. MATCH: *Draw a line to match the suffix with its definition.*

   a. -al   cut into, incision

   b. -scopy   pertaining to

   c. -tomy   visual examination

19. TRANSLATE: *Complete the definitions of the following terms by using the meaning of the word parts to fill in the blanks. Terms built from the combining form **meat/o**, meaning urinary meatus:*

   a. meat/al   _____ to the _____

   b. meat/o/scopy   _____ _____ of the meatus

   c. meat/o/tomy   _____ into the _____ (to enlarge it)

> **FYI**   **Meatus** comes from the Latin **meare**, meaning **to pass** or **to go**. Other anatomic passages share the same name, such as the auditory meatus.

20. READ: **Meatoscopy** (mē-a-TOS-ko-pē) uses a special device to see the urethral meatus. **Meatotomy** (mē-a-TOT-o-mē) is performed when the urinary meatus is too narrow, which may be caused by scarring from injury or from birth defects.

21. MATCH: *Draw a line to match the word part with its definition.*

   a. -gram   one who studies and treats (specialist, physician)

   b. -logist   study of

   c. -logy   record, radiographic image

   d. -stomy   creation of an artificial opening

22. BUILD: *Write word parts to build the following terms using the combining form **ur/o**, meaning urine or urinary tract.*

   a. radiographic image of the urinary tract   _____ / o / _____

                                                   wr   cv   s

   b. physician who studies and treats diseases of the   _____ / o / _____

       urinary tract   wr   cv   s

   c. study of the urinary tract   _____ / o / _____

                                                     wr   cv   s

   d. creation of an artificial opening into the urinary   _____ / o / _____

       tract   wr   cv   s

23. READ: **Urology** (ū-ROL-o-jē) is the study of the urinary tract. A **urologist** (ū-ROL-o-jist) is a surgeon who specializes in diseases of the urinary tract, including bladder cancer, urinary infections, and ureteral stones. A **urogram** (Ū-rō-gram) obtains an image of the entire urinary tract, from the kidneys to the urinary meatus. The surgical creation of a **urostomy** (ū-ROS-tō-mē) allows for diversion of urine around a blocked or missing portion of the urinary tract.

24. LABEL: *Write word parts to complete Figure 5.13.*

—Renal pelvis

—Ureter

—Cystoscope

Figure 5.13 _____ /o/ _____.
                 urinary tract   radiographic image

---

25. TRANSLATE: *Complete the definitions of the following terms by using the meaning of the word parts to fill in the blanks.*

   a. nephr/o/logist   _____ who _____ and _____ _____ of the kidney

   b. nephr/o/logy   _____ of the _____

---

26. READ: **Nephrology** (ne-FROL-o-jē) refers to study of the kidneys and related diseases. A **nephrologist** (ne-FROL-o-jist) is an internal medicine physician who has completed extra years of study to specialize in kidney disease. Nephrologists also treat diseases that affect the kidney, such as hypertension and diabetes.

---

27. REVIEW OF MORE URINARY SYSTEM TERMS BUILT FROM WORD PARTS: *The following is an alphabetical list of terms built and translated in the previous exercises.*

MEDICAL TERMS BUILT FROM WORD PARTS

TERM	DEFINITION	TERM	DEFINITION
1. hydronephrosis (hī-drō-ne-FRŌ-sis)	abnormal condition of water in the kidney (distension of the renal pelvis with urine because of an obstruction) (Figure 5.10)	**4. meatotomy** (mē-a-TOT-o-mē)	incision into the meatus (to enlarge it)
2. meatal (mē-Ā-tal)	pertaining to the meatus	**5. nephrectomy** (ne-FREK-to-mē)	excision of the kidney
3. meatoscopy (mē-a-TOS-ko-pē)	visual examination of the meatus	**6. nephritis** (ne-FRĪ-tis)	inflammation of the kidney

Continued

MEDICAL TERMS BUILT FROM WORD PARTS—cont'd

TERM	DEFINITION	TERM	DEFINITION
7. nephrologist (ne-FROL-o-jist)	physician who studies and treats diseases of the kidney	15. ureterolithotomy (ū-rē-ter-ō-lith-OT-o-mē)	incision into the ureter to remove stone(s)
8. nephrology (ne-FROL-o-jē)	study of the kidney	16. ureteroplasty (ū-RĒ-ter-ō-plas-tē)	surgical repair of the ureter (Figure 5.12)
9. nephrostomy (ne-FROS-to-mē)	creation of an artificial opening into the kidney (Figure 5.11)	17. ureteropyelonephritis (ū-rē-ter-ō-pī-e-lō-ne-FRĪ-tis)	inflammation of the ureter, renal pelvis, and kidney
10. nephrotomy (ne-FROT-o-mē)	incision into the kidney	18. urogram (Ū-rō-gram)	radiographic image of the urinary tract (Figure 5.13)
11. pyelonephritis (pī-e-lō-ne-FRĪ-tis)	inflammation of the renal pelvis and kidney (Figure 5.9)	19. urologist (ū-ROL-o-jist)	physician who studies and treats diseases of the urinary tract
12. renal (RĒ-nal)	pertaining to the kidney	20. urology (ū-ROL-o-jē)	study of the urinary tract
13. ureterectomy (ū-rē-ter-EK-to-mē)	excision of the ureter	21. urostomy (ū-ROS-tō-mē)	creation of an artificial opening in the urinary tract
14. ureterolithiasis (ū-rē-ter-ō-lith-Ī-a-sis)	condition of stone(s) in the ureter		

EXERCISE D   Pronounce and Spell MORE Terms Built from Word Parts

Practice pronunciation and spelling on paper and online.

1. **Practice on Paper**
   a. **Pronounce**: Read the phonetic spelling and say aloud the terms listed in the previous table, Review of MORE Terms Built from Word Parts.
   b. **Spell**: Have a study partner read the terms aloud. Write the spelling of the terms on a separate sheet of paper.

2. **Practice Online** 🌐
   a. **Access** online learning resources. Go to evolve.elsevier.com > Evolve Resources > Practice Student Resources.
   b. **Pronounce**: Select Audio Glossary > Lesson 5 > Exercise D. Select a term to hear its pronunciation and repeat aloud.
   c. **Spell**: Select Activities > Lesson 5 > Spell Terms > Exercise D. Select the audio icon and type the correct spelling of the term.

❏ Check the box when complete.

OBJECTIVE 2

Define, pronounce, and spell medical terms NOT built from word parts.

The terms listed below may contain word parts, but are difficult to translate literally.

MEDICAL TERMS NOT BUILT FROM WORD PARTS

TERM	DEFINITION
1. **chronic kidney disease (CKD)** (KRON-ik) (KID-nē) (di-ZĒZ)	progressive, irreversible loss of kidney function
2. **dialysis** (dī-AL-i-sis)	procedure for removing toxic waste from the blood because of an inability of the kidneys to do so

> **FYI** There are two main types of dialysis. **Hemodialysis** uses an external machine (hemodialyzer) that is connected to the patient's blood vessels via a tube. The hemodialyzer then filters the blood and returns it to the body. In **peritoneal dialysis**, the blood is cleaned inside the body using the abdominal lining as a natural filter. Sterile fluid is put into the abdomen through a catheter, then removed the same way.

TERM	DEFINITION
3. **extracorporeal shock wave lithotripsy (ESWL)** (eks-tra-kor-POR-ē-al) (shok) (wāv) (LITH-ō-trip-sē)	noninvasive surgical procedure to crush stone(s) in the kidney or ureter by administration of repeated shock waves. Stone fragments are eliminated from the body in the urine.

> **FYI** **Extracorporeal** means occurring outside the body

TERM	DEFINITION
4. **incontinence** (in-KON-ti-nens)	inability to control the bladder and/or bowels
5. **renal calculi (*sing.* calculus)** (RĒ-nal) (KAL-kū-lī), (KAL-kū-lus)	stones in the kidney; (also called **nephrolithiasis**)
6. **renal failure** (RĒ-nal) (FĀL-ūr)	loss of kidney function resulting in its inability to remove waste products from the body and maintain fluid balance; can be acute, chronic, or end-stage
7. **renal transplant** (RĒ-nal) (TRANS-plant)	surgical implantation of a donor kidney into a patient with inadequate renal function
8. **urinalysis (UA)** (ū-rin-AL-i-sis)	laboratory test in which multiple routine tests are performed on a urine specimen
9. **urinary catheterization** (Ū-rin-ār-ē) (kath-e-ter-i-ZĀ-shun)	procedure that involves the passage of a catheter into the urinary bladder to withdraw urine
10. **urinary tract infection (UTI)** (Ū-rin-ār-ē) (trakt) (in-FEK-shun)	infection of one or more organs of the urinary tract
11. **void** (voyd)	to pass urine

EXERCISE E   **Label**

Write the medical terms pictured and defined using the previous table of Medical Terms NOT Built from Word Parts. Check your work with the Answer Key in Appendix C.

1. _____

passage of a catheter into the urinary bladder to withdraw urine

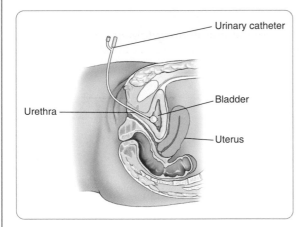

2. _____

_____

noninvasive surgical procedure to crush stone(s) in the kidney or ureter by administration of repeated shock waves

3. _____

procedure for removing toxic waste from the blood because of an inability of the kidneys to do so

4. _____

stones in the kidney; (also called nephrolithiasis)

5. _____

laboratory test in which multiple routine tests are performed on a urine specimen

6. _____

surgical implantation of a donor kidney into a patient with inadequate renal function

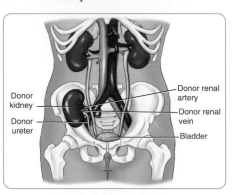

EXERCISE F   **Match**

Match the terms in the first column with their correct descriptions in the second column.

_____ **1.** urinary tract infection
_____ **2.** chronic kidney disease
_____ **3.** void
_____ **4.** renal failure
_____ **5.** incontinence

a. to pass urine
b. progressive, irreversible loss of kidney function
c. inability to control the bladder and/or bowels
d. infection of one or more organs of the urinary tract
e. loss of kidney function resulting in its inability to remove waste products from the body; can be acute, chronic, or end-stage

---

EXERCISE G   **Learn Medical Terms NOT Built from Word Parts**

*Fill in the blanks with medical terms defined in **bold** and abbreviations using the Medical Terms NOT Built from Word Parts table. Check your responses with the Answer Key in Appendix C.*

1. The **inability to control the bladder and/or bowels** is called _____. Urinary incontinence occurs when one loses control over the ability to **pass urine** or _____. This can sometimes be caused by a **UTI** or _____. A **laboratory test that performs multiple routine assessments on a urine specimen**, or _____ (UA), can help to diagnose this. In severe cases of incontinence, a _____ may be performed, which is a **procedure that uses a catheter to withdraw urine from the bladder**.

2. Acute kidney injury (AKI) is the sudden and severe loss of kidney function that leads to a buildup of waste in the body. Prompt treatment can reverse the condition and recovery can occur. **CKD,** or _____ _____, is a **progressive, irreversible loss of kidney function** that leads to the onset of uremia. Dialysis and kidney transplant are used in treating this disease. Chronic renal failure, or CRF, is an older term that has mostly been replaced by CKD. End-stage renal disease (ESRD) refers to _____, or the **loss of kidney function, resulting in its inability to remove waste products from the body and maintain fluid balance,** that has become too severe to sustain life.

3. When kidney failure is advanced, a nephrologist may order _____, a **procedure for removing toxic waste from the blood because of an inability of the kidneys to do so.** This takes over kidney functions by removing waste and extra fluids, helping to keep a safe level of necessary chemicals in the blood, and controlling blood pressure. In some cases, a **surgical implantation of a donor kidney into a patient with inadequate renal function,** or _____, may be performed if a match can be found.

4. Another term for **nephrolithiasis,** which also means **stones in the kidney,** is _____. If stones become large or obstructive, treatment is required. A urologist may order a type of lithotripsy that uses a **noninvasive surgical procedure to crush stone(s) in the kidney or ureter by administration of repeated shock waves** called **ESWL** or _____.

EXERCISE H   Pronounce and Spell Medical Terms NOT Built from Word Parts

Practice pronunciation and spelling on paper with the textbook and online.

1. **Practice on Paper**
   a. **Pronounce:** Read the phonetic spelling and say aloud the terms listed in the previous table, Medical Terms NOT Built from Word Parts.
   b. **Spell:** Have a study partner read the terms aloud. Write the spelling of the terms on a separate sheet of paper.

2. **Practice Online** ⊕
   a. **Access** online learning resources. Go to evolve.elsevier.com > Evolve Resources > Practice Student Resources.
   b. **Pronounce:** Select Audio Glossary > Lesson 5 > Exercise H. Select a term to hear its pronunciation and repeat aloud.
   c. **Spell:** Select Activities > Lesson 5 > Spell Terms > Exercise H. Select the audio icon and type the correct spelling of the term.

❏ Check the box when complete.

OBJECTIVE 3

Write abbreviations.

ABBREVIATIONS RELATED TO THE URINARY SYSTEM

Use the online **flashcards** to familiarize yourself with the following abbreviations.

ABBREVIATION	TERM	ABBREVIATION	TERM
cath	catheterization, catheter	**UA**	urinalysis
CKD	chronic kidney disease	**UTI**	urinary tract infection
ESWL	extracorporeal shock wave lithotripsy	**VCUG**	voiding cystourethrogram
HD	hemodialysis		
OAB	overactive bladder		
PCT	patient care technician		
PKD	polycystic kidney disease		

FYI   **Polycystic kidney disease** (PKD) is an inherited disorder that causes cysts (fluid-filled sacs) to form throughout the kidneys. PKD can range from mild to severe, with the worst cases resulting in renal failure.

EXERCISE I   Abbreviate Medical Terms

Write the correct abbreviation next to its medical term.

1. Diseases and Disorders:

    a. _____ chronic kidney disease

    b. _____ urinary tract infection

    c. _____ polycystic kidney disease

    d. _____ overactive bladder

2. Diagnostic Tests:

    a. _____ urinalysis

    b. _____ voiding cystourethrogram

3. Surgical Procedures:

    a. _____ extracorporeal shock wave lithotripsy

    b. _____ hemodialysis

4. Specialties and Professions:

    _____ (dialysis) patient care technician

5. Related Term:

    _____ catheterization, catheter

OBJECTIVE 4

Identify medical terms by clinical category.

Now that you have worked through the urinary system lesson, review and practice medical terms grouped by clinical category. Categories include signs and symptoms, diseases and disorders, diagnostic tests and equipment, surgical procedures, specialties and professions, and other terms related to the urinary system.

| EXERCISE J | Signs and Symptoms |

Write the medical terms for signs and symptoms next to their definitions.

1. _____ condition of absence of urine

2. _____ condition of difficult or painful urination

3. _____ condition of blood in the urine

4. _____ condition of night urination

5. _____ condition of scanty urine (amount)

6. _____ condition of pus in the urine

7. _____ inability to control the bladder and/or bowels

| EXERCISE K | Diseases and Disorders |

Write the medical terms for diseases and disorders next to their definitions.

1. _____ inflammation of the bladder

2. _____ condition of stone(s) in the bladder

3. _____ abnormal condition of water (urine) in the kidney

4. _____ condition of stone(s) in the kidney

5. _____ inflammation of the kidney

6. _____ inflammation of the renal pelvis and kidney

7. _____ inflammation of the urethra and bladder

8. _____ stones in the kidney

9. _____ loss of kidney function resulting in its inability to remove waste products from the body and maintain fluid balance

10. _____ infection of one or more organs of the urinary tract

11. _____ condition of urine in the blood

12. _____   condition of stone(s) in the ureter

13. _____   inflammation of the ureter, renal pelvis, and kidney

14. _____   progressive, irreversible loss of renal function; leads to the onset of uremia

---

EXERCISE L   Diagnostic Tests and Equipment

Write the medical terms for diagnostic tests and equipment next to their definitions.

1. _____   radiographic image of the bladder

2. _____   radiographic imaging of the bladder

3. _____   instrument used for visual examination of the bladder

4. _____   visual examination of the bladder

5. _____   radiographic imaging of the bladder and urethra

6. _____   visual examination of the meatus

7. _____   instrument used for visual examination of the urethra

8. _____   laboratory test in which multiple routine tests are performed on a urine specimen

9. _____   radiographic image of the urinary tract

EXERCISE M   Surgical Procedures

Write the medical terms for surgical procedures next to their definitions.

1. _____   incision into the bladder to remove stone(s)

2. _____   creation of an artificial opening into the bladder

3. _____   noninvasive surgical procedure to crush stone(s) in the kidney or ureter by administration of repeated shock waves

4. _____   surgical crushing of stone(s)

5. _____   incision into the meatus (to enlarge it)

6. _____   excision of the kidney

7. _____   surgical repair of the ureter

8. _____   creation of an artificial opening into the kidney

9. _____   incision into the kidney

10. _____   incision into the renal pelvis to remove stone(s)

11. _____   surgical implantation of a donor kidney into a patient with inadequate renal function

12. _____ excision of the ureter

13. _____ creation of an artificial opening in the urinary tract

14. _____ incision into the ureter to remove stone(s)

15. _____ surgical repair of the urethra

EXERCISE N **Specialties and Professions**

Write the medical terms for specialties and professions next to their definitions.

1. _____ study of the kidney

2. _____ physician who studies and treats diseases of the kidney

3. _____ study of the urinary tract

4. _____ physician who studies and treats diseases of the urinary tract

---

EXERCISE O **Medical Terms Related to the Urinary System**

Write the medical terms related to the urinary system next to their definitions.

1. _____ pertaining to the (urinary) meatus

2. _____ pertaining to the kidney

3. _____ procedure for removing toxic waste from the blood because of an inability of the kidneys to do so

4. _____ procedure that involves the passage of a catheter into the urinary bladder to withdraw urine

5. _____ to pass urine

OBJECTIVE 5

Use medical language in clinical statements, the case study, and a medical record.

EXERCISE P   **Use Medical Terms in Clinical Statements**

Circle the medical terms and abbreviations defined in the bolded phrases. Answers are listed in Appendix C. For pronunciation practice, read the answers aloud.

1. Mr. Yin was admitted to the medical center for a(n) **excision of a kidney** (nephrostomy, nephrectomy, nephrotomy). The kidney will be used as a donor organ for **pertaining to the kidney** (renal, meatal, ureteral) transplant for his brother, who is suffering from chronic, bilateral (both) **inflammation of the kidneys** (pyelonephritis, ureteropyelonephritis, nephritis).

2. Mr. Garcia was complaining of **difficult or painful urination** (dysuria, anuria, oliguria) and was noted to have **condition of blood in the urine** (pyuria, hematuria, uremia). The **multiple routine tests done on a urine specimen** (urogram, cystoscopy, urinalysis) revealed **condition of pus in the urine** (nocturia, pyuria, incontinence). He was diagnosed and treated for **inflammation of the bladder** (cystitis, nephritis, pyelonephritis).

3. Tassiana Smith, a 10-year-old girl, has had recurrent (chronic) **inflammation of the urethra and bladder** (urethrocystitis, ureteropyelonephritis, hydronephrosis). To determine the cause, the physician ordered a(n) **radiographic image of the urinary tract** (urogram, cystogram, parallelogram) to be followed by **radiographic imaging of the bladder and urethra** (cystourethrography, cystoscopy, urethroscope) if necessary.

4. **Surgical crushing of stone(s)** (Pyelolithotomy, Lithotripsy, Dialysis) was used to treat Mrs. Hand, who was diagnosed as having **condition of stone(s) in the ureter** (ureteropyelonephritis, cystolithiasis, ureterolithiasis).

5. To correct a condition called stress **inability to control the bladder** (incontinence, oliguria, nocturia), a **physician who studies and treats diseases of the urinary tract** (nephrologist, urologist, pulmonologist) may perform a **surgical repair of the urethra** (ureterolithotomy, urethroplasty, ureterectomy).

6. Voiding **radiographic imaging of the bladder and urethra** (urinalysis, cystourethrography, cystography) is performed by instilling radiopaque dye in the bladder. Radiographic images called cystourethrograms are taken of the bladder during voiding of the dye. The test may be performed to find the cause of repeated **infection of one or more organs of the urinary tract** (cystitis, urinary tract infection, uremia).

7. A(n) **physician who studies and treats diseases of the kidney** (dermatologist, oncologist, nephrologist) takes care of patients with **progressive, irreversible loss of kidney function** (UTI, COPD, CKD) and prescribes **procedure for removing toxic waste from the blood because of an inability of the kidneys to do so** (dialysis, incontinence, lithotripsy) therapy. A urologist performs procedures on the male and female urinary systems, including **incision into the ureter to remove stone(s)** (ureteroplasty, ureterolithotomy, ureterectomy) and treats diseases of the male reproductive system, both medically and surgically.

EXERCISE Q **Apply Medical Terms to the Case Study**

Think back to Tyrone, who was introduced in the case study at the beginning of the lesson. After working through Lesson 5 on the urinary system, consider the medical terms that might be used to describe his experience. List two terms relevant to the case study and their meanings. ■

Medical Term   Definition

1. _____   _____

2. _____   _____

EXERCISE R **Use Medical Terms in a Document**

Tyrone went to an urgent care center near his work. A medical assistant saw him, wrote down his problems, and took his vital signs. A physician assistant examined him, ordered tests, then gave him a diagnosis and recommendations for his care. These are documented in the medical record below.

Use the definitions in numbers 1-9 to write medical terms within the following document.

1. condition of blood in the urine

2. stones in the kidney

3. infection of one or more organs of the urinary tract

4. pertaining to the kidney

5. procedure for removing toxic waste from the blood because of an inability of the kidneys to do so

6. laboratory test in which multiple routine tests are performed on a urine specimen

7. condition of pus in the urine

8. condition of stone(s) in the ureter

9. abnormal condition of water (urine) in the kidney

Refer to the medical record to answer questions 10-14.

10. The term **hematuria**, used in the medical record to describe findings on the urinalysis, is also often described as a sign or symptom. Use your knowledge of word parts to review this term.

    ur/o means _____

    -ia means _____

    hem/o, hemat/o means _____

    Thus, **hematuria** means _____ of _____ in the _____

```
0045689 PARKER, Tyrone                                                    _ □ X
File     Patient    Navigate    Custom Fields    Help
  <    >   8   &   □   ▤   ▤   ⊟   Rx  ⊙  ⊘  ✂  ▯  ⊠  ▦  ✔  ⊙  🔍  ?
Chart Review  Encounters   Notes   Labs   Imaging   Procedures   Rx   Documents   Referrals   Scheduling   Billing
Name: PARKER, Tyrone       MR#: 0045689      Sex: M       Allergies: Demerol
                           DOB: 10/17/19XX   Age: 38      PCP: Pearson, Michael, PA-C
```

Urgent Care Visit
Date of visit: 12/15/20XX
Patient Care Provider: Michael Pearson, PA-C

SUBJECTIVE: The patient is a 38-year-old man who was in his usual state of good health when he began to experience left-sided flank pain accompanied by gross (1.) _____ three days ago. He denies chills or fever. He has no prior history of (2.) _____ but was treated for (3.) _____ one year ago. He had an appendectomy as a child. His father had chronic (4.) _____ failure requiring (5.) _____.

OBSERVATION: T 98.6 F, BP 140/80 mm Hg, P 72, R 16. He is oriented and in no acute distress. Abdomen is soft with mild tenderness over the left flank. No organomegaly. (6.) _____ showed hematuria without (7.) _____. CT scan of the abdomen revealed (8.) _____ of the distal left ureter. There is no (9.) _____ of the left kidney.

ASSESSMENT: Left distal ureterolithiasis.

PLAN:　1. Strain urine.
　　　　　2. Increase fluid intake.
　　　　　3. Ketorolac, 60 mg IM was given in the urgent care with good pain relief. He was advised to take over-the-counter ibuprofen or naproxen as needed for pain.
　　　　　4. Return for office visit in one week. Call if pain worsens or fever or chills develop.

Electronically signed: Michael Pearson, PA-C 12/16/20XX 16:15

```
Start   Log On/Off   Print   Edit                                    🖨 ◊ ⅍ 🗛
```

11. List two other terms that use **ur/o** and **–ia** to describe signs or symptoms related to urine:

_____

_____

12. CKD is the abbreviation for _____, which has also been called chronic renal failure.

13. Left distal ureterolithiasis means that a stone is located in the _____ section of the left _____.

14. Identify two new medical terms in the medical record you would like to investigate. Use your medical dictionary or an online resource to look up the definition.

	Medical Term	**Definition**
1.	_____	_____
2.	_____	_____

EXERCISE S   Interpret Language Used in a Medical Record

Read the medical record and answer the questions.

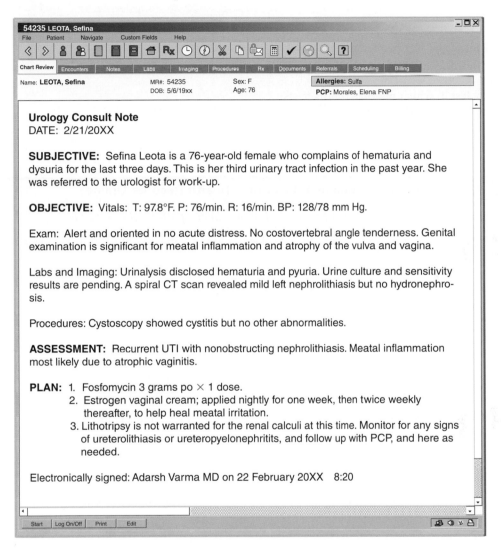

```
54235 LEOTA, Sefina                                                    _ □ ×
File     Patient    Navigate    Custom Fields    Help
《   》  🧍 🧑  ☐  ☐  ☐  📧 Rx ⏱ ⏲ ✂ 📋 📧 🗓 ✓ 🌐 🔍 ?
Chart Review  Encounters  Notes  Labs  Imaging  Procedures  Rx  Documents  Referrals  Scheduling  Billing

Name: LEOTA, Sefina        MR#: 54235       Sex: F       Allergies: Sulfa
                           DOB: 5/6/19xx     Age: 76      PCP: Morales, Elena FNP
```

Urology Consult Note
DATE: 2/21/20XX

SUBJECTIVE: Sefina Leota is a 76-year-old female who complains of hematuria and dysuria for the last three days. This is her third urinary tract infection in the past year. She was referred to the urologist for work-up.

OBJECTIVE: Vitals: T: 97.8°F. P: 76/min. R: 16/min. BP: 128/78 mm Hg.

Exam: Alert and oriented in no acute distress. No costovertebral angle tenderness. Genital examination is significant for meatal inflammation and atrophy of the vulva and vagina.

Labs and Imaging: Urinalysis disclosed hematuria and pyuria. Urine culture and sensitivity results are pending. A spiral CT scan revealed mild left nephrolithiasis but no hydronephrosis.

Procedures: Cystoscopy showed cystitis but no other abnormalities.

ASSESSMENT: Recurrent UTI with nonobstructing nephrolithiasis. Meatal inflammation most likely due to atrophic vaginitis.

PLAN: 1. Fosfomycin 3 grams po × 1 dose.
2. Estrogen vaginal cream; applied nightly for one week, then twice weekly thereafter, to help heal meatal irritation.
3. Lithotripsy is not warranted for the renal calculi at this time. Monitor for any signs of ureterolithiasis or ureteropyelonephritits, and follow up with PCP, and here as needed.

Electronically signed: Adarsh Varma MD on 22 February 20XX   8:20

```
Start   Log On/Off   Print   Edit
```

Circle the letter with the best answer for 1-4 and write your answers for 5.

1. Identify the definition of the symptom the patient did NOT complain of:
   a. condition of absence of urine
   b. condition of blood in the urine
   c. condition of difficult or painful urination

2. The patient was referred to which type of healthcare professional:
   a. physician who studies and treats diseases of the kidney
   b. physician who studies and treats diseases of the urinary tract
   c. physician who studies and treats using x-rays

3. During the exam, inflammation of which structure was identified:
   a. urinary meatus
   b. vulva
   c. kidney

4. Which diagnostic test was performed?
   a. instrument used for visual examination of the urethra
   b. laboratory test in which multiple routine tests are performed on a urine sample
   c. passage of a catheter into the urinary bladder to withdraw urine

5. Identify one new medical term used in the report and research its meaning using a medical dictionary or reliable online source.

   Term: _____

   Definition: _____

   Source: _____

EXERCISE T **Use Medical Language in Electronic Health Records Online**

Select the correct medical terms to complete three medical records in one patient's electronic file.

🌐 Access online resources at evolve.elsevier.com > Evolve Resources > Practice Student Resources > Activities > Lesson 5 > Electronic Health Records

Topic: Renal Calculus
Record 1: Encounter Visit
Record 2: Operative Report
Record 3: Postoperative Office Visit

 OBJECTIVE 6

Recall and assess knowledge of word parts, medical terms, and abbreviations.

EXERCISE U **Online Review of Lesson Content**

🌐 *Recall and assess your learning from working through the lesson by completing online learning activities at evolve. elsevier.com > Evolve Resources > Student Resources.*

❏ Check the box when complete.

EXERCISE V **Lesson Content Quiz**

Test your knowledge of the terms and abbreviations introduced in this lesson. Circle the letter for the medical term or abbreviation related to the words in italics.

1. *Condition of night urination* is more common in men over the age of 50, and may be associated with an enlarged prostate.
   a. oliguria
   b. nocturia
   c. dysuria

2. *Incision into the renal pelvis to remove stone(s)* may be necessary if ESWL is not possible.
   a. pyelolithotomy
   b. cystolithotomy
   c. urereterectomy

3. *Loss of kidney function resulting in its inability to remove waste products from the body and maintain fluid balance* can be due to diabetes, high blood pressure, or a number of other acute and chronic conditions.
   a. renal transplant
   b. renal calculi
   c. renal failure

4. Autosomal dominant *polycystic kidney disease* is the most common type of cystic disease of the kidneys; it usually appears during the third decade of life.
   a. PKD
   b. CKD
   c. PCT

5. Percutaneous *creation of an artificial opening into the kidney* may be necessary if there is blockage that is preventing urine flow from the kidney; *abnormal condition of water (urine) in the kidney* is often present in these cases.
   a. nephrotomy, nephritis
   b. nephroplasty, ureterolithiasis
   c. nephrostomy, hydronephrosis

6. A urologist uses a(n) *instrument used for visual examination of the bladder* to aid in the diagnosis of conditions such as cystolithiasis, cystitis, and bladder cancers.
   a. cystogram
   b. cystoscope
   c. cystoscopy

7. If a patient has a *UTI* in addition to renal calculi, it must be eliminated with antibiotics prior *to noninvasive surgical procedure to crush stone(s) in the kidney or ureter by administration of repeated shock waves.*
   a. urinary tract infection, extracorporeal shock wave lithotripsy
   b. urinalysis, lithotripsy
   c. urogram, ureterolithotomy

8. During voiding *radiographic imaging of the bladder and urethra*, a catheter is passed through the meatal opening, dye is placed into the bladder through this tube, and images are obtained.
   a. cystography
   b. cystourethrography
   c. meatoscopy

9. *Urine in the blood* can be a serious complication of chronic kidney disease, and may require dialysis.
   a. anuria
   b. hematuria
   c. uremia

10. Suprapubic *creation of an artificial opening into the bladder* is used when a patient is unable to empty his or her bladder, and the use of urinary catheterization is either not desirable or not possible.
    a. meatotomy
    b. cystostomy
    c. ureterocutaneostomy

11. Causes of *condition of scanty urine (amount)* may include decreased blood flow to the kidney, kidney damage, or blockage of the lower urinary tract.
    a. oliguria
    b. anuria
    c. pyuria

12. Hydronephrosis may be caused by a ureteral stricture (narrowing). *Surgical repair of the ureter* may be used to open the stricture and restore urine flow.
    a. urethroplasty
    b. ureterectomy
    c. ureteroplasty

LESSON AT A GLANCE | URINARY SYSTEM WORD PARTS

COMBINING FORMS

cyst/o	olig/o
hem/o	pyel/o
hemat/o	py/o
hydr/o	ren/o
lith/o	ur/o
meat/o	ureter/o
nephr/o	urethr/o
noct/i	

SUFFIXES

-emia
-iasis
-plasty
-tripsy

LESSON AT A GLANCE | URINARY SYSTEM MEDICAL TERMS AND ABBREVIATIONS

SIGNS AND SYMPTOMS

anuria
dysuria
hematuria
incontinence
nocturia
oliguria
pyuria

DISEASES AND DISORDERS

chronic kidney disease (CKD)
cystitis
cystolithiasis
hydronephrosis
nephritis
nephrolithiasis
pyelonephritis
renal calculi
renal failure
uremia
ureterolithiasis
ureteropyelonephritis
urethrocystitis
urinary tract infection (UTI)

DIAGNOSTIC TESTS AND EQUIPMENT

cystogram
cystography
cystoscope
cystoscopy
cystourethrography
meatoscopy
urethroscope
urinalysis (UA)
urogram

SURGICAL PROCEDURES

cystolithotomy
cystostomy
extracorporeal shock wave lithotripsy (ESWL)
lithotripsy
meatotomy
nephrectomy
nephrostomy
nephrotomy
pyelolithotomy
renal transplant
ureterectomy
ureterolithotomy
ureteroplasty
urethroplasty
urostomy

SPECIALTIES AND PROFESSIONS

nephrologist
nephrology
urologist
urology

RELATED TERMS

dialysis
meatal
renal
urinary catheterization
void

ABBREVIATIONS

cath	OAB	UTI
CKD	PCT	VCUG
ESWL	PKD	
HD	UA	

Reproductive Systems

Cindy Collier and Rajive Modi

Cindy and Rajive want to have a baby. They have been trying for over a year, but Cindy hasn't gotten pregnant. Cindy worries something is wrong. Even though she has her period every month, it is very painful, and she bleeds a lot. She often has pain low in her belly. She had sexual partners before Rajive, and she is worried that one may have given her a disease. Rajive is also concerned, and wonders if something might be wrong with him that is keeping Cindy from getting pregnant. When he was born only one of his testicles was down, and they had to do surgery to fix the other one. He hasn't had any problems with it since then. He had partners before Cindy. Now he is worried that he may have passed something on to Cindy.

■ *Consider Cindy and Rajive's situation as you work through the lesson on reproductive systems. We will return to this case study and identify medical terms used to describe and document their experiences.*

OBJECTIVES

1 ■ Build, translate, pronounce, and spell medical terms built from word parts (p. 162).

2 ■ Define, pronounce, and spell medical terms NOT built from word parts (p. 177).

3 ■ Write abbreviations (p. 184).

4 ■ Identify medical terms by clinical category (p. 185).

5 ■ Use medical language in clinical statements, the case study, and a medical record (p. 189).

6 ■ Recall and assess knowledge of word parts, medical terms, and abbreviations (p. 192).

INTRODUCTION TO THE REPRODUCTIVE SYSTEMS

Anatomic Structures of the Female Reproductive System	
breasts (brests)	milk-producing glands (also called **mammary glands**)
cervix (SER-vicks)	narrow lower portion of the uterus
endometrium (en-dō-MĒ-trē-um)	inner lining of the uterus
fallopian tubes (fa-LŌ-pē-an (toobz)	tubes attached to the uterus that provide a passageway for the ovum to move from the ovary to the uterus (also called **uterine tubes**)

FYI The **fallopian tube** was named after Gabriele Falloppio, 1523-1562, the Italian anatomist who first described female reproductive organs in detail. Fallopian, an eponym, is often not capitalized because of its common usage.

Continued

Anatomic Structures of the Female Reproductive System—cont'd

ovaries (Ō-var-ēs)	almond-shaped organs located in the pelvic cavity; form and store ova; produce the hormones estrogen and progesterone
ovum (*pl.* ova) (Ō-vum), (Ō-vah)	female reproductive (egg) cell produced by the ovaries
uterus (Ū-ter-us)	pear-sized and -shaped muscular organ that lies in the pelvic cavity, except during pregnancy when it enlarges and extends up into the abdominal cavity; its functions are menstruation, pregnancy, and labor
vagina (va-JĪ-nah)	passageway between the uterus and the outside of the body

Anatomic Structures of the Male Reproductive System

epididymis (*pl.* epididymides) (ep-i-DID-a-mis), (ep-i-DID-i-mē-dēz)	coiled tube attached to each of the testes that provides for storage, transit, and maturation of sperm
penis (PĒ-nis)	male organ of urination and coitus (sexual intercourse)
prostate gland (PROS-tāt) (gland)	encircles the upper end of the urethra; secretes fluid that aids in the movement of sperm and ejaculation
scrotum (SKRŌ-tem)	sac containing the testes and epididymis, suspended on both sides of and just behind the penis
semen (SĒ-men)	composed of sperm, seminal fluids, and other secretions
seminal vesicles (SEM-e-nel) (VES-i-kelz)	main glands located at the base of the urinary bladder that open into the vas deferens; secrete a thick fluid that forms part of the semen
sperm (spurm)	male reproductive cell produced by the testes
testis, testicle (*pl.* testes, testicles) (TES-tis), (TES-ti-kel); (TES-tēs), (TES-ti-kelz)	primary male sex organ; oval-shaped and enclosed within the scrotum; produce sperm and the hormone testosterone
urethra (ū-RĒ-thra)	narrow tube that carries semen from the vas deferens to the outside of the body; also connects to the urinary bladder in the male (a circular muscle constricts during intercourse to prevent urination)
vas deferens (vas) (DEF-ar-enz)	duct carrying the sperm from the epididymis to the urethra

Functions of the Reproductive Systems

- Produce egg and sperm cells
- Secrete hormones
- Provide for conception and pregnancy

How the Reproductive Systems Work

Male and female reproductive organs do not fully develop and begin performing reproductive functions until the individual is approximately 11 years of age. Puberty is the time during which the reproductive organs mature.

Hormones initiate puberty and play a key role in all the reproductive cycles. Hormones secreted by the reproductive systems produce feminine and masculine physical traits.

At birth, the **female reproductive system** (Figure 6.2) contains all the ova that will be produced. Upon puberty, a mature **ovum** is released from an **ovary** in a cyclical manner, usually every 28 days. Once released, the ovum travels through the **fallopian tube** to the **uterus.** Because this is approximately a seven-day journey, conception or fertilization of the ovum with sperm usually occurs in the fallopian tube. If the egg is not fertilized, layers of the endometrium detach and pass through the **vagina** along with blood as menstrual flow. The menstrual cycle occurs from puberty until women reach menopause, the cessation of the female reproductive cycles occurring sometime in middle age.

In contrast, the **male reproductive system** (Figure 6.9) generally remains functional from puberty to the end of life. **Sperm** is produced in the **testes** and passes through the **epididymis, vas deferens,** and **urethra.** The sperm matures as it travels through this series of ducts. Additional fluid, produced by the **prostate gland** and **seminal vesicles,** is contributed along the way to produce **semen.** Semen is ejaculated from the **penis** into the vagina for potential creation of offspring.

CAREER FOCUS | **Professionals Who Work with the Reproductive Systems**

- **Obstetric technicians (OB/GYN tech)** assist during vaginal births, sterilize equipment, and maintain medical records. Training requirements may include certification in nursing assisting and surgical technology.

- **Certified nurse midwives (CNM)** are registered nurses who hold a master's degree in nursing and certification in midwifery. CNMs work closely with gynecologists and specialize in the care of pregnant women, childbirth, and care of infants.

- **Direct-entry midwives** are trained in midwifery but are not nurses. They usually practice in non-hospital settings, including birthing centers and the patient's home.

- **Mammographers,** also called mammography technologists, obtain diagnostic images of breast tissue using special x-ray equipment. They take medical histories, answer questions, and position patients for imaging.

Figure 6.1 A mammographer assisting a patient with her screening exam.

OBJECTIVE 1

Build, translate, pronounce, and spell medical terms built from word parts.

WORD PARTS	Presented with the Reproductive Systems

Use the paper or online **flashcards** to familiarize yourself with the following word parts.

COMBINING FORM (WR + CV)	DEFINITION	COMBINING FORM (WR + CV)	DEFINITION
FEMALE		**MALE**	
cervic/o	cervix (or neck)	**orchi/o**	testis (testicle)
colp/o, vagin/o	vagina	**prostat/o**	prostate gland
endometri/o	endometrium	**scrot/o**	scrotum
gynec/o	woman, female reproductive system	**vas/o**	vessel, duct (vas deferens)
hyster/o	uterus		
mamm/o, mast/o	breast		
men/o	menstruation, menstrual		
oophor/o	ovary		
salping/o	fallopian tube (uterine tube)		

FYI In male reproductive system terms, **vas/o** refers to the **vas deferens**, the duct carrying sperm from the epididymis to the urethra.

SUFFIX (S)	DEFINITION	SUFFIX (S)	DEFINITION
-cele	hernia, protrusion	**-rrhaphy**	suturing, repairing
		-rrhexis	rupture

FYI A **hernia** is the protrusion of an organ through an abnormal opening in a membrane or cavity wall.

-pexy	surgical fixation, suspension		

WORD PARTS PRESENTED IN PREVIOUS LESSONS	Used to Build Terms for the Reproductive Systems

COMBINING FORM (WR + CV)	DEFINITION	COMBINING FORM (WR + CV)	DEFINITION
cyst/o	bladder, sac	**lith/o**	stone(s), calculus (*pl.* calculi)

SUFFIX (S)	DEFINITION	SUFFIX (S)	DEFINITION
-al, -ic	pertaining to	**-itis**	inflammation
-ectomy	surgical removal, excision	**-logist**	one who studies and treats (specialist, physician)
-gram	record, radiographic image	**-logy**	study of
-graphy	process of recording, radiographic imaging	**-osis**	abnormal condition

Continued

WORD PARTS PRESENTED IN PREVIOUS LESSONS		Used to Build Terms for the Reproductive Systems—cont'd	
SUFFIX (S)	**DEFINITION**	**SUFFIX (S)**	**DEFINITION**
-plasty	surgical repair	**-scope**	instrument used for visual examination
-rrhagia	excessive bleeding	**-scopy**	visual examination
-rrhea	flow, discharge	**-tomy**	cut into, incision
PREFIX (P)	**DEFINITION**	**PREFIX (P)**	**DEFINITION**
a-	absence of, without	**dys-**	difficult, painful, abnormal

Refer to Appendix A, Word Parts Used in *Basic Medical Language* for alphabetical lists of word parts and their meanings.

EXERCISE A **Build and Translate Terms Built from Word Parts**

*Use the **Word Parts Tables** to complete the following questions. Check your responses with the Answer Key in Appendix C.*

1. LABEL: *Write the combining forms for anatomic structures of the female reproductive system on Figure 6.2. These anatomic combining forms will be used to build and translate medical terms in Exercise A.*

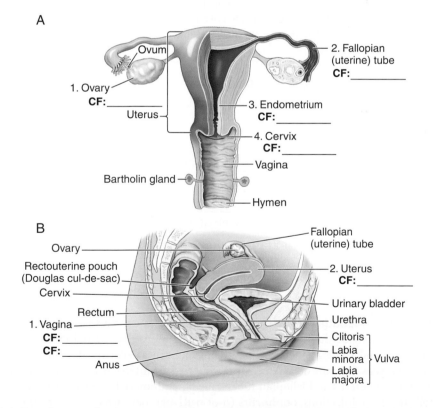

Figure 6.2 Female reproductive system with combining forms. **A,** Frontal view; **B,** Sagittal view.

2. MATCH: *Draw a line to match the suffix with its definition.*

    a. -al   inflammation
    b. -itis   abnormal condition
    c. -osis   pertaining to

---

3. BUILD: *Using the suffix **-itis**, build terms describing inflammation of female reproductive organs. Remember, the definition usually starts with the meaning of the suffix.*

    a. inflammation of the vagina (*Hint:*   _____/_____
        *Use the combining form starting with a **v**.)*   wr   s

    b. inflammation of the fallopian tube   _____/_____
                                                  wr   s

    c. inflammation of an ovary   _____/_____
                                      wr   s

    d. inflammation of the cervix   _____/_____
                                      wr   s

> **FYI**   **Cervic/o** is also used to denote the neck or any part of a body organ resembling a neck. By examining the other word parts in the medical term, you can determine whether the term applies to the cervix of the uterus or another body organ. For example, **cervic/o/thorac/ic** means pertaining to the neck and thorax. Locate **cervic/o** in your medical dictionary or an online source and read the definitions of the many medical terms containing the combining form **cervic/o**.

---

4. TRANSLATE: *Complete the definitions of the following terms by using the meaning of word parts to fill in the blanks. Remember, the definition usually starts with the meaning of the suffix.*

    a. vagin/al   _____ to the _____
    b. cervic/al   pertaining _____ the _____
    c. endometri/al   _____ to the _____
    d. endometr/itis   _____ of the endometrium
    e. endometri/osis   abnormal _____ of the _____
                                 (growth of endometrial tissue outside of the uterus)

> **FYI**   Embedded within the combining form **endometri/o** are the prefix **endo-**, meaning within, and the word root **metr**, meaning uterus.

---

5. READ: Noninfectious **vaginitis** (vaj-i-NĪ-tis) may occur after menopause as a result of dryness caused by reduced estrogen, or may be the result of irritation caused by use of **vaginal** (VAJ-i-nal) sprays, perfumed soap and detergent, and some methods of birth control, such as spermicides. Infectious vaginitis may be caused by bacteria, yeast, or parasites. A **cervical** (SER-vi-kal) infection may cause **cervicitis** (ser-vi-SĪ-tis) and may spread to the uterus and fallopian tubes causing **endometritis** (en-dō-mē-TRĪ-tis) and **salpingitis** (sal-pin-JĪ-tis). In severe infections, **oophoritis** (ō-of-o-RĪ-tis) may also occur. Infections of one or more of the female reproductive organs, including the cervix, uterus, fallopian tubes, and ovaries are called pelvic inflammatory disease (PID).

---

6. LABEL: *Write word parts to complete Figure 6.3.*

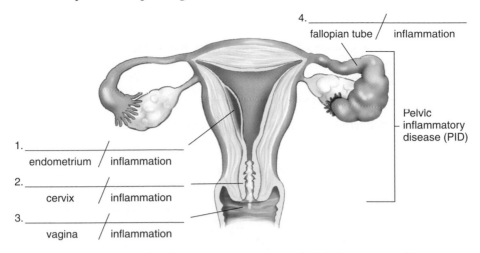

4. _____ / _____
fallopian tube / inflammation

Pelvic inflammatory disease (PID)

1. _____ / _____
endometrium / inflammation

2. _____ / _____
cervix / inflammation

3. _____ / _____
vagina / inflammation

Figure 6.3 Potential infection sites as seen in pelvic inflammatory disease.

7. READ: Endometriosis (en-dō-mē-trē-Ō-sis) is an abnormal condition in which **endometrial** (en-dō-MĒ-trē-l) tissue grows outside of the uterus in various areas of the pelvic cavity, including the surfaces of the ovaries, fallopian tubes, uterus, and intestines.

8. LABEL: *Write word parts to complete Figure 6.4.*

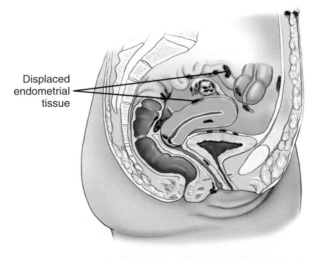

Displaced endometrial tissue

Figure 6.4 _____ / _____ .
endometrium / abnormal condition

9. MATCH: *Draw a line to match the combining form or suffix with its definition.*

a. -logy   woman (women)
b. -logist   visual examination
c. -scope   one who studies and treats (specialist, physician)
d. -scopy   study of
e. gynec/o   instrument used for visual examination

10. BUILD: *Build the following terms, using the word parts from the previous exercise and the combining form* **colp/o** *for vagina:*

a. instrument used for visual examination of the vagina

_____/_o_/_____
wr   cv   s

b. visual examination of the vagina

_____/_o_/_____
wr   cv   s

c. study of women (female reproductive system)

_____/_o_/_____
wr   cv   s

d. physician who studies and treats disease of women
(female reproductive system)

_____/_o_/_____
wr   cv   s

11. READ: **Colposcopy** (kol-POS-ko-pē) is performed by a **gynecologist** (gīn-ek-OL-o-jist) to provide a closer look at vaginal tissue, the vulva, and the cervix. It is performed with a **colposcope** (KOL-pō-skōp) equipped with a light and microscope. A biopsy may be performed during colposcopy if abnormal tissue is present. Colposcopy can be used to diagnose cancers of the vulva, vagina, and cervix, as well as genital warts and cervicitis.

12. MATCH: *Draw a line to match the suffix with its definition.*

a. -cele   surgical fixation
b. -pexy   hernia, protrusion

13. TRANSLATE: *Complete the definitions of the following terms by using the meaning of word parts to fill in the blanks. (Hint: Use the definition that starts with a* **p** *for the first term)*

a. cyst/o/cele   _____ of the (urinary) _____
                        (through anterior vaginal wall)
b. hyster/o/pexy   surgical _____ of the _____

14. READ: Weakening of pelvic muscles and ligaments resulting from traumatic vaginal childbirth, straining during bowel movements, and normal aging can lead to displacement of pelvic organs, as seen in **cystocele** (SIS-tō-sēl) and rectocele. Cystocele refers to the protrusion of the urinary bladder into the vagina through the anterior vaginal wall, while rectocele describes protrusion of the rectum against the posterior wall of the vagina. **Hysteropexy** (HIS-ter-ō-pek-sē) may be performed when the uterus is dropping into the superior portion of the vagina (uterovaginal prolapse).

15. LABEL: *Write word parts to complete Figure 6.5.*

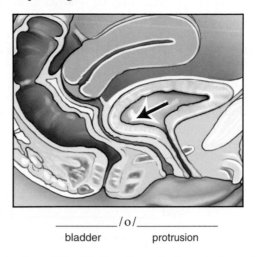

_____/o/_____
bladder   protrusion

Figure 6.5 Protrusion of the bladder through the anterior wall of the vagina.

16. MATCH: *Draw a line to match the suffix with its definition.*

a. -gram   surgical removal, excision
b. -pexy   record, radiographic image
c. -ectomy   suturing, repairing
d. -rrhexis   surgical fixation
e. -rrhaphy   rupture

> **FYI** All four **–rrh** suffixes have now been introduced: **-rrhea, -rrhagia,-rrhaphy**, and **-rrhexis**. Can you recall their definitions?

17. BUILD: *Build the following terms, using the word parts from the previous exercise and the combining forms for the uterus and the ovary:*

a. excision of the uterus   _____/_____
                                          wr   s

b. surgical fixation of the ovary   _____/_o_/_____
                                          wr   cv   s

c. rupture of the uterus   _____/_o_/_____
                                          wr   cv   s

d. suturing of the uterus   _____/_o_/_____
                                          wr   cv   s

18. **READ:** **Hysterorrhexis** (his-ter-ō-REK-sis), while rare, is a risk factor in a vaginal birth after a previous birth by Cesarean section. Any suturing of the uterus may be referred to as **hysterorrhaphy** (his-ter-OR-a-fē). Uterovaginal prolapse may be treated surgically by **hysteropexy** (HIS-ter-ō-pek-sē) or, in more severe cases, by **hysterectomy** (his-te-REK-to-mē). **Oophoropexy** (ō-OF-ō-rō-pek-sē), in which the ovaries are positioned outside the radiation field, may be performed to preserve fertility in cancer patients receiving radiation to the pelvic area.

19. **TRANSLATE:** *Complete the definitions of the following terms by using the meaning of word parts to fill in the blanks.*

   a. cervic/ectomy   _____ of the _____

   b. oophor/ectomy   _____ of the _____

   c. hyster/o/salping/o/–oophor/ectomy   excision of the _____, fallopian _____(s),

   and _____ (plural)

   d. hyster/o/salping/o/gram   _____ image of the _____

   and _____ tubes

> **FYI**   A hyphen is often used between two word parts when one ends and the other begins with the same vowel, as in the term **salpingo-oophoritis**.

20. **READ:** A **hysterosalpingogram** (his-ter-ō-sal-PING-gō-gram), which is often performed in fertility studies, provides a radiographic image of the inside of the uterus and the fallopian tubes. The image is analyzed by a radiologist and may be used to assess the patency (openness) of fallopian tubes and to diagnose uterine abnormalities.

21. **LABEL:** *Write word parts to complete Figure 6.6.*

> **FYI**   Use your medical dictionary or a reliable online source to learn more about **hysterosalpingogram** and the use of **fluoroscopy** in obtaining the image.

Figure 6.6 _____/o/_____/o/_____.
                    uterus   fallopian tube   radiographic image

22. **READ:** **Cervicectomy** (ser-vi-SEK-to-mē), hysterectomy, **oophorectomy** (ō-of-o-REK-to-mē), and **hysterosalpingo-oophorectomy** (his-ter-ō-sal-ping-gō-ō-of-ō-REK-to-mē) are surgical procedures used to treat cancer and other pelvic abnormalities.

23. LABEL: *Write word parts to complete Figure 6.7.*

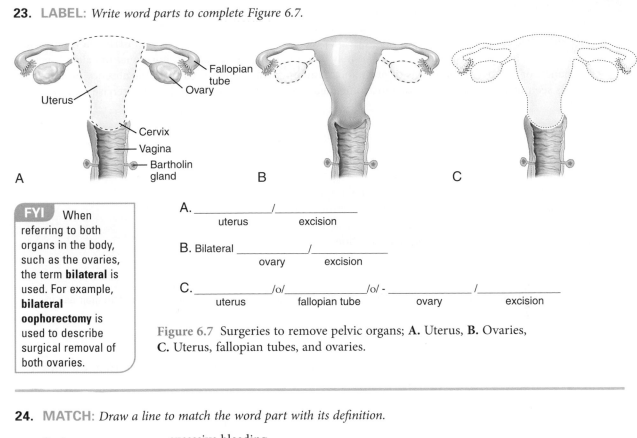

FYI When referring to both organs in the body, such as the ovaries, the term **bilateral** is used. For example, **bilateral oophorectomy** is used to describe surgical removal of both ovaries.

A. _____/_____
         uterus   excision

B. Bilateral _____/_____
               ovary   excision

C. _____/o/_____/o/ - _____/_____
      uterus   fallopian tube   ovary   excision

Figure 6.7 Surgeries to remove pelvic organs; **A.** Uterus, **B.** Ovaries, **C.** Uterus, fallopian tubes, and ovaries.

24. MATCH: *Draw a line to match the word part with its definition.*

    a. a-   excessive bleeding
    b. dys-   flow, discharge
    c. men/o   without, absence of
    d. -rrhea   difficult, painful, abnormal
    e. -rrhagia   menstruation, menstrual

FYI The combining form **men/o** is used in medicine to describe the monthly menstrual cycle in women. It is derived from the Greek word **mene,** or moon, which refers to the lunar month.

25. TRANSLATE: *Complete the definitions of the following terms built from the combining form **men/o**, meaning menstruation, menstrual. Hints: Use **flow** for the definition of -**rrhea**, and begin the definition with the prefix if present.*

    a. a/men/o/rrhea   _____ menstrual _____

    b. dys/men/o/rrhea   _____ flow

    c. men/o/rrhea   flow at _____

    d. men/o/rrhagia   _____ bleeding at _____

26. READ: **Menorrhea** (men-ō-RĒ-a) refers to normal discharge during menstruation. Primary **dysmenorrhea** (dis-men-ō-RĒ-a) refers to pelvic cramping occurring with normal menstruation. Secondary dysmenorrhea refers to pelvic cramping resulting from a disease process, such as endometriosis. **Menorrhagia** (men-ō-RĀ-jea) indicates heavy menstrual bleeding and may be caused by fibroid tumors, hormonal imbalance, ectopic pregnancy, or abnormal conditions of pregnancy. **Amenorrhea** (a-men-ō-RĒ-a) is the absence of menstruation, as seen with pregnancy, menopause, some medications, excessive weight loss or exercise, or stress.

27. MATCH: *Draw a line to match the suffix or combining form with its definition.*

a.	-gram	surgical repair
b.	-graphy	breast
c.	-plasty	record, radiographic image
d.	-ectomy	process of recording, radiographic imaging
e.	mamm/o, mast/o	surgical removal, excision
f.	-pexy	surgical fixation

> **FYI** **Mamm** is of Latin origin, and **mast** is of Greek origin. With practice, you will become familiar with their use in medical terms.

28. BUILD: *Write word parts to build terms describing diagnosis and treatment of the breast. Hint: Use **mast/o** to build the first two terms, and **mamm/o** for any remaining terms that relate to the breast.*

a. excision of the breast

_____/_____
　　　　　　　　　　　wr　　　　　　　　　　s

b. surgical fixation of the breast

_____/_o_/_____
　　　　　　　　　　　wr　　　cv　　　s

c. radiographic image of the breast

_____/_o_/_____
　　　　　　　　　　　wr　　　cv　　　s

d. radiographic imaging of the breast

_____/_o_/_____
　　　　　　　　　　　wr　　　cv　　　s

e. surgical repair of the breast

_____/_o_/_____
　　　　　　　　　　　wr　　　cv　　　s

29. READ: **Mammography** (ma-MOG-ra-fē) is a radiography procedure that uses specialized equipment to obtain an image of the breast for examination. The resulting image is a **mammogram** (MAM-ō-gram). Mammography is used for screening when no symptoms are present and for diagnosis when a lump has been detected, nipple discharge is present, or as warranted based on findings of a screening mammogram. Sonography, also called ultrasonography, can be used to determine whether a lump is cystic (fluid-filled) or solid. **Mastectomy** (mas-TEK-tō-mē) is a surgical procedure used to prevent and treat breast cancer. **Mammoplasty** (MAM-ō-plas-tē) is a surgical procedure to alter the size and shape of the breast through augmentation, reduction, or for reconstruction after mastectomy. **Mastopexy** (MAS-tō-pek-sē), a surgical procedure to lift sagging breast tissue, may be performed after weight loss, pregnancy, or removal of an implant.

30. LABEL: *Write word parts to complete Figure 6.8.*

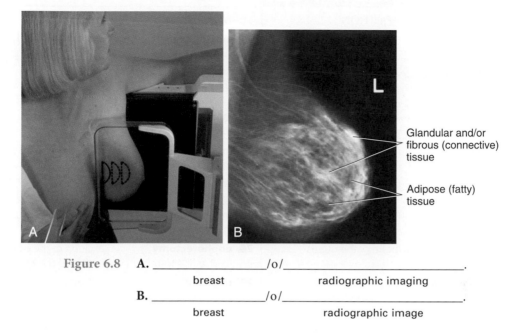

Glandular and/or fibrous (connective) tissue

Adipose (fatty) tissue

Figure 6.8   **A.** _____/o/_____.
                           breast   radiographic imaging

               B. _____/o/_____.
                           breast   radiographic image

31. REVIEW OF FEMALE REPRODUCTIVE SYSTEM TERMS BUILT FROM WORD PARTS: The following is an alphabetical list of terms built and translated in the previous exercises.

MEDICAL TERMS BUILT FROM WORD PARTS

TERM	DEFINITION	TERM	DEFINITION
1. amenorrhea (a-men-ō-RĒ-a)	without menstrual flow	**7. cystocele** (SIS-tō-sēl)	protrusion of the bladder (through anterior vaginal wall) (Figure 6.5)
2. cervical (SER-vi-kal)	pertaining to the cervix	**8. dysmenorrhea** (dis-men-ō-RĒ-a)	painful menstrual flow
3. cervicectomy (ser-vi-SEK-to-mē)	excision of the cervix (also called **trachelectomy**)	**9. endometrial** (en-dō-MĒ-trē-l)	pertaining to the endometrium
4. cervicitis (ser-vi-SĪ-tis)	inflammation of the cervix (Figure 6.3, 2)	**10 endometriosis** (en-dō-mē-trē-Ō-sis)	abnormal condition of the endometrium (growth of endometrial tissue outside of the uterus) (Figure 6.4)
5. colposcope (KOL-pō-skōp)	instrument used for visual examination of the vagina	**11. endometritis** (en-dō-mē-TRĪ-tis)	inflammation of the endometrium (Figure 6.3, 1)
6. colposcopy (kol-POS-ko-pē)	visual examination of the vagina	**12. gynecologist** (gīn-ek-OL-o-jist)	physician who studies and treats diseases of women (female reproductive system)

Continued

MEDICAL TERMS BUILT FROM WORD PARTS—cont'd

TERM	DEFINITION	TERM	DEFINITION
13. gynecology (gīn-ek-OL-o-jē)	study of women (the branch of medicine focused on the health and diseases of the female reproductive system)	**24. mastopexy** (MAS-tō-pek-sē)	surgical fixation of the breast (performed to lift sagging breast tissue or to create symmetry)
14. hysterectomy (his-te-REK-to-mē)	excision of the uterus (Figure 6.7, A)	**25. mastitis** (mas-TĪ-tis)	inflammation of the breast
15. hysteropexy (HIS-ter-ō-pek-sē)	surgical fixation of the uterus	**26. menorrhagia** (men-ō-RĀ-jea)	excessive bleeding at menstruation (heavy bleeding in regular, cyclical pattern)
16. hysterorrhaphy (his-ter-OR-a-fē)	suturing of the uterus	**27. menorrhea** (men-ō-RĒ-a)	flow at menstruation
17. hysterorrhexis (his-ter-ō-REK-sis)	rupture of the uterus	**28. oophorectomy** (ō-of-o-REK-tō-mē)	excision of the ovary (Figure 6.7, B)
18. hysterosalpingogram (his-ter-ō-sal-PING-gō-gram)	radiographic image of the uterus and fallopian tubes (Figure 6.6)	**29. oophoritis** (ō-of-o-RĪ-tis)	inflammation of the ovary
19. hysterosalpingo-oophorectomy (his-ter-ō-sal-ping-gō-ō-of-ō-REK-to-mē)	excision of the uterus, fallopian tubes, and ovaries (Figure 6.7, C)	**30. oophoropexy** (ō-OF-ō-rō-pek-sē)	surgical fixation of the ovary
20. mammogram (MAM-ō-gram)	radiographic image of the breast (Figure 6.8, B)	**31. salpingitis** (sal-pin-JĪ-tis)	inflammation of the fallopian tube (Figure 6.3, 4)
21. mammography (ma-MOG-ra-fē)	radiographic imaging of the breast (Figure 6.8, A)	**32. vaginal** (VAJ-i-nal)	pertaining to the vagina
22. mammoplasty (MAM-ō-plas-tē)	surgical repair of the breast	**33. vaginitis** (vaj-i-NĪ-tis)	inflammation of the vagina (Figure 6.3, 3)
23. mastectomy (mas-TEK-tō-mē)	excision of the breast		

EXERCISE B   Pronounce and Spell Terms Built from Word Parts

Practice pronunciation and spelling on paper and online.

1. Practice on Paper
   a. **Pronounce:** Read the phonetic spelling and say aloud the terms listed in the previous table, Review of Female Reproductive System Terms Built from Word Parts.
   b. **Spell:** Have a study partner read the terms aloud. Write the spelling of the terms on a separate sheet of paper.

2. **Practice Online** 🌐

    a. **Access** online learning resources. Go to evolve.elsevier.com > Evolve Resources > Practice Student Resources.

    b. **Pronounce:** Select Audio Glossary > Lesson 6 > Exercise B. Select a term to hear its pronunciation and repeat aloud.

    c. **Spell:** Select Activities > Lesson 6 > Spell Terms > Exercise B. Select the audio icon and type the correct spelling of the term.

❏ Check the box when complete.

EXERCISE C   **Build and Translate MORE Medical Terms Built from Word Parts**

1. LABEL: *Write the combining forms for anatomic structures of the male reproductive system on Figure 6.9. These anatomic combining forms will be used to build and translate medical terms in Exercise C.*

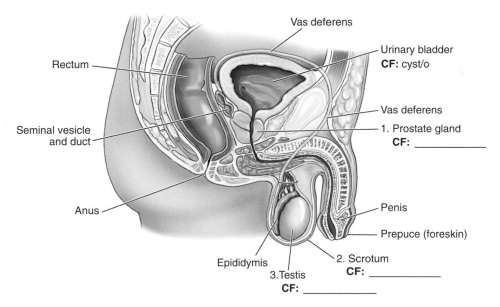

Figure 6.9 Male reproductive system with combining forms.

---

2. MATCH: *Draw a line to match the combining form or suffix with its definition.*

    a. cyst/o   inflammation

    b. lith/o   bladder, sac

    c. -itis   pertaining to

    d. -ectomy   stone(s), calculus (*pl.* calculi)

    e. -ic   surgical removal, excision

3. TRANSLATE: *Complete the definitions of the following terms built from the combining form **prostat/o**, meaning prostate gland.*

a. prostat/itis   _____ of the _____ gland

b. prostat/o/cyst/itis   inflammation of the prostate _____ and the (urinary) _____

c. prostat/ic   _____ to the _____ gland

d. prostat/o/lith   _____(s) in the prostate _____

e. prostat/ectomy   _____ of the prostate gland

---

4. READ: Bacterial **prostatitis** (pros-ta-TĪ-tis) may be acute, characterized by a sudden onset of symptoms, or chronic, as seen with recurring urinary tract infections. In **prostatocystitis** (pros-ta-tō-sis-TĪ-tis) the prostate gland and the bladder are affected. The formation of one or more **prostatoliths** (pros-TAT-ō-liths) may contribute to **prostatic** (pros-TAT-ik) inflammation. **Prostatectomy** (pros-ta-TEK-to-mē) is a surgical procedure used to treat prostate cancer.

---

5. LABEL: *Write word parts to complete Figure 6.10.*

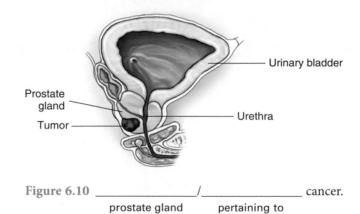

Prostate gland
Tumor
Urinary bladder
Urethra

Figure 6.10 _____/_____ cancer.
            prostate gland   pertaining to

---

6. MATCH: *Draw a line to match the prefix or suffix with its definition.*

a. -itis   surgical fixation
b. -ectomy   inflammation
c. -pexy   surgical removal, excision
d. -al   surgical repair
e. -plasty   pertaining to

7. BUILD: *Write word parts to build the following terms using the combining forms **orchi/o**, meaning testis (testicle), and **scrot/o**, meaning scrotum.*

a. inflammation of the testis _____ / _____
   wr   s

b. surgical fixation of the testis _____ / ___o___ / _____
   wr   cv   s

c. excision of the testis _____ / _____
   wr   s

d. pertaining to the scrotum _____ / _____
   wr   s

e. surgical repair of the scrotum _____ / ___o___ / _____
   wr   cv   s

8. READ: Orchitis (or-KĪ-tis) results from a viral infection, as seen in mumps, or a bacterial infection, as seen in sexually transmitted infections such as gonorrhea and chlamydia. The infection may be unilateral, involving one testicle, or bilateral, involving both testicles. **Orchiopexy** (OR-kē-ō-pek-sē) is a surgical procedure that may be performed to bring an undescended testicle into the scrotum. **Orchiectomy** (or-kē-EK-to-mē) is a surgical procedure performed to treat testicular cancer and may be unilateral or bilateral. **Scrotoplasty** (SKRŌ-tō-plas-tē) describes surgical procedures to repair the **scrotal** (SKRŌT-al) sac, including placement of testicular implants after an orchiectomy.

9. MATCH: *Draw a line to match the combining form or the suffix with its definition.*

a. vas/o   creation of an artificial opening
b. -ectomy   surgical removal, excision
c. -stomy   vessel, duct (refers to vas deferens in the context of the
                     male reproductive system)

10. TRANSLATE: *Complete the definitions of surgical terms by using the meaning of word parts to fill in the blanks:*

a. vas/ectomy   _____ of the _____ (vas deferens)
b. vas/o/vas/o/stomy _____ of an artificial _____ between _____(s)

11. READ: Vasectomy (va-SEK-to-mē) is a surgical procedure to remove a portion of the vas deferens for the purpose of birth control by preventing the flow of sperm to the outside of the body. A **vasovasostomy** (vas-ō-vā-ZOS-to-mē) may be performed at a later time to reverse the vasectomy and to reconnect the vas deferens, potentially returning male fertility.

12. LABEL: *Write word parts to complete Figure 6.11.*

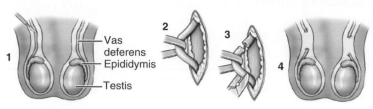

1. incision is made into the covering of the vas deferens
2. vas deferens is exposed
3. segment of vas deferens is excised
4. vas deferens is repositioned and skin is sutured

Figure 6.11 _____ / _____ .

　　　　　　　　　duct (vas deferens)　　　　excision

---

13. REVIEW OF MALE REPRODUCTIVE SYSTEM TERMS BUILT FROM WORD PARTS: The following is an alphabetical list of terms built and translated in the previous exercises.

MEDICAL TERMS BUILT FROM WORD PARTS

TERM	DEFINITION	TERM	DEFINITION
1. orchiectomy (or-kē-EK-to-mē)	excision of the testis	**7. prostatocystitis** (pros-ta-tō-sis-TĪ-tis)	inflammation of the prostate gland and the bladder
2. orchitis (or-KĪ-tis)	inflammation of the testis	**8. prostatolith** (pros-TAT-ō-lith)	stone(s) in the prostate gland
3. orchiopexy (OR-kē-ō-pek-sē)	surgical fixation of the testis	**9. scrotal** (SKRŌT-al)	pertaining to the scrotum
4. prostatectomy (pros-ta-TEK-to-mē)	excision of the prostate gland	**10. scrotoplasty** (SKRŌ-tō-plas-tē)	surgical repair of the scrotum
5. prostatic (pros-TAT-ik)	pertaining to the prostate gland (Figure 6.10)	**11. vasectomy** (va-SEK-to-mē)	excision of the duct (vas deferens) (Figure 6.11)
6. prostatitis (pros-ta-TĪ-tis)	inflammation of the prostate gland	**12. vasovasostomy** (vas-ō-vā-ZOS-to-mē)	creation of an artificial opening between ducts

---

EXERCISE D | **Pronounce and Spell MORE Terms Built from Word Parts**

Practice pronunciation and spelling on paper and online.

1. Practice on Paper

    a. Pronounce: Read the phonetic spelling and say aloud the terms listed in the previous table, Review of Male Reproductive System Terms Built from Word Parts.

    b. Spell: Have a study partner read the terms aloud. Write the spelling of the terms on a separate sheet of paper.

2. **Practice Online** 🌐

    a. **Access** online learning resources. Go to evolve.elsevier.com > Evolve Resources > Practice Student Resources.

    b. **Pronounce:** Select Audio Glossary > Lesson 6 > Exercise D. Select a term to hear its pronunciation and repeat aloud.

    c. **Spell:** Select Activities > Lesson 6 > Spell Terms > Exercise D. Select the audio icon and type the correct spelling of the term.

❏   Check the box when complete.

OBJECTIVE 2

Define, pronounce, and spell medical terms NOT built from word parts.

The terms listed below may contain word parts, but are difficult to translate literally.

FEMALE REPRODUCTIVE SYSTEM TERMS NOT BUILT FROM WORD PARTS

TERM	DEFINITION
1. dilation and curettage (D&C) (dī-LĀ-shun) (and) (kū-re-TAHZH)	surgical procedure to widen the cervix and scrape the endometrium with an instrument called a curette
2. obstetrics (ob-STET-riks)	branch of medicine that deals with the management of pregnancy, labor, and the postpartum period (approximately 6 weeks after giving birth)
3. Pap test (pap) (test)	laboratory test involving cytological study of cervical and vaginal secretions used to determine the presence of abnormal or cancerous cells; primarily used for cervical cancer screening (formerly called **Pap smear**)

FYI   **Pap test** is named after Dr. George N. Papanicolaou (1883–1962), who in 1943 developed the original method of "smearing" cervical cells directly on a microscopic slide to evaluate for the possibility of cancer. More recently, a Pap test has been developed that involves releasing the cells into a vial of liquid preservative, and then transferring them to a microscopic slide in the lab.

TERM	DEFINITION
4. pelvic inflammatory disease (PID) (PEL-vik) (in-FLAM-a-tor-ē) (di-ZĒZ)	inflammation of some or all of the female reproductive organs; can be caused by many different pathogens
5. uterine fibroid (Ū-ter-in) (FĪ-broyd)	benign tumor of the uterine muscle (also called **myoma and leiomyoma**)
6. uterovaginal prolapse (ū-ter-ō-VAG-i-nal) (PRO-laps)	dropping of the uterus (and sometimes vagina) due to weakened pelvic muscles; the uterus moves downward into and is sometimes visible outside the vagina

TABLE 6.1	CANCERS OF THE REPRODUCTIVE SYSTEMS

Cancer can affect organs of the reproductive systems. The anatomic structure affected appears before the term "cancer" as seen in the following examples.

FEMALE REPRODUCTIVE SYSTEM

- breast cancer (can also affect men)
- vulvar cancer
- vaginal cancer
- cervical cancer
- uterine cancer (also called endometrial cancer)
- fallopian tube cancer
- ovarian cancer

MALE REPRODUCTIVE SYSTEM

- penile cancer
- testicular cancer
- prostate cancer

MALE REPRODUCTIVE SYSTEM TERMS NOT BUILT FROM WORD PARTS

TERM	DEFINITION
1. **benign prostatic hyperplasia** (**BPH**) (be-NĪN) (pros-TAT-ik) (hī-per-PLĀ-zha)	nonmalignant enlargement of the prostate gland; as the gland enlarges, it causes narrowing of the urethra, which interferes with the passage of urine. Symptoms include frequency of urination, nocturia, urinary retention, and incomplete emptying of the bladder. (also called **benign prostatic hypertrophy**)
2. **circumcision** (ser-kum-SI-shun)	surgical removal of all or part of the foreskin of the penis
3. **digital rectal examination** (**DRE**) (DIJ-i-tal) (REK-tal) (eg-zam-i-NĀ-shun)	physical examination in which the healthcare provider inserts a gloved finger into the rectum and palpates the size and shape of the prostate gland through the rectal wall; used to screen for BPH and prostate cancer. BPH usually presents as a uniform, nontender enlargement, whereas cancer usually presents as a stony hard nodule.
4. **erectile dysfunction** (**ED**) (e-REK-tīl) (dis-FUNK-shun)	inability of the male to attain or maintain an erection of the penis sufficient to perform sexual acts (formerly called **impotence**)
5. **prostate-specific antigen** (**PSA**) **assay** (PROS-tāt) (spe-SIF-ik) (AN-ti-gen) (AS-ā)	blood test that measures the level of prostate-specific antigen, a protein produced by the prostate gland
6. **semen analysis** (SĒ-men) (a-NAL-i-sis)	laboratory test involving microscopic observation of ejaculated semen, revealing the size, structure, and movement of sperm; used to evaluate male infertility and to determine the effectiveness of a vasectomy (also called **sperm count** and **sperm test**)
7. **sexually transmitted infection** (**STI**) (SEKS-ū-al-ē) (TRANS-mi-ted) (in-FEK-shun)	infection spread through sexual contact; STIs affect both male and female reproductive systems, causing damage to organs and potentially serious health consequences if left untreated (also called **sexually transmitted disease [STD]**)

FYI **Sexually Transmitted Infection (STI) vs. Sexually Transmitted Disease (STD): what's the difference?** Usually, a "disease" refers to a clear medical problem, often with signs or symptoms. But patients with an infection may have no signs or symptoms and still have the problem. While STI is medically more accurate, you will also frequently hear the term STD. These infections affect all genders, causing damage to reproductive organs and potentially serious health consequences if left untreated. Any sexual behavior involving contact with the body fluids of another person puts an individual at risk for infection.

| 8. **transurethral resection of the prostate gland** (**TURP**) (trans-ū-RĒ-thral) (rē-SEK-shun) (of) (the) (PROS-tāt) | surgical removal of pieces of the prostate gland tissue by using an instrument inserted through the urethra |

TABLE 6.2	TYPES OF SEXUALLY TRANSMITTED INFECTIONS

Consult the Centers for Disease Control and Prevention website at cdc.gov/std/ or your medical dictionary for more information about the following types of sexually transmitted infections:

PARASITIC	BACTERIAL	VIRAL
• pubic lice • trichomoniasis	• chlamydia • gonorrhea • syphilis • vaginosis	• genital herpes • hepatitis B • human immunodeficiency virus (HIV)/AIDS • human papillomavirus (HPV)

EXERCISE E	Label

Write the medical terms pictured and defined using the previous tables of Medical Terms NOT Built from Word Parts. Check your work with the Answer Key in Appendix C.

1. _____

laboratory test involving cytological study of cervical and vaginal secretions used to determine the presence of abnormal or cancerous cells

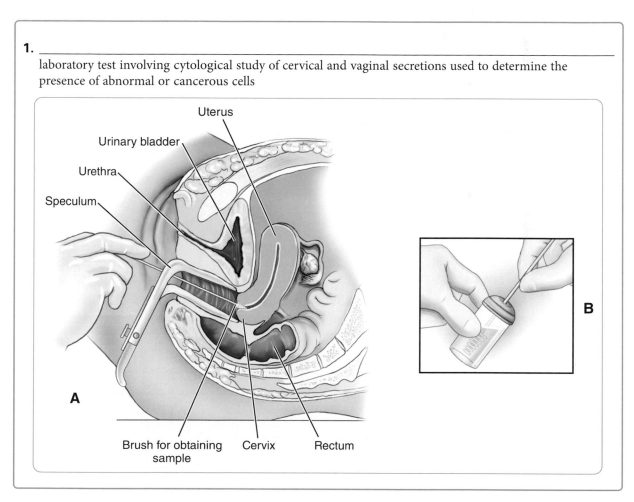

2. _____

surgical procedure to widen the cervix and scrape the endometrium with an instrument called a curette

3. _____

benign tumor of the uterine muscle

4. _____

dropping of the uterus (and sometimes vagina) due to weakened pelvic muscles

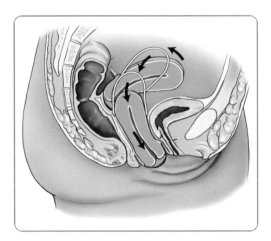

5. _____

inflammation of some or all of the female reproductive organs; can be caused by many different pathogens

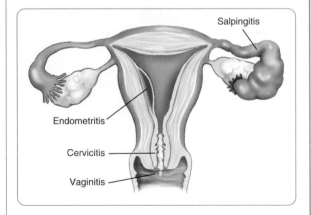

6. _____

branch of medicine that deals with the management of pregnancy, labor, and the post-partum period

7. _____

surgical removal of pieces of the prostate gland tissue by using an instrument inserted through the urethra

8. _____

surgical removal of all or part of the foreskin of the penis

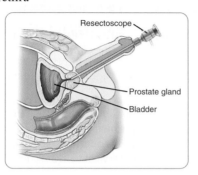

9. _____

nonmalignant enlargement of the prostate gland

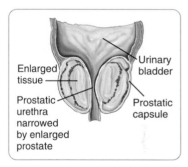

EXERCISE F **Match**

Match the terms in the first column with their correct descriptions in the second column.

_____ **1.** semen analysis

_____ **2.** erectile dysfunction

_____ **3.** digital rectal examination

_____ **4.** sexually transmitted infection

_____ **5.** prostate-specific antigen assay

a. infection spread through sexual contact, which can affect all genders, causing damage to reproductive organs and potentially serious health consequences if left untreated

b. blood test that measures the level of prostate-specific antigen, a protein produced by the prostate gland

c. inability of the male to attain or maintain an erection of the penis sufficient to perform sexual acts

d. laboratory test involving microscopic observation of ejaculated semen, revealing the size, structure, and movement of sperm

e. physical examination in which the healthcare provider inserts a gloved finger into the rectum and palpates the size and shape of the prostate gland through the rectal wall

EXERCISE G   Learn Medical Terms NOT Built from Word Parts

Fill in the blanks with medical terms defined and abbreviated in bold using the Female and Male Reproductive Systems Terms Not Built from Word Parts tables. Check your responses with the Answer Key in Appendix C.

1. A **cytologic study of cervical and vaginal secretions,** or _____, is used to detect cancers of the cervix and is generally recommended for women between the ages of 21 and 65.

2. Human papillomavirus (HPV) is a common **infection spread through sexual contact,** or _____ _____, which is associated with the development of cervical cancer. Penile, anal, vulvar, vaginal, and throat cancers are also linked to HPV infection.

> **FYI**   The Food and Drug Administration (FDA) approved the first vaccine against **human papillomavirus (HPV)** in 2006, directly impacting the prevention of cervical cancer. The vaccine is highly effective in protecting against a majority of forms of HPV as long as it is administered before a male or female becomes sexually active. Because vaccination is not 100% effective, periodic cervical cancer screening is recommended.

3. Although sometimes asymptomatic, **benign tumors of the uterine muscle,** or _____ made up of mainly fibrous tissue may cause pelvic pain, heavy bleeding, miscarriage, or pregnancy loss.

4. **PID,** or _____, characterized by inflammation of some or all of the female reproductive organs, is caused by an infection. The patient may have fever, foul-smelling vaginal discharge, and pain in the lower abdomen. PID may result in infertility if left untreated.

5. A **D&C,** or _____, is performed to diagnose disease, correct bleeding, or empty uterine contents, such as tissue remaining after a miscarriage.

6. A **blood test that measures the level of PSA,** or _____, is used for early detection of prostate cancer along with a **DRE,** or _____. An elevated PSA level or a palpated, stony hard nodule may indicate cancer. The assay is also used to monitor the disease after treatment.

7. A patient with a **nonmalignant enlargement of the prostate gland,** or _____ _____, may have difficulty with urination. As a result, the bladder may retain urine, causing the patient to be more susceptible to bladder infections. Treatment may include **surgical removal of pieces of the prostate gland tissue using an instrument inserted through the urethra,** or _____ _____.

8. **ED,** or _____, is common in men who have undergone prostate surgery. Other causes of ED include diabetes and cardiovascular disease. Medications that work by relaxing smooth muscle cells and increasing the flow of blood to the genital area are the current first-line treatment.

9. **Surgical removal of all or part of the foreskin of the penis,** or _____, is practiced by many cultures throughout the world for religious or health reasons. The Latin term translates as "a cutting around."

10. A laboratory test involving microscopic observation of ejaculated semen, revealing the size, structure, and movement of sperm, or _____, is one of the first steps in evaluating a couple for infertility, which is usually described as a failure to achieve pregnancy after 12 months or more of regular, unprotected sexual intercourse.

11. Branch of medicine that deals with the management of pregnancy, labor, and the postpartum period, or _____, is a field that centers around pregnancy, while gynecology addresses the health and diseases of females outside of pregnancy. An obstetrician/gynecologist specializes in both forms of care.

12. Dropping of the uterus (and sometimes vagina) due to weakened pelvic muscles, or _____, is caused by weakening of the pelvic muscles and ligaments, often due to previous childbirth, straining, or loss of estrogen during normal aging. Nonsurgical treatment may include pelvic strengthening exercises or a pessary (a device inserted into the vagina to keep the uterus in place). Hysteropexy and hysterectomy are surgical treatments for this disorder.

EXERCISE H Pronounce and Spell Terms NOT Built from Word Parts

Practice pronunciation and spelling on paper and online.

1. **Practice on Paper**
   a. **Pronounce:** Read the phonetic spelling and say aloud the terms listed in the previous tables, Medical Terms NOT Built from Word Parts.
   b. **Spell:** Have a study partner read the terms aloud. Write the spelling of the terms on a separate sheet of paper.

2. **Practice Online** ⊕
   a. **Access** online learning resources. Go to evolve.elsevier.com > Evolve Resources > Practice Student Resources.
   b. **Pronounce**: Select Audio Glossary > Lesson 6 > Exercise H. Select a term to hear its pronunciation and repeat aloud.
   c. **Spell**: Select Activities > Lesson 6 > Spell Terms > Exercise H. Select the audio icon and type the correct spelling of the term.

❏ Check the box when complete.

OBJECTIVE 3

Write abbreviations.

ABBREVIATIONS FOR THE REPRODUCTIVE SYSTEMS

Use the online **flashcards** to familiarize yourself with the following abbreviations.

ABBREVIATION	TERM	ABBREVIATION	TERM
BPH	benign prostatic hyperplasia	PID	pelvic inflammatory disease
Cx	cervix	PSA	prostate-specific antigen
D&C	dilation and curettage	RP	radical prostatectomy
DRE	digital rectal examination	STD	sexually transmitted disease
ED	erectile dysfunction	STI	sexually transmitted infection
HPV	human papillomavirus	TAH/BSO	total abdominal hysterectomy/ bilateral salpingo-oophorectomy
HSG	hysterosalpingogram	TRUS	transrectal ultrasound
OB/GYN	obstetrician-gynecologist	TURP	transurethral resection of the prostate gland

EXERCISE I   Abbreviate Medical Terms

Write the correct abbreviation next to its medical term.

1. Diseases and Disorders:

a. _____ sexually transmitted infection

b. _____ sexually transmitted disease

c. _____ pelvic inflammatory disease

d. _____ benign prostatic hyperplasia

e. _____ human papillomavirus

f. _____ erectile dysfunction

2. Diagnostic Tests:

a. _____ digital rectal examination

b. _____ prostate-specific antigen

c. _____ hysterosalpingogram

d. _____ transrectal ultrasound

3. Surgical Procedures:

a. _____   dilation and curettage

b. _____   transurethral resection of the prostate gland

c. _____   total abdominal hysterectomy/bilateral salpingo-oophorectomy

d. _____   radical prostatectomy

4. Specialties and Professions:

_____   obstetrician-gynecologist

5. Related Terms:

_____   cervix

OBJECTIVE 4

Identify medical terms by clinical category.

Now that you have worked through the reproductive systems lesson, review and practice medical terms grouped by clinical category. Categories include signs and symptoms, diseases and disorders, diagnostic tests and equipment, surgical procedures, specialties and professions, and terms related to the female and male reproductive systems. Check your responses with the Answer Key in Appendix C.

EXERCISE J   Signs and Symptoms

Write the medical terms for signs and symptoms next to their definitions.

1. _____   excessive bleeding at menstruation (heavy bleeding in regular, cyclical pattern)

2. _____   without menstrual flow

3. _____   painful menstrual flow

EXERCISE K   Diseases and Disorders

Write the medical terms for diseases and disorders next to their definitions.

1. _____   nonmalignant enlargement of the prostate gland; as the gland enlarges, it causes narrowing of the urethra, which interferes with the passage of urine

2. _____   inability of the male to attain or maintain an erection of the penis sufficient to perform sexual acts (formerly called **impotence**)

3. _____ infection spread through sexual contact; affects both male and female reproductive systems, causing damage to organs and potentially serious health consequences if left untreated

4. _____ inflammation of the cervix

5. _____ protrusion of the bladder (through anterior vaginal wall)

6. _____ inflammation of the endometrium

7. _____ abnormal condition of the endometrium (growth of endometrial tissue outside of the uterus)

8. _____ dropping of the uterus (and sometimes vagina) due to weakened pelvic muscles

9. _____ inflammation of the breast

10. _____ inflammation of the ovary

11. _____ inflammation of the fallopian tube

12. _____ inflammation of the vagina

13. _____ inflammation of the testis

14. _____ inflammation of the prostate gland

15. _____ inflammation of the prostate gland and the bladder

16. _____ stone(s) in the prostate gland

17. _____ inflammation of some or all of the female reproductive organs; can be caused by many different pathogens

18. _____ benign tumor of the uterine muscle (also called **myoma** and **leiomyoma**)

EXERCISE L   Surgical Procedures

Write the medical terms for surgical procedures next to their definitions.

1. _____ excision of the testis

2. _____ surgical fixation of the testis

3. _____ excision of the prostate gland

4. _____ surgical repair of the scrotum

5. _____ excision of the duct (vas deferens)

6. _____ creation of an artificial opening between ducts

7. _____ excision of the cervix (also called **trachelectomy**)

8. _____ excision of the uterus

9. _____ surgical fixation of the uterus

10. _____ suturing of the uterus

11. _____ rupture of the uterus

12. _____ excision of the uterus, fallopian tubes, and ovaries

13. _____ surgical repair of the breast

14. _____ excision of the breast

15. _____ excision of the ovary

16. _____ surgical fixation of the ovary

17. _____ surgical removal of pieces of the prostate gland tissue by using
_____ an instrument inserted through the urethra

18. _____ surgical procedure to widen the cervix and scrape the
endometrium with an instrument called a curette

19. _____ surgical fixation of the breast (performed to lift sagging breast
tissue or to create symmetry)

EXERCISE M **Diagnostic Tests and Equipment**

Write the medical terms for diagnostic tests and equipment next to their definitions.

1. _____ instrument used for visual examination of the vagina

2. _____ visual examination of the vagina

3. _____ radiographic image of the uterus and fallopian tubes

4. _____ radiographic image of the breast

5. _____ radiographic imaging of the breast

6. _____ laboratory test involving cytological study of cervical and
vaginal secretions used to determine the presence of abnormal
or cancerous cells

7. _____ physical examination in which the healthcare provider inserts a
gloved finger into the rectum and palpates the size and shape of
the prostate gland through the rectal wall

8. _____ blood test that measures the level of a protein produced by the
_____ prostate gland

9. _____ laboratory test involving microscopic observation of ejaculated
semen, revealing the size, structure, and movement of sperm

EXERCISE N   Specialties and Professions

Write the medical terms for specialties and professions next to their definitions.

1. _____   study of women (the branch of medicine focused on the health and diseases of the female reproductive system)

2. _____   physician who studies and treats diseases of women (female reproductive system)

3. _____   branch of medicine that deals with the management of pregnancy, labor, and the postpartum period (approximately 6 weeks after giving birth)

EXERCISE O   Medical Terms Related to the Reproductive Systems

Write the medical terms related to the reproductive systems next to their definitions.

1. _____   flow at menstruation

2. _____   pertaining to the vagina

3. _____   pertaining to the cervix

4. _____   pertaining to the endometrium

5. _____   pertaining to the scrotum

6. _____   pertaining to the prostate gland

OBJECTIVE 5

Use medical language in clinical statements, the case study, and a medical record.

EXERCISE P **Use Medical Terms in Clinical Statements**

Circle the medical terms and abbreviations defined in the bolded phrases. Medical terms from previous lessons are included. Answers are listed in Appendix C. For pronunciation practice, read the answers aloud.

1. A **visual examination of the vagina** (hysterosalpingogram, colposcopy, colposcope) is used to further evaluate abnormal **cytologic study of the cervical and vaginal secretions** (Pap test, PSA assay, DRE) results to identify suspicious lesions. A biopsy of the tissue is used to diagnose the condition.

2. Mariana Esteban was experiencing **pertaining to the vagina** (endometrial, cervical, vaginal) itching, burning, and excessive discharge. She was diagnosed with **inflammation of the vagina** (cervicitis, vaginitis, endometritis) caused by *Candida albicans,* a yeastlike fungus.

3. After Lin Xiang's routine **process of radiographic imaging of the breast** (mammogram, mammography) exam, the radiologist discovered a breast lesion on the **radiographic image of the breast** (mammogram, mammography). A biopsy revealed a malignant tumor. A(n) **excision of the breast** (mastectomy, mammoplasty, mastopexy) was performed. The patient is scheduled, at a later date, for reconstructive **surgical repair of the breast** (mastectomy, mammoplasty, mastopexy) with an implant.

4. When **nonmalignant enlargement of the prostate gland** (BPH, PID, ED), chronic **inflammation of the prostate gland** (scrotal, prostatic, prostatitis), or **pertaining to the prostate gland** (prostatolith, prostatitis, prostatic) cancer fails to respond to medical treatment, **excision of the prostate gland** (prostatectomy, scrotoplasty, orchiopexy) may be necessary.

5. A 14-year-old male was admitted to the emergency department with abdominal pain and unilateral **pertaining to the scrotum** (prostatic, scrotoplasty, scrotal) swelling. Testicular torsion was diagnosed; treatment included a unilateral **excision of the testis** (orchitis, orchiopexy, orchiectomy) to remove the damaged testicle and **surgical fixation of the testis** (orchitis, orchiopexy, orchiectomy) of the remaining testicle to prevent future occurrence of testicular torsion.

EXERCISE Q **Apply Medical Terms to the Case Study**

Think back to Cindy and Rajive, introduced in the case study at the beginning of the lesson. After working through Lesson 6 on the reproductive systems, consider the medical terms that might be used to describe their experiences. List three terms relevant to the case study and their meanings. ■

Medical Term   **Definition**

1. _____   _____

2. _____   _____

3. _____   _____

EXERCISE R   Use Medical Terms in a Document

Cindy and Rajive finally had a heart-to-heart talk about their feelings and decided it was time to reach out for help. Cindy checked
in with her gynecologist, who referred the couple to a fertility
clinic at the local hospital.

*Use the definitions in numbers 1-11 to write medical terms within
the following consultation report.*

1. surgical fixation of the testis

2. flow at menstruation

3. painful menstrual flow

4. excessive bleeding at menstruation (heavy bleeding in regular, cyclical pattern)

5. cytological examination of the cervical and vaginal secretions

6. inflammation of the prostate gland

7. infection spread through sexual contact (plural)

8. inflammation of the cervix

9. inflammation of some or all of the female reproductive organs

10. microscopic observation of ejaculated semen, revealing the size, structure, and movement of sperm

11. radiographic image of the uterus and fallopian tubes

Refer to the medical record to answer questions 12-14.

12. The term **scrotocele** appears in the medical record. Use your knowledge of word parts to define the term.

    scrot/o means _____

    -cele means _____

    Remember, most definitions begin with the suffix.

    scrot/o/cele means _____

13. Identify the abbreviations used in the Physical Exam section of the report.

    Abbreviation   Medical Term

    _____   _____

    _____   _____

14. Identify new medical terms in the medical record you would like to investigate. Use your medical dictionary or an online resource to look up the definition.

    Medical Term   **Definition**

    1. _____   _____

    2. _____   _____

    3. _____   _____

```
0120890 COLLIER, Cindy                                          _ □ X
File    Patient    Navigate    Custom Fields    Help
```

Chart Review | Encounters | Notes | Labs | Imaging | Procedures | Rx | Documents | Referrals | Scheduling | Billing

Name: **COLLIER, Cindy**   MR#: 0120890   Gender: F   **Allergies:** None
                            DOB: 05/13/19XX   Age: 31   **PCP:** Alvaro, Belinha MD

Fertility Clinic Consultation
Encounter Date: 11/03/20XX

History:
Cindy, 31-year-old female, and her husband, Rajive, a 32-year-old male, present for workup and treatment for infertility. They have been trying to conceive for 14 months. Cindy has never been pregnant and Rajive has never fathered a child. Prior to 14 months ago they used oral contraceptive pills and condoms as their birth control method. Rajive's past medical history is significant for an undescended testicle at birth; this was repaired by (1.) _____ at age 2. He denies any other significant medical history. Cindy had the onset of (2.) _____ at age 14; she has symptoms of (3.) _____ and (4.) _____, both of which have worsened since discontinuing birth control pills. Her menstrual cycles are approximately 26 days long. She had a normal (5.) _____ approximately 1 year ago. Cindy is taking folic acid but no other medications. Rajive is not taking any medications or supplements. They do not smoke cigarettes, drink alcohol, or use any other drugs.

Physical Examination:
Rajive has previously had a physical examination with his family doctor. According to the records his genitourinary exam revealed an uncircumcised male with normal external genitalia, no evidence of testicular masses, scrotocele, or hernias. DRE revealed no evidence of BPH or (6.) _____.
Cindy's gynecologic exam today reveals normal external genitalia. Examination of the vagina reveals a small amount of discharge and a slightly inflamed cervix. Vaginal and cervical cultures were obtained to test for (7.)_____
Bimanual exam of the uterus and ovaries reveals diffuse tenderness to palpation with slight fullness in the left adnexa.

Diagnostic Studies:
A complete blood count (CBC) was ordered as well as serum tests for thyroid stimulating hormone, follicle stimulating hormone, and prolactin level. A urine pregnancy test was negative.

Impression:
Primary infertility; cause undetermined. Possible chlamydial (8.) _____ and possible (9.) _____.

Recommendation:
We will await culture results and treat both partners with antibiotics if necessary. If labs are normal, we will proceed with a (10.) _____ for Rajive. We should consider a (11.) _____ for Cindy, based on her history and physical exam findings.

Electronically signed: Elyse Conner, MD; Department of Obstetrics and Gynecology

```
Start | Log On/Off | Print | Edit
```

EXERCISE S   **Use Medical Language in Electronic Health Records Online**

Select the correct medical terms to complete three medical records in one patient's electronic file.

Access online resources at evolve.elsevier.com > Evolve Resources > Practice Student Resources > Activities > Lesson 6 > Electronic Health Records

Topic: Prostate Cancer
Record 1: Office Visit
Record 2: Pathology Report
Record 3: Progress Note

OBJECTIVE 6

Recall and assess knowledge of word parts, medical terms, and abbreviations.

EXERCISE T   **Online Review of Lesson Content**

Recall and assess your learning from working through the lesson by completing online learning activities at evolve. elsevier.com > Evolve Resources > Student Resources.

❏   Check the box when complete.

EXERCISE U   **Lesson Content Quiz**

Test your knowledge of the terms and abbreviations introduced in this lesson. Circle the letter for the medical term or abbreviation related to the words in italics.

1. *Surgical removal of all or part of the foreskin of the penis* may be performed for cultural or health purposes.
   a. scrotoplasty
   b. circumcision
   c. cervicectomy

2. A *surgical repair of the breast* to reduce size is called reduction:
   a. mammoplasty
   b. mastopexy
   c. mastectomy

3. A *laboratory test involving microscopic observation of ejaculated semen* was ordered after the patient's *excision of a duct (vas deferens)* to evaluate the success of the procedure.
   a. prostate-specific antigen, vasovasostomy
   b. digital rectal examination, orchiopexy
   c. semen analysis, vasectomy

4. Radical *excision of the prostate gland* is used to treat prostate cancer.
   a. prostatectomy
   b. orchiectomy
   c. vasectomy

5. The *surgical procedure to widen the cervix and remove contents from the uterus* can be used for treatment and for diagnostics.
   a. D&C
   b. DRE
   c. HSG

6. *Inflammation of some or all of the female reproductive organs* is often the result of an STI.
   a. endometritis
   b. prostatitis
   c. pelvic inflammatory disease

7. *Surgical fixation of the testis* may be necessary in cases of testicular torsion, in which the spermatic cord becomes twisted, depriving the testicle of its blood supply.
   a. oophoropexy
   b. orchiopexy
   c. hysteropexy

8. For a *cytological study of cervical and vaginal secretions to detect abnormal and cancerous cells*, a scraping of cells from the *pertaining to the cervix* area is obtained for evaluation
   a. Pap test, cervical
   b. mammogram, vaginal
   c. colposcopy, endometrial

9. *Surgical removal of pieces of the prostate gland tissue by using an instrument inserted through the urethra* is associated with a small risk of *inability of the male to attain or maintain an erection sufficient to perform sexual intercourse.*
   a. digital rectal examination; benign prostatic hyperplasia
   b. transurethral resection of the prostate gland (TURP); erectile dysfunction
   c. hysterectomy; hysterorrhexis

10. *Painful menstrual flow* is a common symptom of *abnormal condition of the endometrium (growth of endometrial tissue outside of the uterus).*
    a. amenorrhea; uterine fibroid
    b. menorrhagia; hysterorrhexis
    c. dysmenorrhea; endometriosis

11. *Inflammation of the breast*, most commonly occurring with breast-feeding, is an infection characterized by pain in the breast, edema, warmth, and erythema.
    a. cervicitis
    b. mastitis
    c. oophoritis

12. Upon diagnosis of an intratesticular mass, a radical inguinal *excision of the testis* was recommended as a diagnostic and therapeutic procedure.
    a. orchiectomy
    b. prostatectomy
    c. vasectomy

LESSON AT A GLANCE   **REPRODUCTIVE SYSTEMS WORD PARTS**

COMBINING FORMS

cervic/o	oophor/o
colp/o	orchi/o
endometri/o	prostat/o
gynec/o	salping/o
hyster/o	scrot/o
mamm/o	vagin/o
mast/o	vas/o
men/o	

SUFFIXES
-cele
-pexy
-rrhaphy
-rrhexis

LESSON AT A GLANCE | **REPRODUCTIVE SYSTEMS MEDICAL TERMS AND ABBREVIATIONS**

SIGNS AND SYMPTOMS
amenorrhea
dysmenorrhea
menorrhagia

DISEASE AND DISORDERS
benign prostatic hyperplasia (BPH)
cervicitis
cystocele
endometriosis
endometritis
erectile dysfunction (ED)
hysterorrhexis
mastitis
oophoritis
orchitis
pelvic inflammatory disease (PID)
prostatitis
prostatocystitis
prostatolith
salpingitis
sexually transmitted infection (STI)
uterine fibroid
uterovaginal prolapse
vaginitis

SURGICAL PROCEDURES
cervicectomy
circumcision
dilation and curettage (D&C)
hysterectomy
hysteropexy
hysterorrhaphy
hysterosalpingo-oophorectomy
mammoplasty
mastectomy
mastopexy
oophorectomy
oophoropexy
orchiectomy
orchiopexy
prostatectomy
scrotoplasty
transurethral resection of the
    prostate gland (TURP)
vasectomy
vasovasostomy

DIAGNOSTIC TESTS AND EQUIPMENT
colposcope
colposcopy
digital rectal examination (DRE)
hysterosalpingogram
mammogram
mammography
Pap test
prostate-specific antigen (PSA) assay
semen analysis

SPECIALTIES AND PROFESSIONS
gynecologist
gynecology
obstetrics

RELATED TERMS
cervical
endometrial
menorrhea
prostatic
scrotal
vaginal

ABBREVIATIONS

BPH	ED	PID	STI
Cx	HPV	PSA	TAH/BSO
DRE	HSG	RP	TRUS
D&C	OB/GYN	STD	TURP

CASE STUDY **Natalia Krouse**

Natalia has not been feeling well lately. She seems to feel "wiped out" most of the time. She wonders if maybe her blood pressure medicine isn't working as well as it used to. Tonight she went for her usual walk with her dogs after dinner. She had barely made it down the driveway when she started to feel pressure in her chest. It felt like something pushing down on her and squeezing her. She noticed pain in her left arm and even in her jaw. She noticed her heart was racing, and she was breathing faster than usual. She was also feeling dizzy at the same time and was afraid she might pass out. She stopped to sit down, and after about 5 minutes she started to feel a little better. Her neighbor saw her and called 911. An ambulance came and took her to the Emergency Department of her local hospital.

■ *Consider Natalia's situation as you work through the lesson on the cardiovascular and lymphatic systems. At the end of the lesson, we will return to this case study and identify medical terms used to document Natalia's experience and the care she receives.*

OBJECTIVES

1 ■ Build, translate, pronounce, and spell medical terms built from word parts (p. 199).

2 ■ Define, pronounce, and spell medical terms NOT built from word parts (p. 214).

3 ■ Write abbreviations (p. 221).

4 ■ Identify medical terms by clinical category (p. 222).

5 ■ Use medical language in clinical statements, the case study, and a medical record (p. 225).

6 ■ Recall and assess knowledge of word parts, medical terms, and abbreviations (p. 229).

INTRODUCTION TO THE CARDIOVASCULAR AND LYMPHATIC SYSTEMS

Anatomic Structures of the Cardiovascular System	
arteries (AR-te-rēs)	blood vessels that carry blood away from the heart
blood (blud)	fluid circulated through the heart, arteries, capillaries, and veins; composed of plasma and formed elements such as erythrocytes, leukocytes, and thrombocytes (platelets) (Figure 7.1)
blood vessels (blud) (VES-els)	tubelike structures that carry blood throughout the body, including arteries, veins, and capillaries
capillaries (KAP-i-lar-ēs)	microscopic blood vessels; materials are passed between blood and tissues through capillary walls
heart (hart)	muscular, cone-shaped organ the size of a fist, located behind the sternum (breastbone) and between the lungs; pumping action circulates blood throughout the body

Continued

Anatomic Structures of the Cardiovascular System—cont'd

plasma (PLAZ-ma)	clear, straw-colored liquid portion of blood in which cells are suspended; composed of approximately 90% water and is about 55% of total blood volume
veins (vānz)	blood vessels that carry blood back to the heart

Functions of the Cardiovascular System

- Pumps blood
- Transports oxygen, nutrients, immune substances, hormones, and other chemicals to and from organs
- Carries waste products away from tissues

Anatomic Structures of the Lymphatic System

lymph (limf)	transparent, colorless tissue fluid; contains white blood cells and flows in a one-way direction to the heart
lymph nodes (limf) (nōdz)	small, spherical bodies composed of lymphoid tissue; may be singular or grouped together along the path of lymphatic vessels; filter lymph to keep bacteria and other foreign agents from entering blood
lymphatic vessels (lim-FAT-ik) (VES-els)	transport lymph from body tissues to a large vein in the chest
spleen (splēn)	lymphatic organ located in the upper left abdominal cavity between the stomach and the diaphragm; filters blood and acts as a blood reservoir
thymus (THĪ-mus)	lymphatic organ with two lobes located behind the sternum between the lungs; plays an important role in development of the body's immune system, particularly from infancy to puberty

Functions of the Lymphatic System

- Returns excess fluid from tissues to blood
- Helps maintain blood volume and pressure
- Absorbs fats and fat-soluble vitamins from the small intestine and transports them to the blood
- Filters lymph, trapping and destroying harmful cells
- Generates disease-fighting cells

Figure 7.1 Composition of blood.

How the Cardiovascular and Lymphatic Systems Work

The cardiovascular and lymphatic systems are closely related. They work together to maintain an internal balance in the body—transporting nutrients and waste, protecting against infection, and regulating fluid and electrolyte levels. Each system circulates fluid: blood in the cardiovascular system, and lymph in the lymphatic system.

Blood is composed of plasma and formed elements (Figure 7.1). Plasma is the liquid portion of the blood in which the cells are suspended. The formed elements include erythrocytes (red blood cells), leukocytes (white blood cells), and thrombocytes (platelets).

The cardiovascular system (Figure 7.2) pumps blood from the heart through a closed system of vessels composed of arteries, capillaries, and veins. The heart functions as two pumps operating simultaneously. The left side of the heart pumps blood to the arteries, which carry blood rich in oxygen and other nutrients to replenish organs, tissues, and cells. The exchange of gases, nutrients, and waste between the blood and body tissues takes place in the capillaries. Along the way, blood passes through the organs of other body systems, transporting chemical substances, such as hormones, that are essential for body functioning. Veins carry blood back to the right side of the heart, which pumps blood containing carbon dioxide to the lungs to be replenished with oxygen. This oxygen-rich blood then returns from the lungs to the left side of the heart, to begin the process again.

Figure 7.2 Cardiovascular System.

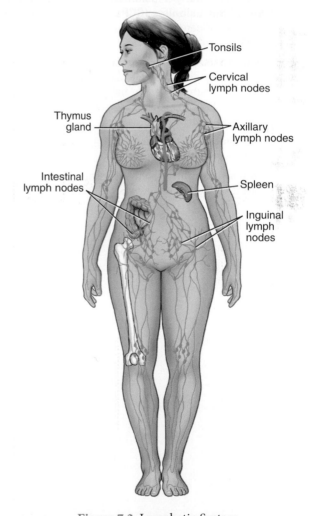

Figure 7.3 Lymphatic System.

The lymphatic system (Figure 7.3) does not have a pump; it passively absorbs fluid called lymph (composed of fluid that passes from capillaries into tissue) and passes it through lymphatic vessels, whose duty it is to return lymph to the blood. Lymph nodes, which filter lymphatic fluid, are located along the paths of these collecting vessels. Infectious agents, cancerous cells, and other debris may be trapped and destroyed. The thymus, a lymphatic organ, generates disease-fighting white blood cells and releases them into the blood for delivery to the specific body site in need. The spleen filters blood, much like lymph nodes filter lymph, and acts as a reservoir.

CAREER FOCUS Professionals Who Work with the Cardiovascular and Lymphatic Systems

- **Phlebotomists** draw blood from patients using a process called venipuncture to collect the blood into special tubes, which is then processed and tested using specialized machines (Figure 7.4). Phlebotomists can also sample blood through a skin puncture, such as pricking a finger to test a patient's blood sugar.

- **Cardiovascular perfusionists,** also called **certified clinical perfusionists (CCPs),** operate the heart-lung machine for cardiopulmonary bypass during open-heart surgery.

- **Cardiovascular technologists** are trained to prepare patients and assist physicians during procedures such as cardiac catheterization, balloon angioplasty, and open-heart surgery. They also monitor patients' blood pressure and heart rate.

Figure 7.4 Phlebotomist performing venipuncture to withdraw blood from a patient.

- **Cardiovascular technicians** conduct electrocardiograms (ECG) and assist with cardiac stress tests and other monitoring.

- **Echocardiography technicians** are specialized cardiovascular technicians who perform ultrasounds of the heart. The ultrasound collects reflected echoes and Doppler signals from images and spectral tracings of the heart.

OBJECTIVE 1

Build, translate, pronounce, and spell medical terms built from word parts.

WORD PARTS	Presented with the Cardiovascular and Lymphatic Systems

Use the paper or online **flashcards** to familiarize yourself with the following word parts.

COMBINING FORM (WR + CV)	DEFINITION	COMBINING FORM (WR + CV)	DEFINITION
aden/o	gland(s); (nodes when combined with lymph/o)	**lymph/o**	lymph, lymphatic tissue
angi/o	blood vessel(s)	**phleb/o**	vein(s)
arteri/o	artery (s.), arteries (pl.)	**splen/o**	spleen
cardi/o	heart	**thromb/o**	blood clot
ech/o	sound	**ven/o**	vein(s)
electr/o	electrical activity		
SUFFIX (S)	**DEFINITION**	**SUFFIX (S)**	**DEFINITION**
-ac	pertaining to	**-penia**	abnormal reduction (in number)
-graph	instrument used to record	**-sclerosis**	hardening
PREFIX (P)	**DEFINITION**	**PREFIX (P)**	**DEFINITION**
brady-	slow	**tachy-**	rapid, fast

WORD PARTS PRESENTED IN PREVIOUS LESSONS	Used to Build Cardiovascular and Lymphatic System Terms

COMBINING FORM (WR + CV)	DEFINITION	COMBINING FORM (WR + CV)	DEFINITION
cyt/o	cell(s)	**my/o**	muscle
hem/o, hemat/o	blood	**path/o**	disease
SUFFIX (S)	**DEFINITION**	**SUFFIX (S)**	**DEFINITION**
-a, -e, -y	no meaning	**-lysis**	dissolution, separating
-al, -ous	pertaining to	**-megaly**	enlargement
-ectomy	surgical removal, excision	**-oma**	tumor
-gram	record, radiographic image	**-osis**	abnormal condition
-graphy	process of recording, radiographic imaging	**-plasty**	surgical repair
-ia	diseased state, condition of	**-pnea**	breathing
-itis	inflammation	**-stasis**	control, stop
-logist	one who studies and treats (specialist, physician)	**-tomy**	cut into, incision
-logy	study of		
PREFIX (P)	**DEFINITION**	**PREFIX (P)**	**DEFINITION**
a-, an-	absence of, without	**endo-**	within

Refer to Appendix A, Word Parts Used in *Basic Medical Language*, for alphabetical lists of word parts and their meanings.

EXERCISE A **Build and Translate Medical Terms Built from Word Parts**

*Use the **Word Parts Tables** to complete the following questions. Check your responses with the Answer Key in Appendix C.*

1. LABEL: *Write the combining forms for anatomic structures of the cardiovascular system on Figure 7.5. These anatomic combining forms will be used to build and translate medical terms in Exercise A.*

Vein

1. Artery

CF: _____

2. Heart

CF: _____

Capillaries

3. Blood vessels

CF: _____

Figure 7.5 Heart and blood vessels with combining forms.

2. MATCH: *Draw a line to match the word part with its definition.*

    a. -logist   enlargement
    b. -logy   study of
    c. -ac   one who studies and treats (specialist, physician)
    d. -megaly   pertaining to

3. BUILD: *Using the combining form **cardi/o** and the word parts reviewed in the previous exercise, build the following terms related to the heart. Remember, the definition usually starts with the meaning of the suffix.*

    a. pertaining to the heart

                                             _____/_____
                                                wr   **s**

    b. study of the heart

                                             _____/_o_/_____
                                                wr   **cv**   **s**

    c. physician who studies and treats diseases of the heart

                                             _____/_o_/_____
                                                wr   **cv**   **s**

    d. enlargement of the heart

                                             _____/_o_/_____
                                                wr   **cv**   **s**

4. **READ: Cardiology** (kar-dē-OL-o-jē) is the field of medicine related to the study of the heart. A **cardiologist** (kar-dē-OL-o-jist) is a physician with special training to diagnose and treat heart disease. **Cardiomegaly** (kar-dē-ō-MEG-a-lē) may be caused by high blood pressure or other **cardiac** (KAR-dē-ak) disorders.

5. **MATCH:** *Draw a line to match the word part with its definition.*

   a. -gram   process of recording, radiographic imaging
   b. -graph   record, radiographic image
   c. -graphy   instrument used to record

6. **TRANSLATE:** *Complete the definitions of the following terms built from the combining form **electr/o**, meaning electrical activity. Use the meaning of word parts to fill in the blanks. Remember, the definition usually starts with the meaning of the suffix.*

   a. electr/o/cardi/o/gram   _____ of the electrical activity of the _____
   b. electr/o/cardi/o/graph   instrument used to record the _____ of the heart
   c. electr/o/cardi/o/graphy   _____ of _____ the electrical activity of the heart

7. **READ:** An **electrocardiogram** (ē-lek-trō-KAR-dē-ō-gram) may be ordered by the physician when a patient has chest pain, a symptom of cardiac disease. **Electrocardiography** (ē-lek-trō-kar-dē-OG-ra-fē) records electrical currents generated by the heart and is frequently used for cardiac assessment. Cardiac technicians are trained to use the **electrocardiograph** (ē-lek-trō-KAR-dē-ō-graf); they place sensors on the patient to record these electrical impulses.

> **FYI**   Compare the three suffixes **-gram**, **-graph**, and **-graphy**. The suffix **-gram** is the record. It may be a paper record or radiographic image. The suffix **-graph** is the machine or instrument used to make the record. The suffix **-graphy** is the process of recording.

8. **LABEL:** *Write word parts to complete Figure 7.6.*

Figure 7.6 _____/o/_____/o/_____.
            electrical activity   heart   record

9. MATCH: *Draw a line to match the word part with its definition.*

    a. my/o   no meaning
    b. ech/o   breathing
    c. tachy-   muscle
    d. brady-   sound
    e. -pnea   rapid, fast
    f. path/o   slow
    g. -a, -y   disease

---

10. BUILD: *Using the combining form **cardi/o** and the word parts reviewed in the previous exercise, build the following terms related to the heart:*

    a. record of the heart using sound   _____/ o /_____/ o /_____
                                                     wr   cv   wr   cv   s

    b. slow heart rate   _____/_____/a
                                                p   wr   s

    c. disease of the heart muscle   _____/ o /_____/ o /_____/y
                                              wr   cv   wr   cv   wr   s

---

11. READ: Bradycardia (brad-ē-KAR-dē-a) may be caused by medications that slow the heart rate, or by diseases that affect the electrical impulses in the heart. In dilated **cardiomyopathy** (kar-dē-ō-mī-OP-a-thē) the heart muscle stretches and becomes thinner, and the heart doesn't pump as well. An **echocardiogram** (ek-ō-KAR-dē-ō-gram) uses sound waves to show the structure and motion of the heart, and is often used to diagnose cardiomyopathies.

---

12. LABEL: *Write word parts to complete Figure 7.7.*

Figure 7.7 _____/o/_____/o/_____ in a patient with cardiomyopathy.
             sound   heart   record

13. TRANSLATE: *Complete the definitions of the following terms:*

    a. my/o/cardi/al   pertaining to the _____ of the heart

    b. tachy/cardi/a   rapid _____ rate

    c. tachy/pnea   _____ breathing

14. READ: Tachycardia (tak-i-KAR-dē-a) can be detected either by a physical exam or by electrocardiography. **Tachypnea** (tak-IP-nē-a) occurs when an adult takes more than 20 breaths in 1 minute. **Myocardial** (mī-ō-KAR-dē-al) events can cause both tachycardia and tachypnea.

15. MATCH: *Draw a line to match the word part with its definition.*

    a. -ectomy   record, radiographic image

    b. -al   hardening

    c. -gram   within

    d. -sclerosis   surgical removal, excision

    e. endo-   pertaining to

16. BUILD: *Using the combining form **arteri/o** and the word parts reviewed in the previous exercise, build the following terms related to arteries:*

    a. excision within the artery   _____ / _____ / _____
                                                p   wr   s

    b. pertaining to the arteries   _____ / _____
                                             wr   s

    c. hardening of the arteries   _____ / o / _____
                                             wr   cv   s

    d. radiographic image of the arteries   _____ / o / _____
                                             wr   cv   s

17. READ: In **arteriosclerosis** (ar-tēr-ē-ō-skle-RŌ-sis), the **arterial** (ar-TĒ-rē-al) walls become thickened and lose their elasticity. This is usually due to plaque formation. An **arteriogram** (ar-TĒR-ē-ō-gram), which uses injected contrast media to outline arteries, may be performed to determine the extent of disease. An **endarterectomy** (end-ar-ter-EK-to-mē) is a procedure performed to remove plaque from the interior wall of a diseased artery.

18. LABEL: *Write word parts to complete Figures 7.8 and 7.9.*

Right
main
pulmonary
artery

Figure 7.8 _____/o/_____
　　　　　　artery　　　radiographic image
　　　showing the right main pulmonary artery.

Figure 7.9 _____/_____/_____.
　　　　　within　　artery　　excision

19. MATCH: *Draw a line to match the word part with its definition.*

a. -graphy　　　surgical repair
b. -plasty　　　process of recording, radiographic imaging

20. TRANSLATE: *Complete the definitions of the following terms using the word root **angi/o** meaning blood vessel.*

a. angi/o/graphy　　_____ imaging of the blood _____
b. angi/o/plasty　　surgical _____ of the blood _____

21. READ: Coronary **angiography** (an-jē-OG-ra-fē) is an invasive procedure in which a catheter is inserted into a vessel in the arm or groin and passed all the way into the coronary arteries. Contrast media is injected and images are recorded. **Angioplasty** (AN-jē-ō-plas-tē) is a procedure to restore blood flow through blocked vessels. Coronary angioplasty can be done at the same time as coronary angiography.

FYI　In **percutaneous transluminal coronary angioplasty** (PTCA), also called balloon angioplasty, a balloon is passed through a blood vessel into the coronary artery. Inflation of the balloon compresses the obstructing plaque against the vessel wall, expands the inner diameter of the blood vessel, and allows the blood to circulate more freely.

22. **LABEL:** *Write word parts to complete Figure 7.10.*

A   Balloon catheter positioned
in stenotic area

Inflated balloon presses
plaque against arterial wall,
expanding the size of
vessel opening

Balloon is deflated and
blood flow reestablished

B

C

Figure 7.10 Percutaneous transluminal coronary _____/o/_____ (PTCA).
blood vessel   surgical repair

A, Balloon dilation. **B,** Coronary arteriogram before PTCA. The arrow indicates the area with approximately 95% blockage. **C,** Coronary arteriogram after PTCA in the same patient, now showing increased blood flow through the previously blocked area.

---

23. **REVIEW OF CARDIOVASCULAR AND LYMPHATIC SYSTEM TERMS BUILT FROM WORD PARTS:** *The following is an alphabetical list of terms built and translated in the previous exercises.*

MEDICAL TERMS BUILT FROM WORD PARTS

TERM	DEFINITION	TERM	DEFINITION
1. angiography (an-jē-OG-ra-fē)	radiographic imaging of the blood vessels	**5. arteriosclerosis** (ar-tēr-ē-ō-skle-RŌ-sis)	hardening of the arteries
2. angioplasty (AN-jē-ō-plas-tē)	surgical repair of the blood vessels (Figure 7.10)	**6. bradycardia** (brad-ē-KAR-dē-a)	slow heart rate
3. arterial (ar-TĒ-rē-al)	pertaining to the arteries	**7. cardiac** (KAR-dē-ak)	pertaining to the heart
4. arteriogram (ar-TĒR-ē-ō-gram)	radiographic image of the arteries (after an injection of contrast media) (Figure 7.8)	**8. cardiologist** (kar-dē-OL-o-jist)	physician who studies and treats diseases of the heart

Continued

MEDICAL TERMS BUILT FROM WORD PARTS—cont'd

TERM	DEFINITION	TERM	DEFINITION
9. **cardiology** (kar-dē-OL-o-jē)	study of the heart	15. **electrocardiography** (ē-lek-trō-kar-dē-OG-ra-fē)	process of recording electrical activity of the heart
10. **cardiomegaly** (kar-dē-ō-MEG-a-lē)	enlargement of the heart	16. **endarterectomy** (end-ar-ter-EK-to-mē)	excision within the artery (excision of plaque from the arterial wall) (Figure 7.9)
11. **cardiomyopathy** (kar-dē-ō-mī-OP-a-thē)	disease of the heart muscle	17. **myocardial** (mī-ō-KAR-dē-al)	pertaining to the muscle of the heart
12. **echocardiogram (ECHO)** (ek-ō-KAR-dē-ō-gram)	record of the heart using sound (Figure 7.7)	18. **tachycardia** (tak-i-KAR-dē-a)	rapid heart rate
13. **electrocardiogram (ECG/EKG)** (ē-lek-trō-KAR-dē-ō-gram)	record of electrical activity of the heart (Figure 7.6)	19. **tachypnea** (tak-IP-nē-a)	rapid breathing
14. **electrocardiograph** (ē-lek-trō-KAR-dē-ō-graf)	instrument used to record electrical activity of the heart		

EXERCISE B   **Pronounce and Spell Terms Built from Word Parts**

Practice pronunciation and spelling on paper and online.

1. **Practice on Paper**
    a. **Pronounce:** Read the phonetic spelling and say aloud the terms listed in the previous table, Review of Terms Built from Word Parts.
    b. **Spell:** Have a study partner read the terms aloud. Write the spelling of the terms on a separate sheet of paper.

2. **Practice Online** 🌐
    a. **Access** online learning resources. Go to evolve.elsevier.com > Evolve Resources > Practice Student Resources.
    b. **Pronounce:** Select Audio Glossary > Lesson 7 > Exercise B. Select a term to hear its pronunciation and repeat aloud.
    c. **Spell:** Select Activities > Lesson 7 > Spell Terms > Exercise B. Select the audio icon and type the correct spelling of the term.

❏   Check the box when complete.

EXERCISE C   Build and Translate MORE Medical Terms Built from Word Parts

*Use the **Word Parts Tables** near the beginning of the lesson to complete the following questions. Check your responses with the Answer Key in Appendix C.*

1. **LABEL:** *Write the combining forms for anatomic structures of the cardiovascular system on Figure 7.11. These anatomic combining forms will be used to build and translate medical terms in Exercise C.*

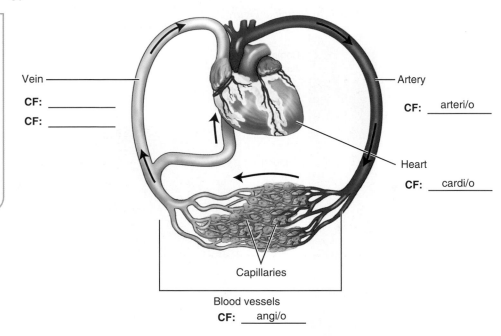

> **FYI** Though the combining form **angi/o** usually refers to blood vessels, it can also refer to lymphatic vessels. In these instances **lymph/o** appears before **angi/o** to specify the lymphatic vessels. Examples include lymphangitis and lymphangioma.

Vein —
CF: _____
CF: _____

Artery —
CF: ___arteri/o___

Heart —
CF: ___cardi/o___

Capillaries

Blood vessels
CF: ___angi/o___

Figure 7.11 Heart and blood vessels with combining forms.

2. **MATCH:** *Draw a line to match the word part with its definition.*

   a. -ous   within
   b. -gram   pertaining to
   c. intra-   record, radiographic image

3. **BUILD:** *Using the combining form **ven/o** and the word parts reviewed in the previous exercise, build the following terms related to veins.*

   a. pertaining to within the veins   _____/_____/_____
                                                   p   wr   s

   b. radiographic image of the veins   _____/_o_/_____
                                                  wr   cv   s

4. READ: An **intravenous** (in-tra-VĒ-nus) catheter is used to inject substances directly into a vein. This may be done for therapy (such as the injection of medications) or for diagnostic procedures (such as the injection of radiographic dyes). During a leg **venogram** (VĒ-nō-gram), contrast media is injected intravenously into a vein in the foot. The radiograph (x-ray) captures images of the contrast media traveling through the leg veins. This allows the physician to see if there is any blockage or other damage to the veins.

5. LABEL: *Write word parts to complete Figure 7.12, A and B.*

Common
iliac vein

External
iliac vein

Femoral
vein

Popliteal
vein

Figure 7.12 A. _____/o/_____ of the left leg.
                              vein   radiographic image

B. Patient's arm with an _____/_____/_____ (IV) catheter.
                                              within   vein   pertaining to

6. MATCH: *Draw a line to match the word part with its definition.*

a. -itis   cut into, incision
b. -tomy   blood clot
c. thromb/o   inflammation
d. -osis   abnormal condition

7. TRANSLATE: *Complete the definitions of the following terms by using the meaning of the word parts to fill in the blanks. Terms built from the combining form* **phleb/o,** *meaning vein:*

a. phleb/itis   _____ of the veins

b. phleb/o/tomy   incision into the _____ (with a needle to remove or instill fluid)

c. thromb/osis   _____ of a blood clot

d. thromb/o/phleb/itis   inflammation of the veins associated with _____

---

8. READ: **Phlebotomy** (fle-BOT-o-mē), also called **venipuncture,** is a method of obtaining blood for laboratory testing. **Phlebitis** (fle-BĪ-tis) occurs when a vein becomes inflamed and can cause pain and swelling. Superficial phlebitis occurring in veins close to the skin is usually not dangerous. **Thrombophlebitis** (throm-bō-fle-BĪ-tis) that occurs in the deeper veins can be dangerous, especially if a blood clot breaks off the venous wall and travels through the bloodstream into the lungs. **Thrombosis** (throm-BŌ-sis) refers to the formation of blood clots in the blood vessels.

---

9. LABEL: *Write word parts to complete Figure 7.13.*

Figure 7.13 A. Healthy artery with smooth blood flow.

B. Blocked artery due to: _____/_____ and atherosclerosis.
                                   blood clot   abnormal condition

10. **MATCH:** *Draw a line to match the word part with its definition.*

   a. cyt/o   abnormal reduction (in number)
   b. -e   blood clot
   c. -penia   cell
   d. leuk/o   no meaning
   e. thromb/o   white

---

11. **TRANSLATE:** *Complete the definitions of the following terms by using the meaning of the word parts to fill in the blanks.*

   a. thromb/o/cyt/e   blood clotting _____
   b. thromb/o/cyt/o/penia   _____ of blood clotting cells
   c. leuk/o/cyt/o/penia   abnormal reduction of _____ blood cells

---

12. **READ:** A **thrombocyte** (THROM-bō-sīt) is also called a **platelet**. These blood cells aid in the normal clotting process. If **thrombocytopenia** (throm-bō-sī-tō-PĒ-nē-a) becomes severe, spontaneous bleeding can occur. **Leukocytopenia** (lū-kō-sī-tō-PĒ-nē-a) can be caused by diseases of the bone marrow, where leukocytes are produced. It can also be caused by infections, drugs, or autoimmune diseases, all of which destroy the white cells once they are circulating.

---

13. **LABEL:** *Write the combining forms for anatomic structures of the lymphatic system on Figure 7.14.*

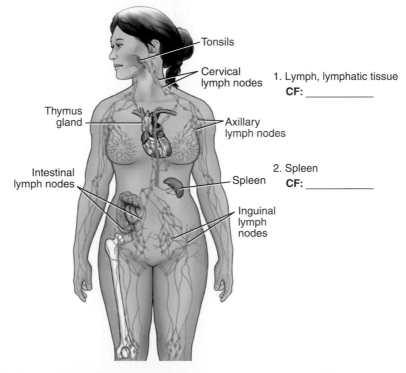

Tonsils

Cervical lymph nodes

1. Lymph, lymphatic tissue
   CF: _____

Thymus gland

Axillary lymph nodes

Intestinal lymph nodes

Spleen

2. Spleen
   CF: _____

Inguinal lymph nodes

Figure 7.14 Lymphatic system and combining forms for lymph nodes and spleen.

14. MATCH: *Draw a line to match the word part with its definition.*

    a. -ectomy   enlargement
    b. -megaly   surgical removal, excision

15. BUILD: *Use the combining form **splen/o** along with the word parts reviewed in the previous exercise, to build terms related to the spleen. Note that the medical term spleen has two e's; the combining form **splen/o** has one.*

    a. enlargement of the spleen   _____ / o / _____
                                                                       wr   cv   s

    b. excision of the spleen   _____ / _____
                                                                       wr   s

16. READ: The spleen is the largest lymphatic organ. It filters and stores blood. **Splenomegaly** (splē-nō-MEG-a-lē) may be caused by infections such as mononucleosis, cancers such as lymphoma, or other diseases that cause the spleen to retain blood. This can occasionally lead to splenic rupture, which usually requires a **splenectomy** (splē-NEK-to-mē). While people can live without their spleens, their risk of infection is increased.

17. MATCH: *Draw a line to match the word part with its definition.*

    a. -itis   no meaning
    b. path/o   gland(s); node(s)
    c. -oma   disease
    d. aden/o   inflammation
    e. -y   tumor

> **FYI**   When the combining forms **lymph/o** and **aden/o** are used together (**lymph/aden/o**), it refers to a collection of tissue called a lymph node, rather than a lymph gland.

18. TRANSLATE: *Complete the definitions of the following terms by using the meaning of the word parts to fill in the blanks.*

    a. lymph/aden/o/path/y   _____ of the lymph nodes
    b. lymph/aden/itis   inflammation of the _____
    c. lymph/oma   _____ of lymphatic tissue

19. READ: Lymph nodes trap and filter bacteria, viruses, cancer cells, and other unwanted substances. **Lymphadenopathy** (lim-fad-e-NOP-a-thē), or swollen lymph nodes, can be caused by infection, autoimmune diseases, or (infrequently) cancer. When swollen lymph nodes are caused by an infection, this is known as **lymphadenitis** (lim-fad-e-NĪ-tis). **Lymphoma** (lim-FŌ-ma) is a cancer that begins in the lymphatic system. Hodgkin lymphoma is a type of lymphatic cancer.

20. MATCH: *Draw a line to match the word part with its definition.*

    a. -logist   tumor
    b. -logy   control, stop
    c. -oma   dissolution, separating
    d. -stasis   one who studies and treats (specialist, physician)
    e. -lysis   study of

21. BUILD: *Use the combining forms **hem/o**, **hemat/o** (hint: **hem/o** for d and e) along with the word parts reviewed in the previous exercise to build terms related to blood.*

    a. study of blood

                        _____ / o / _____
                              wr   cv   s

    b. physician who studies and treats diseases of the blood

                        _____ / o / _____
                              wr   cv   s

    c. tumor of blood (usually a collection of blood)

                        _____ / _____
                              wr   s

    d. stopping (the flow of) blood

                        _____ / o / _____
                              wr   cv   s

    e. dissolution of (red) blood (cells)

                        _____ / o / _____
                            wr   cv   s

22. READ: The specialty of **hematology** (hē-ma-TOL-o-jē) concerns the study of the blood, bone marrow, and lymphatic system. A **hematologist** (hē-ma-TOL-o-jist) treats disorders of abnormal blood cells, as well as bleeding and clotting disorders. The ability to stop bleeding is known as **hemostasis** (hē-mō-STĀ-sis). A **hematoma** (hē-ma-TŌ-ma) is a condition in which blood has leaked out of a broken vessel into the surrounding tissue. **Hemolysis** (hē-MOL-i-sis) refers to the abnormal destruction of erythrocytes, which can lead to anemia.

23. LABEL: *Write word parts to complete Figure 7.15*

Figure 7.15 Postsurgical site displaying swelling and formation of a _____ / _____ .
                                                            blood   tumor

24. **REVIEW OF MORE CARDIOVASCULAR AND LYMPHATIC SYSTEM TERMS BUILT FROM WORD PARTS:** *The following is an alphabetical list of terms built and translated in the previous exercises.*

MEDICAL TERMS BUILT FROM WORD PARTS

TERM	DEFINITION	TERM	DEFINITION
1. **hematologist** (hē-ma-TOL-o-jist)	physician who studies and treats diseases of the blood	11. **phlebitis** (fle-BĪ-tis)	inflammation of the veins
2. **hematology** (hē-ma-TOL-o-jē)	study of blood	12. **phlebotomy** (fle-BOT-o-mē)	incision into the vein (with a needle to remove blood or instill fluid); (also called **venipuncture**)
3. **hemolysis** (hē-MOL-i-sis)	dissolution of (red) blood (cells)	13. **splenectomy** (splē-NEK-to-mē)	excision of the spleen
4. **hematoma** (hē-ma-TŌ-ma)	tumor of blood (collection of blood that has leaked out of a broken vessel into the surrounding tissue) (Figure 7.15)	14. **splenomegaly** (splē-nō-MEG-a-lē)	enlargement of the spleen
		15. **thrombocyte** (THROM-bō-sīt)	blood clotting cell (also called **platelet**)
5. **hemostasis** (hē-mō-STĀ-sis)	stopping (the flow of) blood	16. **thrombocytopenia** (throm-bō-sī-tō-PĒ-nē-a)	abnormal reduction in number of blood clotting cells
6. **intravenous (IV)** (in-tra-VĒ-nus)	pertaining to within the veins (Figure 7.12, *B*)	17. **thrombophlebitis** (throm-bō-fle-BĪ-tis)	inflammation of the veins associated with blood clots
7. **leukocytopenia** (lū-kō-sī-tō-PĒ-nē-a)	abnormal reduction of white (blood) cells	18. **thrombosis** (throm-BŌ-sis)	abnormal condition of a blood clot (Figure 7.13, *B*)
8. **lymphadenitis** (lim-fad-e-NĪ-tis)	inflammation of the lymph nodes	19. **venogram** (VĒ-nō-gram)	radiographic image of the veins (after an injection of contrast media) (Figure 7.12, *A*)
9. **lymphadenopathy** (lim-fad-e-NOP-a-thē)	disease of the lymph nodes		
10. **lymphoma** (lim-FŌ-ma)	tumor of the lymphatic tissue		

EXERCISE D Pronounce and Spell MORE Terms Built from Word Parts

Practice pronunciation and spelling on paper and online.

1. **Practice on Paper**
   a. **Pronounce**: Read the phonetic spelling and say aloud the terms listed in the previous table, Review of MORE Cardiovascular and Lymphatic System Terms Built from Word Parts.
   b. **Spell**: Have a study partner read the terms aloud. Write the spelling of the terms on a separate sheet of paper.

2. **Practice Online** ⊕

    a. **Access** online learning resources. Go to evolve.elsevier.com > Evolve Resources > Practice Student Resources.

    b. **Pronounce:** Select Audio Glossary > Lesson 7 > Exercise D. Select a term to hear its pronunciation and repeat aloud.

    c. **Spell:** Select Activities > Lesson 7 > Spell Terms > Exercise D. Select the audio icon and type the correct spelling of the term.

❏ Check the box when complete.

OBJECTIVE 2

Define, pronounce, and spell medical terms NOT built from word parts.

The terms listed below may contain word parts, but are difficult to translate literally.

MEDICAL TERMS NOT BUILT FROM WORD PARTS

TERM	DEFINITION
1. **anemia** (a-NĒ-mē-a)	condition in which there is a reduction in the number of erythrocytes (RBCs). Anemia may be caused by blood loss, by decreased production of RBCs, or by increased destruction of RBCs.
2. **aneurysm** (AN-ū-rizm)	condition in which there is a ballooning of a weakened portion of the arterial wall (Figure 7.17)
3. **blood pressure (BP)** (blud) (PRES-ūr)	pressure exerted by the blood against the blood vessel walls; a blood pressure measurement written as systolic pressure (120) and diastolic pressure (80) is commonly recorded as 120/80 mm Hg
4. **cardiac catheterization** (KAR-dē-ak) (kath-e-ter-i-ZĀ-shun)	diagnostic procedure performed by passing a catheter into the heart from a blood vessel in the groin or arm to examine the condition of the heart and surrounding blood vessels (Figure 7.16)
5. **cardiopulmonary resuscitation (CPR)** (kar-dē-ō-PUL-mo-nar-ē) (rē-sus-i-TĀ-shun)	emergency procedure consisting of artificial ventilation and external cardiac compressions
6. **complete blood count (CBC)** (com-PLĒT) (blud) (kownt)	laboratory test for basic blood screening that measures various aspects of erythrocytes, leukocytes, and thrombocytes (platelets); this automated test quickly provides a tremendous amount of information about the blood
7. **coronary artery bypass graft (CABG)** (KOR-o-nar-ē) (AR-ter-ē) (BĪ-pas) (graft)	surgical technique to bring a new blood supply to the heart muscle (myocardium) by detouring around blocked arteries
8. **coronary artery disease (CAD)** (KOR-o-nar-ē) (AR-ter-ē) (di-ZĒZ)	condition that reduces the flow of blood through the coronary arteries to the heart muscle (myocardium) that may progress to depriving the heart tissue of sufficient oxygen and nutrients to function normally
9. **embolus (*pl.* emboli)** (EM-bō-lus), (EM-bō-lī)	blood clot or foreign material, such as air or fat, that enters the bloodstream and moves until it lodges at another point in the circulation
10. **heart failure (HF)** (hart) (FĀL-ūr)	condition in which there is an inability of the heart to pump enough blood through the body to supply the tissues and organs with nutrients and oxygen (also called **congestive heart failure [CHF]**)

Continued

MEDICAL TERMS NOT BUILT FROM WORD PARTS—cont'd

TERM	DEFINITION
11. **hemorrhage** (HEM-ō-rij)	excessive flow of blood (bleeding internally or externally)
12. **hypertension (HTN)** (hī-per-TEN-shun)	blood pressure that is above normal (generally greater than 130/80 mm Hg in adults)
13. **hypotension** (hī-pō-TEN-shun)	blood pressure that is below normal (generally less than 90/60 mm Hg in adults)
14. **leukemia** (lū-KĒ-mē-a)	malignant disease characterized by excessive increase in abnormal leukocytes formed in the bone marrow
15. **myocardial infarction (MI)** (mī-ō-KAR-dē-al) (in-FARK-shun)	death (necrosis) of a portion of the heart muscle caused by lack of oxygen resulting from an interrupted blood supply (also called **heart attack**)
16. **pulse (P)** (puls)	contraction of the heart, which can be felt with a fingertip. The pulse is most commonly felt over the radial artery (in the wrist); however, the pulsations can be felt over a number of sites, including the femoral (groin) and carotid (neck) arteries.
17. **sphygmomanometer** (sfig-mō-ma-NOM-e-ter)	device used for measuring blood pressure
18. **stethoscope** (STETH-ō-skōp)	instrument used to hear internal body sounds; used for performing auscultation and blood pressure measurement
19. **varicose veins** (VAR-i-kōs) (vānz)	condition demonstrated by distended or tortuous veins; usually found in the lower extremities

EXERCISE E Label

Write the medical terms pictured and defined using the previous table of Medical Terms NOT Built from Word Parts. Check your work with the Answer Key in Appendix C.

1. _____

diagnostic procedure performed by passing a catheter into the heart from a blood vessel in the groin or arm to examine the condition of the heart and surrounding blood vessels

2. _____

surgical technique to bring a new blood supply to the heart muscle by detouring around blocked arteries

Blockage in coronary artery

Bypass graft

3. _____

distended or tortuous veins

4. _____

laboratory test for basic blood screening that measures various aspects of erythrocytes, leukocytes, and thrombocytes (platelets)

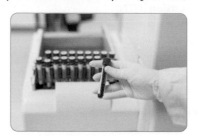

5. _____

ballooning of a weakened portion of the arterial wall

Ballooning

6. _____

emergency procedure consisting of artificial ventilation and external cardiac compressions

7. _____

instrument used to hear internal body sounds

8. _____

pressure exerted by the blood against the blood vessel walls; measurement is written as systolic pressure (120) and diastolic pressure (80), commonly recorded as 120/80 mm Hg

Sphygmomanometer

EXERCISE F   Match

Match the terms in the first column with their correct descriptions in the second column. Answers are listed in Appendix C.

_____ **1.** heart failure
_____ **2.** leukemia
_____ **3.** coronary artery bypass graft
_____ **4.** myocardial infarction
_____ **5.** pulse

a. also called heart attack
b. brings a new blood supply to the heart muscle by detouring around blocked arteries
c. malignant disease characterized by excessive increase in abnormal leukocytes formed in the bone marrow
d. contraction of the heart, which can be felt with a fingertip
e. inability of the heart to pump enough blood through the body to supply the tissues and organs with nutrients and oxygen

EXERCISE G   Match

Match the terms in the first column with their correct descriptions in the second column. Answers are listed in Appendix C.

_____ **1.** embolus
_____ **2.** hypertension
_____ **3.** coronary artery disease
_____ **4.** hemorrhage
_____ **5.** anemia
_____ **6.** hypotension

a. condition in which there is a reduction in the number of erythrocytes
b. blood pressure that is below normal
c. blood pressure that is above normal
d. condition that reduces the flow of blood through the coronary arteries to the heart muscle
e. excessive flow of blood (bleeding internally or externally)
f. blood clot or foreign material that enters the bloodstream and moves until it lodges at another point in the circulation

EXERCISE H   Learn Medical Terms NOT Built from Word Parts

Fill in the blanks with medical terms defined in bold using the Medical Terms NOT Built from Word Parts table. Answers are listed in Appendix C.

1. To evaluate the extent of a hemorrhage, a physician may order a **basic blood screening that measures aspects of erythrocytes, leukocytes, and thrombocytes (platelets)**, or _____ _____ _____ abbreviated as _____. This basic blood test will help determine whether a blood transfusion is necessary.

FYI **Hemorrhage** is a commonly misspelled word. Think of the word part **hem** for blood and the -rrh suffix **-rrhagia**. Change the suffix -ia to -e and you have the term **hem/o/rrhag/e**.

2. In a physical exam, **pressure exerted by the blood against the blood vessel walls**, or _____ _____, abbreviated as _____, is usually measured when vital signs are assessed. Vital signs include the measurement of temperature, respiration rate, and **contraction of the heart that can be felt with a fingertip**, or _____, abbreviated as ____. The pulse can be felt through the skin at many points, including the wrist, neck, or groin.

3. Tools needed to evaluate blood pressure include an **instrument used to hear internal body sounds, which is used for performing auscultation and blood pressure measurement**, or_____, and a **device used for measuring blood pressure**, or _____. To record a blood pressure measurement, the systolic (when the ventricles are contracting) pressure is listed over the diastolic (when the ventricles are relaxing) pressure, such as in a normal blood pressure of 120/80 mm Hg. A reading greater than 130/80 mm Hg generally signifies **blood pressure that is above normal**, or_____, abbreviated _____. A reading less than 90/60 mm Hg generally signifies **blood pressure that is below normal**, or _____.

4. A patient with a **condition that reduces the flow of blood through the coronary arteries to the heart muscle (myocardium)**, or _____ _____ _____, abbreviated as _____, may have angina pectoris, pain in the thoracic region sometimes radiating to the left arm and neck. This can be a warning sign for an upcoming **death of a portion of the heart muscle caused by an interrupted blood supply (also called heart attack)** _____ _____, abbreviated as _____. A physician may order a **diagnostic procedure performed by passing a catheter into the heart from a blood vessel in the groin or arm to examine the condition of the heart and surrounding blood vessels**, or _____ _____ (Figure 7.16).

Left ventricle   Aorta

Radial artery   Catheter inserted in femoral artery

Figure 7.16 Cardiac catheterization.

5. The most common site for **ballooning of a weakened portion of the arterial wall**, or _____, is the abdominal aorta, the main blood vessel that transports blood away from the heart (Figure 7.17). While surgery may be needed for larger abdominal aortic aneurysms (AAA), many patients with smaller ones may never need surgery, and are periodically monitored to make sure the aneurysms don't get larger.

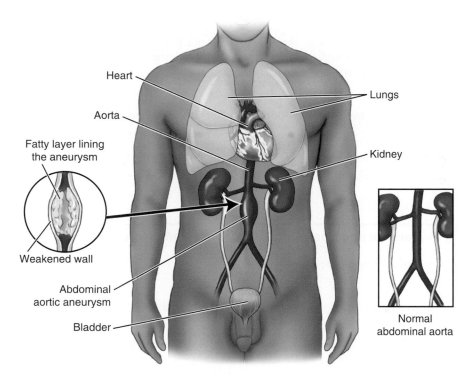

Figure 7.17 Abdominal aortic aneurysm.

6. A **reduction in the number of erythrocytes**, or _____, can be caused by low production in the bone marrow, destruction of circulating red blood cells, or **excessive flow of blood, or _____. Malignant disease characterized by excessive increase in abnormal leukocytes formed in the bone marrow**, or _____, can also cause anemia by replacing normal red cells with abnormal white cells.

7. In extreme cases, **condition in which there is an inability of the heart to pump enough blood through the body to supply the tissues and organs with nutrients and oxygen**, or _____ _____, abbreviated as _____, can lead to cardiac arrest, in which the heart stops beating. If recognized quickly, **emergency procedure consisting of artificial ventilation and external cardiac compressions**, or _____ _____, abbreviated as _____, can be performed and the heart may start beating again.

8. **A blood clot or foreign material, such as air or fat, that enters the bloodstream and moves until it lodges at another point in the circulation** is called a(n) _____. If it travels to the coronary arteries, a **surgical technique to bring a new blood supply to the heart muscle (myocardium) by detouring around blocked arteries,** or _____ _____ _____ _____, abbreviated as _____, may be necessary.

> **FYI**   Do you remember that thrombosis is an abnormal condition of a blood clot? A **thrombus** is attached to the interior wall of a vessel. If it breaks away and circulates in the bloodstream, it becomes known as an **embolus**. The condition of an embolus blocking an artery is referred to as an **embolism**.

9. **Distended or tortuous veins usually found in the lower extremities,** or _____ _____, usually occur in the superficial veins of the legs. One-way valves in veins help move blood upward. When these valves fail or veins lose their elasticity because of heredity, obesity, pregnancy, or illness, the blood flows backward, pools, and then forms varicose veins. A varicose vein in the rectal area is called a hemorrhoid.

EXERCISE I   Pronounce and Spell Terms NOT Built from Word Parts

Practice pronunciation and spelling on paper and online.

1. **Practice on Paper**
   a. **Pronounce:** Read the phonetic spelling and say aloud the terms listed in the previous table, Medical Terms NOT Built from Word Parts.
   b. **Spell:** Have a study partner read the terms aloud. Write the spelling of the terms on a separate sheet of paper.

2. **Practice Online** ⊕
   a. **Access** online learning resources. Go to evolve.elsevier.com > Evolve Resources > Practice Student Resources.
   b. **Pronounce:** Select Audio Glossary > Lesson 7 > Exercise I. Select a term to hear its pronunciation and repeat aloud.
   c. **Spell:** Select Activities > Lesson 7 > Spell Terms > Exercise I. Select the audio icon and type the correct spelling of the term.

❏ Check the box when complete.

OBJECTIVE 3

Write abbreviations.

ABBREVIATIONS RELATED TO THE CARDIOVASCULAR AND LYMPHATIC SYSTEMS

Use the online **flashcards** to familiarize yourself with the following abbreviations.

ABBREVIATION	TERM	ABBREVIATION	TERM
BP	blood pressure	HF	heart failure
CABG	coronary artery bypass graft	HHD	hypertensive heart disease
CAD	coronary artery disease	HTN	hypertension
CBC	complete blood count	IV	intravenous
CPR	cardiopulmonary resuscitation	MI	myocardial infarction
DSA	digital subtraction angiography	P	pulse
DVT	deep vein thrombosis	PAD	peripheral artery disease
ECHO	echocardiogram	PTCA	percutaneous transluminal coronary angioplasty
ECG, EKG	electrocardiogram	VS	vital signs

EXERCISE J   Abbreviate Medical Terms

Write the correct abbreviation next to its medical term. Check your responses with the answer key in Appendix C.

1. Diseases and Disorders:

a. _____ coronary artery disease

b. _____ heart failure

c. _____ myocardial infarction

d. _____ hypertension

e. _____ peripheral artery disease

f. _____ hypertensive heart disease

g. _____ deep vein thrombosis

2. Diagnostic Tests and Equipment:

a. _____ blood pressure

b. _____ complete blood count

c. _____ echocardiogram

d. _____ electrocardiogram
   _____

e. _____ vital signs

f. _____ pulse

g. _____ digital subtraction angiography

3. Surgical Procedures:

a. _____ coronary artery bypass graft

b. _____ percutaneous transluminal coronary angioplasty

4. Related Terms:

a. _____ cardiopulmonary resuscitation

b. _____ intravenous

OBJECTIVE 4

Identify medical terms by clinical category.

Now that you have worked through the cardiovascular and lymphatic systems lesson, review and practice medical terms grouped by clinical category. Categories include signs and symptoms, diseases and disorders, diagnostic tests and equipment, surgical procedures, specialties and professions, and other terms related to the cardiovascular and lymphatic systems.

EXERCISE K   **Signs and Symptoms**

Write the medical terms for signs and symptoms next to their definitions.

1. _____   slow heart rate

2. _____   enlargement of the heart

3. _____   excessive flow of blood (bleeding internally or externally)

4. _____   blood pressure that is above normal (generally greater than 130/80 mm Hg in adults)

5. _____   blood pressure that is below normal (generally less than 90/60 mm Hg in adults)

6. _____   enlargement of the spleen

7. _____   rapid heart rate

8. _____   rapid breathing

EXERCISE L   **Diseases and Disorders**

Write the medical terms for diseases and disorders next to their definitions.

1. _____   condition in which there is a reduction in the number of erythrocytes (RBC)

2. _____   condition in which there is a ballooning of a weakened portion of the arterial wall

3. _____   hardening of the arteries

4. _____   disease of the heart muscle

5. _____   condition that reduces the flow of blood through the coronary arteries to the heart muscle (myocardium) that may progress to depriving the heart tissue of sufficient oxygen and nutrients to function normally

6. _____   blood clot or foreign material, such as air or fat, that enters the bloodstream and moves until it lodges at another point in the circulation

7. _____ condition in which there is an inability of the heart to pump enough blood through the body to supply the tissues and organs with nutrients and oxygen

8. _____ tumor of blood (collection of blood that has leaked out of a broken vessel into the surrounding tissue)

9. _____ dissolution of (red) blood (cells)

10. _____ malignant disease characterized by excessive increase in abnormal leukocytes formed in the bone marrow

11. _____ abnormal reduction of white (blood) cells

12. _____ inflammation of the lymph nodes

13. _____ disease of the lymph nodes

14. _____ tumor of the lymphatic tissue

15. _____ death (necrosis) of a portion of the heart muscle caused by lack of oxygen resulting from an interrupted blood supply (also called **heart attack**)

16. _____ inflammation of the veins

17. _____ abnormal reduction in number of blood clotting cells

18. _____ inflammation of the veins associated with blood clots

19. _____ abnormal condition of a blood clot

20. _____ condition demonstrated by distended or tortuous veins; usually found in the lower extremities

---

EXERCISE M   **Diagnostic Tests and Equipment**

Write the medical terms for diagnostic tests and equipment next to their definitions.

1. _____ radiographic imaging of the blood vessels

2. _____ radiographic image of the arteries (after an injection of contrast media)

3. _____ pressure exerted by the blood against the blood vessel walls

4. _____ diagnostic procedure performed by passing a catheter into the heart from a blood vessel in the groin or arm to examine the condition of the heart and surrounding blood vessels

5. _____ laboratory test for basic blood screening that measures various aspects of erythrocytes, leukocytes, and thrombocytes (platelets)

6. _____   record of the heart using sound

7. _____   record of electrical activity of the heart

8. _____   instrument used to record electrical activity of the heart

9. _____   process of recording electrical activity of the heart

10. _____   contraction of the heart, which can be felt with a fingertip

11. _____   device used for measuring blood pressure

12. _____   instrument used to hear internal body sounds; used for performing auscultation and blood pressure measurement

13. _____   radiographic image of the veins (after an injection of contrast media)

EXERCISE N   **Surgical Procedures**

Write the medical terms for surgical procedures next to their definitions.

1. _____   surgical repair of a blood vessel

2. _____   surgical technique to bring a new blood supply to the heart muscle (myocardium) by detouring around blocked arteries

3. _____   excision within the artery (excision of plaque from the arterial wall)

4. _____   incision into the vein (with a needle to remove blood or instill fluid); (also called **venipuncture**)

5. _____   excision of the spleen

EXERCISE O   **Specialties and Professions**

Write the medical terms for specialties and professions next to their definitions.

1. _____   physician who studies and treats diseases of the heart

2. _____   study of the heart

3. _____   physician who studies and treats diseases of the blood

4. _____   study of blood

EXERCISE P **Medical Terms Related to Cardiovascular and Lymphatic Systems**

Write the medical terms related to the cardiovascular and lymphatic systems next to their definitions.

1. _____ pertaining to the arteries

2. _____ pertaining to the heart

3. _____ emergency procedure consisting of artificial ventilation and
   _____ external cardiac compressions

4. _____ stopping (the flow of) blood

5. _____ pertaining to within a vein

6. _____ pertaining to the muscle of the heart

7. _____ blood clotting cell (also called **platelet**)

 OBJECTIVE 5

Use medical language in clinical statements, the case study, and a medical record.

Check responses for the following exercises in Appendix C.

EXERCISE Q **Use Medical Terms in Clinical Statements**

Circle the medical terms defined in the bolded phrases. For pronunciation practice, read the answers aloud.

1. Mr. Lauer went to his doctor for follow-up on his **condition in which there is an inability of the heart to pump enough blood through the body to supply the tissues and organs with nutrients and oxygen** (hemostasis, hypertension, heart failure). He had **process of recording the electrical activity of the heart** (electrocardiography, echocardiogram, angiography) performed to help evaluate his **pertaining to the heart** (arterial, myocardial, cardiac) status.

2. Following a trans-Pacific airline flight, Kenji Makoto developed **inflammation of the vein associated with a blood clot** (tachypnea, thrombophlebitis, lymphadenitis). After evaluation by Doppler ultrasound, anticoagulant therapy was ordered for treatment. The goal was prevention of a(n) **blood clot or foreign material, such as air or fat, that enters the bloodstream and moves until it lodges at another point in the circulation** (embolus, thrombosis, myocardial infarction).

3. **Abnormal reduction of blood clotting cells** (Leukocytopenia, Leukemia, Thrombocytopenia) can contribute to **excessive flow of blood** (hemorrhage, aneurysm, thrombosis). If **stopping the flow of blood** (hematoma, hemostasis, hematology) can be achieved quickly, **condition in which there is a reduction in the number of erythrocytes** (anemia, leukemia, hypotension) may be avoided.

4. **Rapid heart rate** (Tachypnea, Hypertension, Tachycardia) may be noted by measuring the **contraction of the heart, which can be felt with a fingertip** (blood pressure, hemostasis, pulse) and may also be accompanied **by blood pressure that is below normal** (hypertension, heart failure, hypotension).

5. **Hardening of the arteries** (Heart failure, Cardiomyopathy, Arteriosclerosis) is a common disorder characterized by thickening, calcification, and loss of elasticity of the **pertaining to the artery** (cardiac, arterial, myocardial) walls.

6. Utilizing a **basic blood screening that measures aspects of erythrocytes, leukocytes, and thrombocytes (platelets)** (stethoscope, venogram, complete blood count) and a bone marrow biopsy, it was determined that Sophia Tompkins had **malignant disease characterized by excessive increase in abnormal leukocytes formed in the bone marrow** (lymphoma, leukemia, hematoma). She was referred to a **physician who studies and treats diseases of the blood** (hematologist, cardiologist, phlebotomist) for consultation and treatment.

7. **Condition that reduces the flow of blood through the coronary arteries to the heart muscle (myocardium)** (Thrombosis, Arteriosclerosis, Coronary artery disease) may eventually lead to an MI. Treatment includes restoring blood supply to the heart. **Surgical repair of the blood vessel** (Angiography, Arteriogram, Angioplasty) is used in some cases, and for more severe blockage, the cardiac surgeon will perform a **surgical technique to bring a new blood supply to the heart muscle (myocardium) by detouring around blocked arteries** (coronary artery bypass graft, cardiac catheterization, cardiopulmonary resuscitation).

EXERCISE R   **Apply Medical Terms to the Case Study**

Think back to Natalia, who was introduced in the case study at the beginning of the lesson. After working through Lesson 7 on the cardiovascular and lymphatic systems, consider the medical terms that might be used to describe her experience. List two terms relevant to the case study and their meaning. ■

Medical Term   **Definition**

1. _____   _____

2. _____   _____

EXERCISE S   **Use Medical Terms in a Document**

Natalia was brought to the emergency department and was admitted to the cardiology unit of the hospital. Her care is documented in the following medical record.

Use the definitions in numbers 1-9 to write medical terms within the document.

1. blood pressure that is above normal (generally greater than 130/80 mm Hg in adults)

2. distended or tortuous veins usually found in the lower extremities

3. physician who studies and treats diseases of the heart

4. surgical technique to bring a new blood supply to the heart muscle (myocardium) by detouring around blocked arteries

5. ballooning of a weakened portion of the arterial wall

6. incision into the vein (with a needle to remove blood or instill fluid)

7. record of the electrical activity of the heart

8. death (necrosis) of a portion of the heart muscle caused by lack of oxygen resulting from an interrupted blood supply

9. diagnostic procedure performed by passing a catheter into the heart from a blood vessel in the groin or arm to examine the condition of the heart and surrounding blood vessels

Refer to the medical record to answer questions 10-13.

10. The term **atherogenic** is used in the medical record to describe her risk factors for coronary artery disease. Ather/o means a fatty plaque deposited on a vessel wall. Use your knowledge of other word parts to review this term.

    ather/o means _____ _____ deposited on a _____ _____.

    -genic means _____, _____, _____.

    Thus, **ather/o/genic** means _____ a _____ _____ deposit on a _____ _____.

31733 KROUSE, Natalia

File | Patient | Navigate | Custom Fields | Help

Chart Review | Encounters | Notes | Labs | Imaging | Procedures | Rx | Documents | Referrals | Scheduling | Billing

Name: **KROUSE, Natalia**
MR#: **31733**
DOB: 2/21/19XX
Sex: F
Age: 76
Allergies: None known
PCP: Lopez, Angelica DO

Cardiology Admission Report
Encounter Date: 05 March 20XX

Chief Complaint: Natalia Krouse is a 76-year-old woman who was admitted to the hospital for chest pain.

History of Present Illness: The patient has an extensive history of chronic cardiovascular issues. Atherogenic risk factors include (1.)_____ and hypercholesterolemia. She also has extensive (2.)_____ of the lower extremities bilaterally. Her family physician referred her to a (3.)_____ in 2016 for medical management of these complications. She smokes one pack of cigarettes a day and has previously declined participation in a smoking cessation program. She is not diabetic. Family history reveals a brother who has had (4.)_____ and a mother deceased from abdominal aortic (5.)_____ rupture.

Over the last 5 days, the patient reports that she has felt "very wiped out," with episodes of nausea and indigestion. This evening while taking a short walk she experienced severe chest pressure, pain radiating to left arm and jaw, and dizziness that lasted 5 minutes. Neighbors called 911 and she was admitted to this hospital for evaluation through the emergency department.

Physical Exam: On exam, blood pressure is 139/86 mm Hg with a pulse of 120. Oxygen saturation is 94% on room air. Lungs are clear to auscultation. She has a regular heart rhythm without murmur. She appears fatigued, but in no acute distress.

Plan:
(6.)_____ to withdraw blood for CPK and troponin values. (7.)_____ will be obtained to rule out (8.)_____.
(9.) _____ with possible coronary stent if necessary.

Electronically signed: DeRouge, Marguerite MD on 05 March 20XX 21:27

Start | Log On/Off | Print | Edit

11. _____ is the abbreviation for heart failure, which is also sometimes referred to as congestive heart failure, or CHF.

12. **Coronary** is derived from the Latin **coronalis**, meaning crown or wreath. It describes the arteries encircling the heart. A stent is a supportive tubular device placed in the _____ (**referring to the arteries circling the heart**) artery; it is used to prevent closure of the artery after angioplasty (Figure 7.18).

Figure 7.18 Coronary stent. **A,** Stent at the site of plaque formation. **B,** Inflated balloon and expanded stent. **C,** Expanded stent with balloon removed.

13. Identify two new medical terms in the medical record you would like to investigate. Use your medical dictionary or an online reference to look up the definition.

Medical Term   **Definition**

a. _____   _____

b. _____   _____

EXERCISE T   **Use Medical Language in Electronic Health Records Online**

Select the correct medical terms to complete three medical records in one patient's electronic file.

⊕ Access online resources at evolve.elsevier.com > Evolve Resources > Practice Student Resources > Activities > Lesson 7 > Electronic Health Records

Topic: Coronary Artery Disease
Record 1: Echocardiogram Report
Record 2: Cardiovascular Operative Report
Record 3: Discharge Summary

❏   Check the box when complete.

OBJECTIVE 6

Recall and assess knowledge of word parts, medical terms, and abbreviations.

EXERCISE U Online Review of Lesson Content

🌐 *Recall and assess your learning from working through the lesson by completing online learning activities at evolve. elsevier.com > Evolve Resources > Student Resources.*

❑ Check the box when complete.

EXERCISE V Lesson Content Quiz

Test your knowledge of the terms and abbreviations introduced in this lesson. Circle the letter for the medical term or abbreviation related to the words in italics.

1. The *record of the heart using sound* showed evidence for moderately severe mitral regurgitation.
   a. echocardiogram
   b. electrocardiogram
   c. angiography

2. A patient with hypothyroidism may present with *slow heart rate.*
   a. hypotension
   b. cardiomegaly
   c. bradycardia

3. *Rapid breathing* was noted in the patient suffering from acute heart failure.
   a. tachycardia
   b. tachypnea
   c. hypertension

4. Symptoms of a pulmonary *blood clot that enters the bloodstream and moves until it lodges at another point in the circulation* include shortness of breath, tachycardia, and chest pain.
   a. thrombosis
   b. phlebitis
   c. embolus

5. *Emergency procedure consisting of artificial ventilation and external cardiac compressions* can be lifesaving in a patient with acute cardiac arrest.
   a. CBC
   b. CABG
   c. CPR

6. A *pressure exerted by blood against the blood vessel walls* of 120/80 mm Hg is normal.
   a. pulse
   b. blood pressure
   c. stethoscope

7. A patient with strep throat can present with cervical *disease of the lymph nodes.*
   a. lymphadenopathy
   b. lymphadenitis
   c. lymphoma

8. A right carotid *excision within the artery* was performed following a transient ischemic attack.
   a. angiography
   b. angioplasty
   c. endarterectomy

9. A chest radiograph showed *enlargement of the heart* in a patient with heart failure.
   a. cardiomegaly
   b. cardiopathy
   c. cardiology

10. Deep vein *abnormal condition of blood clots* can cause pain and swelling of the lower extremities.
    a. phlebitis
    b. embolus
    c. thrombosis

11. Use of a(n) *instrument used to hear internal body sounds* would be the best method for listening to a heart murmur.
    a. sphygmomanometer
    b. stethoscope
    c. electrocardiograph

12. *Condition in which there is an inability of the heart to pump enough blood through the body to supply the tissues and organs with nutrients and oxygen* may be caused by chronic HTN, an MI, or CAD.
    a. HF
    b. HHD
    c. DVT

LESSON AT A GLANCE **CARDIOVASCULAR AND LYMPHATIC SYSTEMS WORD PARTS**

COMBINING FORMS

aden/o	electr/o
angi/o	lymph/o
arteri/o	phleb/o, ven/o
cardi/o	splen/o
ech/o	thromb/o

SUFFIXES
-ac
-graph
-penia
-sclerosis

PREFIXES
brady-
tachy-

LESSON AT A GLANCE **CARDIOVASCULAR AND LYMPHATIC SYSTEMS MEDICAL TERMS AND ABBREVIATIONS**

SIGNS AND SYMPTOMS
bradycardia
cardiomegaly
hemorrhage
hypertension (HTN)
hypotension
splenomegaly
tachycardia
tachypnea

DISEASES AND DISORDERS
anemia
aneurysm
arteriosclerosis
cardiomyopathy
coronary artery disease (CAD)
embolus *pl.* emboli
heart failure (HF)
hematoma
hemolysis
leukemia
leukocytopenia
lymphadenitis
lymphadenopathy
lymphoma
myocardial infarction (MI)
phlebitis

thrombocytopenia
thrombophlebitis
thrombosis
varicose veins

DIAGNOSTIC TESTS AND EQUIPMENT
angiography
arteriogram
blood pressure (BP)
cardiac catheterization
complete blood count (CBC)
echocardiogram (ECHO)
electrocardiogram (ECG, EKG)
electrocardiograph
electrocardiography
pulse (P)
sphygmomanometer
stethoscope
venogram

SURGICAL PROCEDURES
angioplasty
coronary artery bypass graft (CABG)
endarterectomy
phlebotomy
splenectomy

SPECIALTIES AND PROFESSIONS
cardiologist
cardiology
hematologist
hematology

RELATED TERMS
arterial
cardiac
cardiopulmonary resuscitation (CPR)
hemostasis
intravenous (IV)
myocardial
thrombocyte

ABBREVIATIONS

BP	ECHO	MI
CABG	ECG	P
CAD	EKG	PAD
CBC	HF	PTCA
CPR	HHD	VS
DSA	HTN	
DVT	IV	

Digestive System

CASE STUDY
 Ruth Clifton

Ruth is worried about her stomach. She has been having pain on and off for about 3 months. At first it was just once in a while, but now it seems to be every day. Her pain seems to be worse when she hasn't eaten for a while, and after she eats something bland, it usually gets a bit better. She bought some antacids at the pharmacy, and chewing those also seems to help. Lately the pain in her stomach has been waking her up at night. A glass of milk usually helps with that. The last few days, though, she has had nausea and vomiting and is finding it difficult to eat. Her friend recommends that she see a stomach doctor, who helped her when she had similar problems.

■ *Consider Ruth's situation as you work through the lesson on the digestive system. At the end of the lesson, we will return to this case study and identify medical terms used to document Ruth's experience and the care she receives.*

OBJECTIVES

1 ■ Build, translate, pronounce, and spell medical terms built from word parts (p. 234).

2 ■ Define, pronounce, and spell medical terms NOT built from word parts (p. 254).

3 ■ Write abbreviations (p. 260).

4 ■ Identify medical terms by clinical category (p. 261).

5 ■ Use medical language in clinical statements, the case study, and a medical record (p. 265).

6 ■ Recall and assess knowledge of word parts, medical terms, and abbreviations (p. 268).

INTRODUCTION TO THE DIGESTIVE SYSTEM

Anatomic Structures of the Digestive System	
abdomen (AB-duh-men)	portion of the body between the thorax and the pelvis
anus (Ā-nus)	sphincter muscle (ringlike band of muscle fiber that keeps an opening tight) at the end of the digestive tract, connected to the rectum
appendix (a-PEN-diks)	small, wormlike pouch attached to the cecum (the beginning of the large intestine)
colon (KŌ-lun)	major component of the large intestine, which is divided into four parts: ascending colon, transverse colon, descending colon, and sigmoid colon
esophagus (e-SOF-a-gus)	tube that transports food from the pharynx to the stomach

Continued

Anatomic Structures of the Digestive System—cont'd

gallbladder (GAWL-blad-er)	small, saclike structure that stores bile produced by the liver
gums (gumz)	pale pink tissue that is attached to jawbones and teeth; provides supporting structure for the mouth
large intestine (larj) (in-TES-tin)	approximately 5-foot canal extending from the ileum to the anus
liver (LIV-er)	organ that produces bile for the digestion of fats; performs many other functions that support digestion and metabolism
mouth (mouth)	opening through which food passes into the body; breaks food into small particles by mastication (chewing) and mixing with saliva; (also called the **oral cavity**)
pancreas (PAN-kre-us)	organ that secretes multiple enzymes necessary for digestion; also secretes insulin for carbohydrate metabolism
pharynx (FAR-inks)	performs swallowing action that passes food from the mouth into the esophagus
rectum (REK-tum)	last part of the large intestine, connecting to the anus
sigmoid colon (SIG-moyd) (KŌ-lun)	S-shaped section of the large intestine leading into the rectum
small intestine (smal) (in-TES-tin)	20-foot tube extending from the stomach to the large intestine, where most of the nutrients are absorbed; has three sections: duodenum, jejunum, ileum
stomach (STUM-ek)	J-shaped sac that mixes and stores food; secretes substances that aid digestion
tongue (tung)	organ in mouth composed of skeletal muscle; responsible for movement of food from mouth to pharynx, and is also important for taste and speech

Functions of the Digestive System

- **Ingestion:** taking in nutrients through the mouth
- **Digestion:** mechanical and chemical breakdown of food for use by body cells
- **Absorption:** transfer of nutrients (from digested food) from the small intestine to the bloodstream
- **Elimination:** removal of solid waste from the body

How the Digestive System Works

The digestive tract, also known as the **alimentary canal** or **gastrointestinal (GI) tract**, is a continuous passageway from the mouth to the anus (Figure 8.1). The lips, cheeks, tongue, gums, teeth, and palate form the **oral cavity (mouth)**, where food is ingested and masticated (chewed), and enzymes are released to help break it down. Swallowing occurs in the **pharynx**; then masticated food and liquid are moved into the **esophagus**, which transports its contents to the **stomach**. The stomach secretes chemicals for digestion and also churns food, then passes it into the **small intestine**. Absorption, the passage of nutrients into the bloodstream, occurs here. Remaining materials are then emptied into the **large intestine** for the formation of feces, which are then stored in the **rectum** and eliminated through the **anus**. Accessory organs of the digestive system include the salivary glands, pancreas, liver, and gallbladder, which produce various chemicals that assist in various aspects of the digestive process.

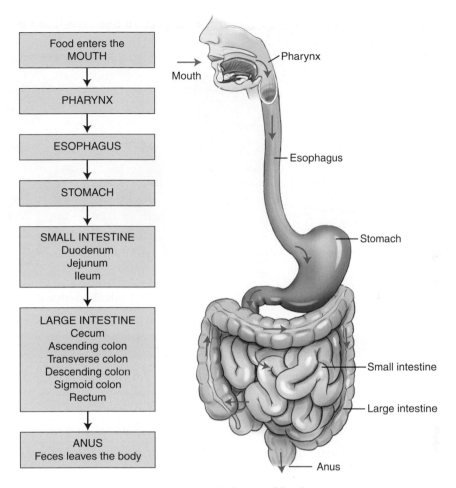

Figure 8.1 Pathway of food.

CAREER FOCUS   **Professionals Who Work with the Digestive System**

- **Registered dietitians** (RD) are food and nutrition experts who have earned a bachelor's degree and met professional requirements to qualify for the credential RD. They may work in hospitals or other healthcare facilities, in the community, or in public health settings.

- **Dietetic technicians** assist in providing food service and nutritional programs under the supervision of a dietitian. They may plan and produce meals based on established guidelines, teach principles of food and nutrition, or counsel patients.

Continued

CAREER FOCUS | **Professionals Who Work with the Digestive System—cont'd**

- **Dental hygienists** work with dentists to meet the oral health needs of patients. They clean teeth by removing plaque deposits and apply sealants and fluoride for preventative care. They also teach patients about appropriate oral hygiene, including toothbrushing, flossing, and nutritional counseling.

- **Dental assistants** assist dentists during many different treatment procedures (Figure 8.2). They may also take dental radiographs (x-rays) and help obtain impressions of patients' teeth for plaster casts. They also provide instructions to patients after their treatment. In addition, they prepare and sterilize equipment and assist with infection control.

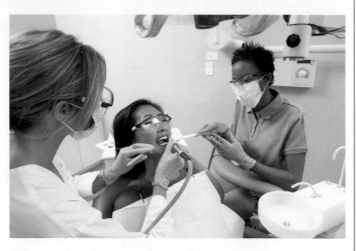

Figure 8.2 A dentist and a dental assistant work on a patient.

 OBJECTIVE 1

Build, translate, pronounce, and spell medical terms built from word parts.

WORD PARTS | Use the paper or online **flashcards** to familiarize yourself with the following word parts.

COMBINING FORM (WR + CV)	DEFINITION	COMBINING FORM (WR + CV)	DEFINITION
abdomin/o, lapar/o	abdomen, abdominal cavity	**gloss/o, lingu/o**	tongue
an/o	anus	**hepat/o**	liver
append/o, appendic/o	appendix	**ile/o**	ileum (3rd portion of the small intestine)
chol/e	gall, bile	**jejun/o**	jejunum (2nd portion of the small intestine)
col/o, colon/o	colon (large intestine)	**or/o**	mouth
duoden/o	duodenum (1st portion of the small intestine)	**pancreat/o**	pancreas
enter/o	intestines (usually the small intestine)	**peps/o**	digestion
esophag/o	esophagus	**phag/o**	swallowing, eating
gastr/o	stomach	**proct/o, rect/o**	rectum
gingiv/o	gums	**sigmoid/o**	sigmoid colon
SUFFIX (S)	DEFINITION		
-algia	pain		

WORD PARTS PRESENTED IN PREVIOUS LESSONS		Used to Build Terms for the Digestive System	
COMBINING FORM (WR + CV)	**DEFINITION**	**COMBINING FORM (WR + CV)**	**DEFINITION**
cyst/o	bladder, sac	**lith/o**	stone(s), calculus (*pl.* calculi)
SUFFIX (S)	**DEFINITION**	**SUFFIX (S)**	**DEFINITION**
-al, -eal, -ic	pertaining to	**-logy**	study of
-cele	hernia, protrusion	**-megaly**	enlargement
-centesis	surgical puncture to remove fluid	**-oma**	tumor
		-osis	abnormal condition
-ectomy	surgical removal, excision	**-plasty**	surgical repair
-graphy	process of recording, radiographic imaging	**-scope**	instrument used for visual examination
-ia	diseased state, condition of	**-scopic**	pertaining to visual examination
		-scopy	visual examination
-iasis	condition	**-stomy**	creation of an artificial opening
-itis	inflammation	**-tomy**	cut into, incision
-logist	one who studies and treats (specialist, physician)	**-y**	no meaning
PREFIX (P)	**DEFINITION**	**PREFIX (P)**	**DEFINITION**
a-, an-	absence of, without	**sub-**	below, under
dys-	difficult, painful, abnormal		

Refer to Appendix A, Word Parts Used in *Basic Medical Language*, for alphabetical lists of word parts and their meanings.

EXERCISE A   Build and Translate Medical Terms Built from Word Parts

*Use the **Word Parts Tables** to complete the following questions. Check your responses with the Answer Key in Appendix C.*

1. **LABEL:** *Write the combining forms for anatomic structures of the digestive system on Figure 8.3. These anatomic combining forms will be used to build and translate medical terms in Exercise A.*

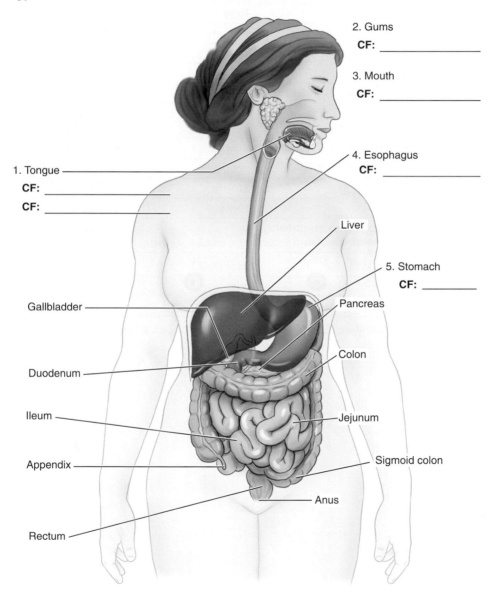

2. Gums
  CF: _____

3. Mouth
  CF: _____

4. Esophagus
  CF: _____

1. Tongue
  CF: _____
  CF: _____

Liver

5. Stomach
  CF: _____

Gallbladder

Pancreas

Duodenum

Colon

Ileum

Jejunum

Appendix

Sigmoid colon

Anus

Rectum

Figure 8.3 The digestive system and related combining forms.

2. MATCH: *Draw a line to match the word part with its definition.*

   a. -algia   inflammation
   b. -itis   pain

3. BUILD: *Using the combining form **gingiv/o** and the word parts reviewed in the previous exercise, build the following terms related to the gums. Remember, the definition usually starts with the meaning of the suffix.*

   a. pain in the gums   _____/_____
                                                       wr   s

   b. inflammation of the gums   _____/_____
                                                       wr   s

4. READ: Gingivitis (jin-ji-VĪ-tis) is frequently caused by poor oral hygiene that allows plaque to form. Plaque is a sticky substance that occurs when mouth bacteria combine with sugars and starches in food. Toothbrushing prevents the buildup of plaque. If plaque is allowed to remain, it causes tartar at the gumline, which is not easily removed. This irritates the gums, causing them to become swollen and bleed easily. Other symptoms of gingivitis include **gingivalgia** (jin-ji-VAL-jē-a), bad breath, and a change in color of the gums from pink to dusky red.

5. LABEL: *Write word parts to complete Figure 8.4.*

Figure 8.4 Severe _____/_____.
                                     gums   inflammation

6. MATCH: *Draw a line to match the word part with its definition.*

   a. -itis   below, under
   b. -al   inflammation
   c. sub-   pertaining to

7. TRANSLATE: *Complete the definitions of the following terms built from the combining forms **gloss/o** or **lingu/o,** meaning tongue. Use the meaning of word parts to fill in the blanks. Remember, the definition usually starts with the meaning of the suffix.*

   a. gloss/itis   _____ of the tongue

   b. sub/lingu/al   pertaining to _____ the _____

---

8. BUILD: *Using the combining form **or/o,** meaning mouth, and the word parts reviewed in the matching exercise, build the following term:*

pertaining to the mouth   _____/_____
                                              wr   **s**

---

9. READ: **Glossitis** (glos-Ī-tis) may be caused by a variety of conditions, including infections, allergic reactions, dry mouth, trauma, or low iron levels. **Oral** (OR-al) examination usually reveals swelling of the tongue, with color and texture changes. It is important to inspect the **sublingual** (sub-LING-gwal) surface to look for leukoplakia (white patches) that could indicate cancer or other diseases.

---

10. LABEL: *Write word parts to complete Figure 8.5.*

Figure 8.5 _____/_____/_____ leukoplakia.
                   below   tongue   pertaining to

---

11. MATCH: *Draw a line to match the word part with its definition.*

   a. peps/o   swallowing, eating
   b. phag/o   no meaning
   c. enter/o   intestines (usually the small intestine)
   d. -ia   digestion
   e. -y   diseased state, condition of
   f. a-   without

12. BUILD: *Use the prefix **dys-**, meaning difficult, painful, or abnormal, and the word parts reviewed in the previous exercise to build the following terms:*

a. painful intestines   _____ / _____ / _____ y _____
                                         p   wr   s

b. condition of difficult digestion   _____ / _____ / _____
                                         p   wr   s

c. condition of difficult swallowing   _____ / _____ / _____
                                         p   wr   s

13. TRANSLATE: *Complete the definition.*

a/phag/ia   _____ of without _____

14. READ: Dyspepsia (dis-PEP-sē-a) is also referred to as indigestion or upset stomach, and refers to a discomfort in the upper abdomen or chest that may be accompanied by burping, bloating, or feeling full. **Dysentery** (DIS-en-ter-ē) symptoms often include fever, abdominal pain, and bloody diarrhea. In the United States it is frequently caused by *Shigella* and *E. coli* bacteria in contaminated food or water. **Dysphagia** (dis-FĀ-ja) is often caused by problems with the esophagus, while **aphagia** (a-FĀ-ja), the loss of the ability to swallow, can be caused by either anatomic or psychological factors.

15. MATCH: *Draw a line to match the word part with its definition.*

a. -eal   inflammation
b. -itis   pertaining to

16. BUILD: *Using the combining form **esophag/o**, meaning esophagus, and the word parts reviewed in the previous exercise, build the following terms:*

a. pertaining to the esophagus   _____ / _____
                                         wr   s

b. inflammation of the esophagus   _____ / _____
                                         wr   s

17. READ: Esophagitis (e-sof-a-JĪ-tis) is frequently caused by acid reflux, a condition that occurs when the **esophageal** (e-sof-a-JĒ-al) sphincter (a valvelike structure between the esophagus and stomach) doesn't close properly. This allows stomach contents to back up into the esophagus, causing irritation to the esophageal lining.

18. LABEL: *Write word parts to complete Figure 8.6.*

← Damage caused by acid reflux

Figure 8.6 Linear streaks visible by endoscopy in _____/_____.

esophagus   inflammation

---

19. MATCH: *Draw a line to match the word part with its definition.*

   a. enter/o   one who studies and treats (specialist, physician)
   b. -itis   study of
   c. -logist   intestines (usually the small intestine)
   d. -logy   inflammation

---

20. BUILD: *Using the combining form **gastr/o** and the word parts reviewed in the previous exercise, build the following terms related to the stomach.*

   a. physician who studies and treats diseases   _____/ o /_____/ o /_____
       of the stomach and intestines   wr   cv   wr   cv   s

   b. study of the stomach and intestines   _____/ o /_____/ o /_____
                                            wr   cv   wr   cv   s

   c. inflammation of the stomach and intestines   _____/ o /_____/_____
                                       wr   cv   wr   s

---

21. MATCH: *Draw a line to match the word part with its definition.*

   a. -ectomy   pertaining to
   b. -itis   excision
   c. -eal, -ic   inflammation

22. TRANSLATE: *Complete the definitions of the following terms using the combining form **gastr/o**.*

   a. gastr/itis   _____ of the stomach

   b. gastr/ic   pertaining to the _____

   c. gastr/ectomy   _____ of the stomach

   d. gastr/o/esophag/eal   _____ to the _____ and _____

23. READ: Gastroenteritis (gas-trō-en-te-RĪ-tis) is often caused by a virus and will resolve on its own. **Gastritis** (gas-TRĪ-tis) can be caused by bacteria, certain medications (such as aspirin and ibuprofen), or excessive alcohol use. A **gastroenterologist** (gas-trō-en-ter-OL-o-jist) often treats this condition. If left untreated, it may lead to stomach ulcers and bleeding. In severe cases, a partial **gastrectomy** (gas-TREK-to-mē) may be required. A complete gastrectomy may be required with certain types of **gastric** (GAS-trik) cancer, in which case the stomach is removed at the **gastroesophageal** (gas-trō-e-sof-a-JĒ-al) junction and the esophagus is connected directly to the jejunum.

24. LABEL: *Write word parts to complete Figure 8.7.*

Esophagus

Stomach

Duodenum

Figure 8.7 A partial _____/_____ may be performed to remove chronic gastric ulcers.
                        stomach   excision

25. MATCH: *Draw a line to match the word part with its definition.*

   a. -scope   creation of an artificial opening

   b. -stomy   visual examination

   c. -scopy   instrument used for visual examination

26. BUILD: *Using the combining form **gastr/o** and the word parts reviewed in the previous exercise, build the following terms.*

   a. instrument used for visual examination of the stomach   _____/_o_/_____
                                                                        wr   cv   s

   b. visual examination of the stomach   _____/_o_/_____
                                                                     wr   cv   s

   c. creation of an artificial opening into the stomach   _____/_o_/_____
                                                                      wr   cv   s

27. **READ:** Percutaneous endoscopic **gastrostomy** (gas-TROS-to-mē), or **PEG**, is one of the most common endoscopic procedures performed. It provides a route to administer nutrition for those who are unable to eat for a long period of time. During **gastroscopy** (gas-TROS-ko-pē), the gastroenterologist inserts the **gastroscope** (GAS-trō-skōp) into the mouth, through the esophagus, and into the stomach. The gastroscope is then directed anteriorly so that the light can be seen through the skin. A small incision is made and then the gastroscope is advanced through this hole, allowing it to grab the gastrostomy tube and bring it into the stomach. This tube is secured to the skin and the gastroscope is removed.

28. **LABEL:** *Write word parts to complete Figure 8.8.*

Light

A

B

Figure 8.8 A. _____/o/_____.
                      stomach   visual examination

B. Fiberoptic _____/o/_____, which has glass fibers
                          stomach   instrument used for visual examination

in a flexible tube, allowing light and images to be transmitted back to the examiner.

29. **MATCH:** *Draw a line to match the word part with its definition.*

a. -scope   pertaining to visual examination
b. -scopic   instrument used for visual examination
c. -scopy   abdomen, abdominal cavity
d. abdomin/o, lapar/o   visual examination

30. TRANSLATE: *Use the combining form **lapar/o,** meaning abdominal cavity, to complete the definitions of the following terms.*

    a. lapar/o/scope   _____ used for visual examination of the _____ _____

    b. lapar/o/scopic   pertaining to _____ _____ of the abdominal cavity

    c. lapar/o/scopy   _____ _____ of the _____ _____

31. READ: Laparoscopic (lap-ar-ō-SKOP-ik) surgery can be performed through small incisions in the abdomen, rather than a large, open incision. It is sometimes referred to as videoscopic surgery because the surgeon performs the surgery by viewing a video screen that is connected to the **laparoscope** (LAP-a-rō-skōp). **Laparoscopy** (lap-a-ROS-ko-pē) reduces cost and trauma to the patient.

32. LABEL: *Write word parts to complete Figure 8.9.*

Figure 8.9 A. _____/o/_____ surgical setup. B. Laparoscopic surgery.
               abdominal cavity   pertaining to visual examination

33. MATCH: *Draw a line to match the word part with its definition.*

    a. -centesis   incision

    b. -tomy   surgical puncture to remove fluid

34. TRANSLATE: *Complete the definitions of the following terms.*

    a. abdomin/o/centesis   surgical _____ to remove _____ from

                         the abdominal _____

    b. lapar/o/tomy   _____ into the _____ cavity

35. READ: In an emergency, a general surgeon will often choose to perform a **laparotomy** (lap-a-ROT-o-mē) rather than a laparoscopy because the long, open incision provides a much larger view of the area in question and can be performed much more quickly. **Abdominocentesis** (ab-dom-i-nō-sen-TĔ-sis) is also known as **abdominal paracentesis**, and is often performed in people with excesses of fluid in their abdominal cavities due to liver disease, cancer, or other disorders.

36. REVIEW OF DIGESTIVE SYSTEM TERMS BUILT FROM WORD PARTS: *The following is an alphabetical list of terms built and translated in the previous exercises.*

MEDICAL TERMS BUILT FROM WORD PARTS

TERM	DEFINITION	TERM	DEFINITION
1. **abdominocentesis** (ab-dom-i-nō-sen-TĔ-sis)	surgical puncture to remove fluid from the abdominal cavity (also called **abdominal paracentesis**)	14. **gastroesophageal** (gas-trō-e-sof-a-JĔ-al)	pertaining to the stomach and esophagus
2. **aphagia** (a-FĀ-ja)	condition of without swallowing	15. **gastroscope** (GAS-trō-skōp)	instrument used for visual examination of the stomach (Figure 8.8, *B*)
3. **dysentery** (DIS-en-ter-ē)	painful intestines	16. **gastroscopy** (gas-TROS-ko-pē)	visual examination of the stomach (Figure 8.8, *A*)
4. **dyspepsia** (dis-PEP-sē-a)	condition of difficult digestion	17. **gastrostomy** (gas-TROS-to-mē)	creation of an artificial opening into the stomach
5. **dysphagia** (dis-FĀ-ja)	condition of difficult swallowing	18. **gingivalgia** (jin-ji-VAL-jē-a)	pain in the gums
6. **esophageal** (e-sof-a-JĔ-al)	pertaining to the esophagus	19. **gingivitis** (jin-ji-VĪ-tis)	inflammation of the gums (Figure 8.4)
7. **esophagitis** (e-sof-a-JĪ-tis)	inflammation of the esophagus (Figure 8.6)	20. **glossitis** (glos-Ī-tis)	inflammation of the tongue
8. **gastrectomy** (gas-TREK-to-mē)	excision of the stomach (Figure 8.7)	21. **laparoscope** (LAP-a-rō-skōp)	instrument used for visual examination of the abdominal cavity
9. **gastric** (GAS-trik)	pertaining to the stomach	22. **laparoscopic** (lap-ar-ō-SKOP-ik)	pertaining to visual examination of the abdominal cavity (Figure 8.9)
10. **gastritis** (gas-TRĪ-tis)	inflammation of the stomach	23. **laparoscopy** (lap-a-ROS-ko-pē)	visual examination of the abdominal cavity
11. **gastroenteritis** (gas-trō-en-te-RĪ-tis)	inflammation of the stomach and intestines	24. **laparotomy** (lap-a-ROT-o-mē)	incision into the abdominal cavity
12. **gastroenterologist** (gas-trō-en-ter-OL-o-jist)	physician who studies and treats diseases of the stomach and intestines	25. **oral** (OR-al)	pertaining to the mouth
13. **gastroenterology** (gas-trō-en-ter-OL-o-jē)	study of the stomach and intestines	26. **sublingual** (sub-LING-gwal)	pertaining to under the tongue (Figure 8.5)

EXERCISE B	**Pronounce and Spell Terms Built from Word Parts**

Practice pronunciation and spelling on paper and online.

1. **Practice on Paper**
   a. **Pronounce**: Read the phonetic spelling and say aloud the terms listed in the previous table, Review Terms Built from Word Parts.
   b. **Spell**: Have a study partner read the terms aloud. Write the spelling of the terms on a separate sheet of paper.

2. **Practice Online** ⊕
   a. **Access** online learning resources. Go to evolve.elsevier.com > Evolve Resources > Practice Student Resources.
   b. **Pronounce:** Select Audio Glossary > Lesson 8 > Exercise B. Select a term to hear its pronunciation and repeat aloud.
   c. **Spell:** Select Activities > Lesson 8 > Spell Terms > Exercise B. Select the audio icon and type the correct spelling of the term.

❏ Check the box when complete.

EXERCISE C	**Build and Translate MORE Medical Terms Built from Word Parts**

*Use the **Word Parts Tables** to complete the following questions. Check your responses with the Answer Key in Appendix C.*

1. **LABEL:** *Write the combining forms for anatomic structures of the digestive system on Figure 8.10. These anatomic combining forms will be used to build and translate medical terms in Exercise C.*

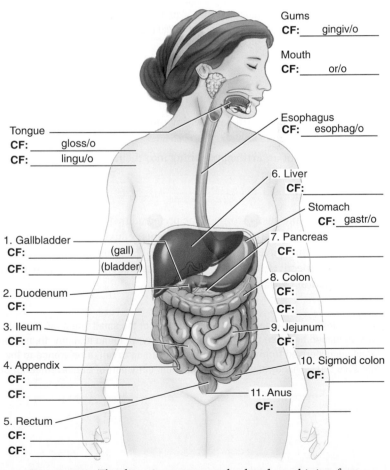

Gums
CF: _____gingiv/o_____

Mouth
CF: _____or/o_____

Esophagus
CF: ___esophag/o___

Tongue
CF: _____gloss/o_____
CF: _____lingu/o_____

6. Liver
   CF: _____

Stomach
CF: ___gastr/o___

1. Gallbladder
   CF: _____ (gall)
   CF: _____ (bladder)

7. Pancreas
   CF: _____

2. Duodenum
   CF: _____

8. Colon
   CF: _____
   CF: _____

3. Ileum
   CF: _____

9. Jejunum
   CF: _____

4. Appendix
   CF: _____
   CF: _____

10. Sigmoid colon
   CF: _____

11. Anus
   CF: _____

5. Rectum
   CF: _____
   CF: _____

Figure 8.10 The digestive system and related combining forms.

2. MATCH: *Draw a line to match the word part with its definition.*

    a. -stomy   visual examination
    b. -al   creation of an artificial opening
    c. -scopy   pertaining to

---

3. TRANSLATE: *Complete the definitions of the following terms by using the meaning of the word parts to fill in the blanks.*

    a. esophag/o/gastr/o/duoden/o/scopy   _____ _____ of the esophagus,

                                 _____, and duodenum

    b. duoden/al   pertaining to the _____

---

4. READ: **Esophagogastroduodenoscopy** (e-sof-a-gō-gas-trō-dū-od-e-NOS-ko-pē), or **EGD**, is used to diagnose peptic ulcers and other conditions of the esophagus, stomach, and duodenum. Peptic ulcers may be found in the stomach and duodenum. They are called **gastric** ulcers and **duodenal** (dū-o-DĒ-nal) ulcers, respectively.

> **FYI**   **Duodenum**, the name for the 1st portion of the small intestine, is derived from the Latin **duodeni**, meaning **12 each**, a reference to its length. It was named in 240 BC by a Greek physician.

---

5. BUILD: *Using the combining form and the word parts reviewed in the previous exercise, build the following terms.*

    a. creation of an artificial opening into the ileum   _____ / o / _____
                                                         wr   **cv**   **s**

    b. creation of an artificial opening into the jejunum   _____ / o / _____
                                                          wr   **cv**   **s**

---

6. READ: While gastrostomy is the preferred method for those who cannot ingest food by mouth, a patient who is at risk of aspiration (stomach contents refluxing up the esophagus and then entering the lungs through the bronchi) may have a **jejunostomy** (je-jū-NOS-te-mē) instead. G-tubes and J-tubes (gastrostomy and jejunostomy, respectively) provide nutrients for patients, while **ileostomy** (il-lē-OS-to-mē) outlets are used for the elimination of waste.

> **FYI**   **Jejunum**, the name for the 2nd portion of the small intestine, is derived from the Latin **jejunus**, meaning **empty**; it was so named because the early anatomists always found it empty. **Ileum**, the name for the 3rd portion of the small intestine, is derived from the Greek **eilein**, meaning **to roll**, a reference to the peristaltic waves that move food along the digestive tract. This term was first used in the early part of the seventeenth century.

7. MATCH: *Draw a line to match the word part with its definition.*

   a. -oma   enlargement
   b. -itis   tumor
   c. -megaly   inflammation

8. TRANSLATE: *Complete the definitions of the following terms built from the combining form **hepat/o**, meaning liver.*

   a. hepat/itis   inflammation of the _____
   b. hepat/oma   _____ of the liver
   c. hepat/o/megaly   _____ of the _____

9. READ: One highly contagious form of **hepatitis** (hep-a-TĪ-tis) is hepatitis A, which is found worldwide but is more common in areas with poor sanitation and low socioeconomic status. A **hepatoma** (hep-a-TŌ-ma) is usually a malignant tumor of the liver; risk factors include hepatitis B and hepatitis C. All forms of hepatitis can cause **hepatomegaly** (hep-a-tō-MEG-a-lē); other causes include alcohol use, metastases from cancer, and heart failure.

10. LABEL: *Write word parts to complete Figure 8.11.*

Figure 8.11 CT scan revealing a _____/_____.
                                  liver   tumor

11. MATCH: *Draw a line to match the word part with its definition.*

   a. -itis   bladder, sac
   b. -ectomy   stone(s), calculus (*pl.* calculi)
   c. cyst/o   excision
   d. lith/o   inflammation

12. TRANSLATE: *Complete the definitions of the following terms built from the combining form chol/e, meaning gall and bile. Hint: The **e** in chol/e/cyst is a combining vowel, and in this textbook it will only be used with the word root **chol**.*

a. chol/e/cyst/itis   _____ of the gallbladder

b. chol/e/cyst/ectomy   excision of the _____

c. chol/e/lith/iasis   condition of gall _____ (s)

> **FYI**   The combining form for gall and bile, **chol/e**, and the combining form for bladder, **cyst/o**, together mean **gallbladder**.

13. READ: The liver, bile ducts, and gallbladder comprise the biliary system, which creates, transports, stores, and releases bile into the small intestine to facilitate the absorption of fat. **Cholelithiasis** (kō-le-li-THĪ-a-sis) may occur when the composition of bile becomes unbalanced or when there is blockage in the bile ducts, trapping the bile and causing it to thicken. Many people have no symptoms with gallstones, but some go on to develop **cholecystitis** (kō-le-sis-TI-tis), which can be very painful and can occasionally lead to rupture of the gallbladder if left untreated. A **cholecystectomy** (kō-le-sis-TEK-to-mē) is the most common treatment for this disease.

> **FYI**   **Cholecystectomy** was first performed in 1882 by a German surgeon. Laparoscopic cholecystectomy was first performed in 1987 in France.

14. LABEL: *Write word parts to complete Figure 8.12.*

Figure 8.12 Abdominal ultrasound showing _____/e/_____/_____.
                                                    gall   stone   condition

15. MATCH: *Draw a line to match the word part with its definition.*

    a. -ic   inflammation

    b. -itis   pertaining to

---

16. BUILD: *Use the combining form **pancreat/o**, meaning pancreas, along with the word parts reviewed in the previous exercise to build the following terms.*

    a. pertaining to the pancreas   _____ / _____

                                                        wr   s

    b. inflammation of the pancreas   _____ / _____

                                                        wr   s

> **FYI** **Pancreas** is derived from the Greek **pan**, meaning **all**, and **krea**, meaning **flesh**. The pancreas was first described in 300 BC. It was so named because of its fleshy appearance.

---

17. READ: The pancreas secretes enzymes necessary for digestion, and also produces insulin, which regulates glucose (sugar) levels in the body. In diabetes mellitus type 1, **pancreatic** (pan-krē-AT-ik) production of insulin is greatly decreased, leading to high glucose levels. **Pancreatitis** (pan-krē-a-TĪ-tis) may be caused by blockage of the common bile duct, excessive alcohol use, cigarette smoking, and a variety of other factors.

---

18. MATCH: *Draw a line to match the word part with its definition.*

    a. -itis   excision

    b. -ectomy   inflammation

---

19. TRANSLATE: *Complete the definitions of the following terms built from the combining forms **append/o** and **appendic/o**, meaning appendix.*

    a. append/ectomy   excision of the _____

    b. appendic/itis   _____ of the _____

---

20. READ: The appendix is a small pouch attached to the cecum (the first part of the large intestine); its function remains unknown. It is susceptible to inflammation and infection, resulting in **appendicitis** (a-pen-di-SĪ-tis). Acute appendicitis is a surgical emergency requiring immediate **appendectomy** (ap-en-DEK-to-mē).

---

21. LABEL: *Write word parts to complete Figure 8.13.*

Figure 8.13 A. Normal appendix.

    B. _____ / _____ .

                appendix   inflammation

A   B

22. MATCH: *Draw a line to match the word part with its definition.*

a. -itis   visual examination
b. -stomy   process of recording, radiographic imaging
c. -ectomy   creation of an artificial opening
d. -graphy   inflammation
e. -scopy   excision

23. BUILD: *Use the combining form **colon/o**, along with the word parts reviewed in the previous exercise, to build terms related to the colon.*

a. visual examination of the colon   _____ / o / _____
                                            wr   cv   s

b. radiographic imaging of the colon   CT _____ / o / _____
   (using a CT scanner and software)   wr   cv   s

24. READ: A common screening method for colon cancer is **colonoscopy** (kō-lon-OS-kō-pē), which allows the gastroenterologist to see lesions directly and biopsy or remove them as indicated. **CT colonography** (C-T) (kō-lon-OG-ra-fē), also called **virtual colonoscopy**, is especially useful in cases where a mass is present that will not allow a colonoscope to pass through; the radiologist can visualize the colon beyond the lesion.

25. LABEL: *Write word parts to complete Figure 8.14.*

Figure 8.14   Image of the large intestine produced by CT _____ / o / _____.
                                                              colon   radiographic imaging

26. BUILD: *Now use the combining form **col/o**, along with the word parts reviewed in the previous matching exercise, to build more terms related to the colon.*

a. inflammation of the colon   _____ / _____
                                            wr   s

b. creation of an artificial opening into the colon _____ / o / _____
                                            wr   cv   s

c. excision of the colon   _____ / _____
                                            wr   s

27. READ: Antibiotic-associated **colitis** (kō-LĪ-tis), which is caused by a bacterium called *Clostridium difficile* *(C. difficile)*, was traditionally found in hospitalized patients; however, it is also now occurring more frequently in the general community. It is usually treated with medicines, but in severe cases, a partial **colectomy** (kō-LEK-to-mē) may be required. If needed, a **colostomy** (ko-LOS-to-mē) may be created to allow the passage of stool.

28. LABEL: *Write word parts to complete Figure 8.15.*

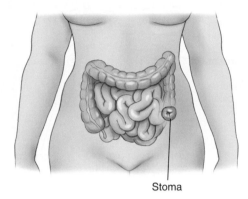

Stoma

Figure 8.15 _____/o/_____ following a partial colectomy.

                   colon   creation of an artifical opening

29. MATCH: *Draw a line to match the word part with its definition.*

    a. -scopy   instrument used for visual examination
    b. -cele   visual examination
    c. -al   pertaining to
    d. -scope   hernia, protrusion

30. TRANSLATE: *Complete the definitions of the following terms.*

    a. sigmoid/o/scopy   visual _____ of the sigmoid _____
    b. proct/o/scope   _____ used for visual examination of the rectum
    c. proct/o/scopy   visual examination of the _____

31. READ: Sigmoidoscopy (sig-moy-DOS-ko-pē) visualizes the rectum and sigmoid colon and stops at the transverse colon. Because it is less involved than colonoscopy, less anesthesia is required for this procedure. In cases of rectal bleeding, a **proctoscope** (PROK-tō-skōp) may be used to examine the rectum just inside the anus. **Proctoscopy** (prok-TOS-ko-pē) is a useful method for diagnosing internal hemorrhoids and anal fissures.

32. LABEL: *Write word parts to complete Figure 8.16.*

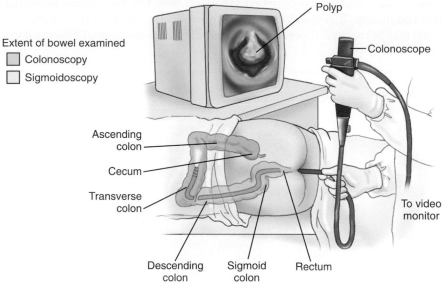

Polyp

Extent of bowel examined
- [ ] Colonoscopy
- [ ] Sigmoidoscopy

Colonoscope

Ascending colon

Cecum

Transverse colon

To video monitor

Descending colon

Sigmoid colon

Rectum

Figure 8.16 _____ /o/_____ and colonoscopy showing a polyp in
                sigmoid colon   visual examination
the transverse colon.

---

33. BUILD: *Use the combining form* **rect/o**, *along with the word parts reviewed in the previous exercise, to build terms related to the rectum.*

a. hernia of the rectum   _____ / o / _____
                                           wr   cv   s

b. pertaining to the rectum   _____ / _____
                                           wr   s

---

34. TRANSLATE: *Complete the definition.*

an/al   _____ to the _____

---

35. READ: **Rectocele** (REK-tō-sēl), also called **posterior prolapse**, occurs when the thin layer of tissue between the vagina and the anterior **rectal** (REK-tal) wall weakens (such as after childbirth or with chronic constipation), causing the rectum to bulge into the vagina. Chronic constipation can also cause **anal** (Ā-nal) fissures, which are tiny tears that are often accompanied by pain and bleeding with bowel movements.

36. **REVIEW OF MORE DIGESTIVE SYSTEM TERMS BUILT FROM WORD PARTS:** *The following is an alphabetical list of terms built and translated in the previous exercises.*

MEDICAL TERMS BUILT FROM WORD PARTS

TERM	DEFINITION	TERM	DEFINITION
1. **anal** (Ā-nal)	pertaining to the anus	13. **esophagogastroduo-denoscopy (EGD)** (e-sof-a-gō-gas-trō-dū-od-e-NOS- ko-pē)	visual examination of the esophagus, stomach, and duodenum
2. **appendectomy** (ap-en-DEK-to-mē)	excision of the appendix	14. **hepatitis** (hep-a-TĪ-tis)	inflammation of the liver
3. **appendicitis** (a-pen-di-SĪ-tis)	inflammation of the appendix (Figure 8.13, *B*)	15. **hepatoma** (hep-a-TŌ-ma)	tumor of the liver (Figure 8.11)
4. **cholecystectomy** (kō-le-sis-TEK-to-mē)	excision of the gallbladder	16. **hepatomegaly** (hep-a-tō-MEG-a-lē)	enlargement of the liver
5. **cholecystitis** (kō-le-sis-TĪ-tis)	inflammation of the gallbladder	17. **ileostomy** (il-lē-OS-to-mē)	creation of an artificial opening into the ileum
6. **cholelithiasis** (kō-le-li-THĪ-a-sis)	condition of gallstone(s) (Figure 8.12)	18. **jejunostomy** (je-jū-NOS-te-mē)	creation of an artificial opening into the jejunum
7. **colectomy** (kō-LEK-to-mē)	excision of the colon	19. **pancreatic** (pan-krē-AT-ik)	pertaining to the pancreas
8. **colitis** (kō-LĪ-tis)	inflammation of the colon	20. **pancreatitis** (pan-krē-a-TĪ-tis)	inflammation of the pancreas
9. **colonoscopy** (kō-lon-OS-kō-pē)	visual examination of the colon	21. **proctoscope** (PROK-tō-skōp)	instrument used for visual examination of the rectum
10. **colostomy** (ko-LOS-to-mē)	creation of an artificial opening into the colon (Figure 8.15)	22. **proctoscopy** (prok-TOS-ko-pē)	visual examination of the rectum
11. **CT colonography (CTC)** (C-T) (kō-lon-OG-ra-fē)	radiographic imaging of the colon (using a CT scanner and software); (also called **virtual colonoscopy**) (Figure 8.14)	23. **rectal** (REK-tal)	pertaining to the rectum
12. **duodenal** (dū-o-DĒ-nal)	pertaining to the duodenum	24. **rectocele** (REK-tō-sēl)	hernia of the rectum (also called **posterior prolapse**)
		25. **sigmoidoscopy** (sig-moy-DOS-ko-pē)	visual examination of the sigmoid colon (Figure 8.16)

EXERCISE D   **Pronounce and Spell MORE Terms Built from Word Parts**

Practice pronunciation and spelling on paper and online.

1. | Practice on Paper |
   a. **Pronounce**: Read the phonetic spelling and say aloud the terms listed in the previous table, Review of MORE Terms Built from Word Parts.
   b. **Spell**: Have a study partner read the terms aloud. Write the spelling of the terms on a separate sheet of paper.

2. | Practice Online ⊕ |
   a. **Access** online learning resources. Go to evolve.elsevier.com > Evolve Resources > Practice Student Resources.
   b. **Pronounce:** Select Audio Glossary > Lesson 8 > Exercise D. Select a term to hear its pronunciation and repeat aloud.
   c. **Spell:** Select Activities > Lesson 8 > Spell Terms > Exercise D. Select the audio icon and type the correct spelling of the term.

❏   Check the box when complete.

  OBJECTIVE 2

Define, pronounce, and spell medical terms NOT built from word parts.

The terms listed below may contain word parts, but are difficult to translate literally.

MEDICAL TERMS NOT BUILT FROM WORD PARTS	
TERM	**DEFINITION**
1. bariatric surgery (bar-ē-AT-trik) (SUR-jer-ē)	surgical reduction of gastric capacity to treat morbid obesity, a condition that can cause serious illness
FYI **Bariatric** contains the word roots **bar**, meaning **weight**, and **iatr**, meaning **treatment**.	
2. barium enema (BE) (BAR-ē-um) (EN-e-ma)	diagnostic procedure in which a series of radiographic images is taken of the large intestine after the rectal administration of the contrast agent barium; (also called **lower GI series**)
3. celiac disease (SĒ-lē-ak) (di-ZĒZ)	malabsorption syndrome caused by an immune reaction to gluten (a protein in wheat, rye, and barley); it may damage the lining of the small intestine, which is responsible for absorption of food into the bloodstream; (also called **gluten enteropathy**)
4. cirrhosis (sir-RŌ-sis)	chronic disease of the liver with gradual destruction of cells and formation of scar tissue; commonly caused by alcoholism and certain types of viral hepatitis
5. constipation (kon-sti-PĀ-shun)	infrequent or difficult evacuation of stool
6. Crohn disease (krōn) (di-ZĒZ)	chronic inflammation of the intestinal tract, usually affecting the ileum and colon; characterized by cobblestone ulcerations and the formation of scar tissue that may lead to intestinal obstruction

Continued

MEDICAL TERMS NOT BUILT FROM WORD PARTS—cont'd

TERM	DEFINITION
7. diarrhea (dī-a-RĒ-a)	frequent discharge of liquid stool
8. endoscopic retrograde cholangiopancreatography (ERCP) (en-dō-SKOP-ic) (RET-rō-grād) (kō-lan-jē-ō-pan-krē-a-TOG-rah-fē)	endoscopic procedure involving radiographic imaging of the biliary ducts and pancreatic ducts

FYI | The **angi/o** in cholangiopancreatography refers not to blood vessels, but to bile ducts.

TERM	DEFINITION
9. gastroesophageal reflux disease (GERD) (gas-trō-e-sof-a-JĒ-al) (RĒ-fluks) (di-ZĒZ)	disorder characterized by the abnormal backward flow of the gastrointestinal contents into the esophagus
10. hemorrhoids (HEM-o-roydz)	swollen or distended veins in the rectal area, which may be internal or external and can be a source of rectal bleeding and pain
11. irritable bowel syndrome (IBS) (IR-i-ta-bl) (BOW-el) (SIN-drōm)	periodic disturbances of bowel function, such as diarrhea and/or constipation, usually associated with abdominal pain
12. parenteral (pah-REN-ter-al)	pertaining to treatment other than through the digestive system
13. peptic ulcer (PEP-tik) (UL-ser)	erosion of the mucous membrane of the stomach or duodenum associated with increased secretion of acid from the stomach, bacterial infection (*Helicobacter pylori*), or use of nonsteroidal antiinflammatory drugs (often referred to as **gastric** or **duodenal ulcer**, depending on its location)
14. polyp (POL-ip)	tumorlike growth extending outward from a mucous membrane
15. stoma (STŌ-ma)	surgical opening between an organ and the surface of the body, such as the opening established in the abdominal wall by colostomy, ileostomy, or a similar operation
16. ulcerative colitis (UC) (UL-ser-a-tiv) (kō-LĪ-tis)	disease characterized by inflammation of the colon with the formation of ulcers, which can cause bloody diarrhea
17. upper GI series (UGI series) (UP-er) (G-Ī) (SĒR-ēz)	diagnostic procedure in which a series of radiographic images is taken of the pharynx, esophagus, stomach, and duodenum after oral administration of the contrast agent barium

EXERCISE E **Label**

Write the medical terms pictured and defined using the previous table of Medical Terms NOT Built from Word Parts.
Check your work with the Answer Key in Appendix C.

1. _____

endoscopic procedure involving radiographic
imaging of the biliary ducts and pancreatic ducts

2. _____

erosion of the mucous membrane of the stomach
or duodenum

3. _____

disorder characterized by the abnormal backward
flow of the gastrointestinal contents into the
esophagus

4. _____

diagnostic procedure in which a series of
radiographic images is taken of the large intestine
after the rectal administration of the contrast
agent barium

5. _____

tumorlike growth extending outward from a mucous membrane

6. _____

surgical opening between an organ and the surface of the body.

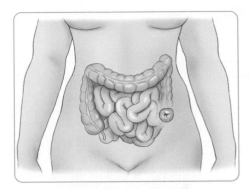

7. _____

surgical reduction of gastric capacity to treat morbid obesity, a condition that can cause serious illness

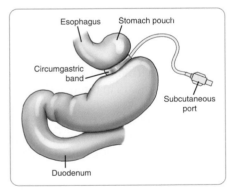

8. _____

swollen or distended veins in the rectal area

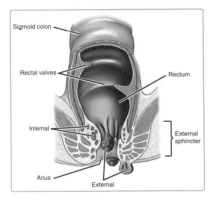

9. _____

chronic disease of the liver with gradual destruction of cells and formation of scar tissue

10. _____

periodic disturbances of bowel function, such as diarrhea and/or constipation, usually associated with abdominal pain

---

EXERCISE F **Match**

Match the terms in the first column with their correct descriptions in the second column.

_____ **1.** parenteral

_____ **2.** celiac disease

_____ **3.** Crohn disease

_____ **4.** ulcerative colitis

_____ **5.** diarrhea

_____ **6.** constipation

_____ **7.** upper GI series

a. malabsorption syndrome caused by an immune reaction to gluten

b. infrequent or difficult evacuation of stool

c. pertaining to treatment other than through the digestive system

d. frequent discharge of liquid stool

e. disease characterized by inflammation of the colon with the formation of ulcers, which can cause bloody diarrhea

f. series of radiographic images of the pharynx, esophagus, stomach, and duodenum after oral administration of the contrast agent barium

g. chronic inflammation of the intestinal tract, usually affecting the ileum and colon

---

EXERCISE G **Learn Medical Terms NOT Built from Word Parts**

Fill in the blanks with medical terms defined in bold using the Medical Terms NOT Built from Word Parts table. Answers are listed in Appendix C.

1. The **disorder characterized by the abnormal backward flow of the gastrointestinal contents into the esophagus**, or _____, abbreviated as _____, causes heartburn and the gradual breakdown of the mucous barrier of the esophagus.

2. Periodic disturbances of bowel function, usually associated with abdominal pain, or _____ _____, abbreviated as _____, can be of three different types: **infrequent or difficult evacuation of stool** _____ type (IBS-C), **frequent discharge of liquid stool** _____ type (IBS-D), or mixed-type IBS with alternating constipation and diarrhea.

3. A **tumorlike growth extending outward from a mucous membrane**, or _____, may be diagnosed from the results of a **series of radiographic images taken after the rectal administration of a contrast agent** _____. Polyps are usually benign and are commonly found in the intestines as well as in the nose and throat.

4. Abdominal sonography is commonly used to visualize organs such as the liver, gallbladder, bile ducts, and pancreas. While not as frequently used for diagnosis, **endoscopic procedure involving radiographic imaging of the biliary ducts and pancreatic ducts**, or _____ _____, abbreviated ERCP, is an excellent method for treating abnormalities of the biliary and pancreatic ducts, including the removal of stones.

5. Bloody diarrhea is the main symptom of **inflammation of the colon with the formation of ulcers** _____, abbreviated UC. UC is usually resolved with a colectomy and with the creation of a **surgical opening between an organ and the surface of the body**, or _____. **Chronic inflammation of the intestinal tract usually affecting the ileum and colon and characterized by cobblestone ulcerations and the formation of scar tissue that may lead to intestinal obstruction**, or _____, can actually occur anywhere in the gastrointestinal tract and can only be controlled, not cured.

6. Chronic alcoholism is a cause of **chronic disease of the liver with gradual destruction of cells and formation of scar tissue**, or _____. The amount of alcohol that causes this disease is different for every person.

7. A(n) **erosion of the mucous membrane of the stomach or duodenum**, or _____, may be diagnosed by a **series of radiographic images taken of the pharynx, esophagus, stomach, and duodenum after the oral administration of the contrast agent barium**, or _____.

8. **Malabsorption syndrome caused by an immune reaction to gluten, which may damage the lining of the small intestine that is responsible for absorption of food into the bloodstream**, or _____, is caused by an interaction among genes, gluten intake, and environment. In very severe cases, patients may require **pertaining to treatment other than through the digestive system**, or _____, fluid replacement and nutritional support.

9. **Surgical reduction of gastric capacity to treat morbid obesity**, or _____, may be performed to treat patients with morbid obesity (BMI greater than 40) or those with a lower BMI and serious medical conditions. During surgery, a small stomach pouch is created for the purpose of restricting the amount of food an individual can eat.

10. Chronic constipation, straining during bowel movements, and pregnancy can increase pressure in the anal vessels, resulting in the formation of **swollen or distended veins in the rectal area**, or _____.

EXERCISE H   Pronounce and Spell Terms NOT Built from Word Parts

Practice pronunciation and spelling on paper and online.

1. Practice on Paper

    a. Pronounce: Read the phonetic spelling and say aloud the terms listed in the previous table, Medical Terms NOT Built from Word Parts.

    b. Spell: Have a study partner read the terms aloud. Write the spelling of the terms on a separate sheet of paper.

2. Practice Online 🌐

    a. Access online learning resources. Go to evolve.elsevier.com > Evolve Resources > Practice Student Resources.

    b. Pronounce: Select Audio Glossary > Lesson 8 > Exercise H. Select a term to hear its pronunciation and repeat aloud.

    c. Spell: Select Activities > Lesson 8 > Spell Terms > Exercise H. Select the audio icon and type the correct spelling of the term.

❏   Check the box when complete.

OBJECTIVE 3

Write abbreviations.

ABBREVIATIONS RELATED TO THE DIGESTIVE SYSTEM

Use the online **flashcards** to familiarize yourself with the following abbreviations.

ABBREVIATION	TERM	ABBREVIATION	TERM
BE	barium enema	GI	gastrointestinal
BM	bowel movement	IBS	irritable bowel syndrome
CTC	computed tomography colonography	PEG	percutaneous endoscopic gastrostomy
EGD	esophagogastroduodenoscopy	TPN	total parenteral nutrition
ERCP	endoscopic retrograde cholangiopancreatography	UC	ulcerative colitis
GERD	gastroesophageal reflux disease	UGI series	upper GI series

EXERCISE I   Abbreviate Medical Terms

Write the correct abbreviation next to its medical term.

1. Diseases and Disorders:

    a. _____   gastroesophageal reflux disease

    b. _____   irritable bowel syndrome

    c. _____   ulcerative colitis

2. Diagnostic Tests and Equipment:

a. _____ barium enema

b. _____ esophagogastroduodenoscopy

c. _____ endoscopic retrograde cholangiopancreatography

d. _____ upper GI series

e. _____ computed tomography colonography

3. Surgical Procedures:

_____ percutaneous endoscopic gastrostomy

4. Related Terms:

a. _____ bowel movement

b. _____ gastrointestinal

c. _____ total parenteral nutrition

OBJECTIVE 4

Identify medical terms by clinical category.

Now that you have worked through the digestive system lesson, review and practice medical terms grouped by clinical category. Categories include signs and symptoms, diseases and disorders, diagnostic tests and equipment, surgical procedures, specialties and professions, and other terms related to the digestive system.

EXERCISE J   Signs and Symptoms

Write the medical terms for signs and symptoms next to their definitions.

1. _____ condition of without swallowing

2. _____ infrequent or difficult evacuation of stool

3. _____ frequent discharge of liquid stool

4. _____ condition of difficult digestion

5. _____ condition of difficult swallowing

6. _____ pain in the gums

7. _____ enlargement of the liver

EXERCISE K   Diseases and Disorders

Write the medical terms for diseases and disorders next to their definitions.

1. _____ inflammation of the appendix

2. _____ inflammation of the gallbladder

3. _____ condition of gallstone(s)

4. _____ inflammation of the colon

5. _____ chronic inflammation of the intestinal tract usually affecting the ileum and colon; characterized by cobblestone ulcerations and the formation of scar tissue that may lead to intestinal obstruction

6. _____ painful intestines

7. _____ inflammation of the esophagus

8. _____ inflammation of the stomach

9. _____ inflammation of the stomach and intestines

10. _____ disorder characterized by the abnormal backward flow of the gastrointestinal contents into the esophagus
   _____

11. _____ inflammation of the gums

12. _____ inflammation of the tongue

13. _____ swollen or distended veins in the rectal area, which may be internal or external and can be a source of rectal bleeding and pain

14. _____ inflammation of the liver

15. _____ tumor of the liver

16. _____ malabsorption syndrome caused by an immune reaction to gluten; it may damage the lining of the small intestine, which is responsible for absorption of food into the bloodstream

17. _____ periodic disturbances of bowel function, such as diarrhea and/or constipation, usually associated with abdominal pain

18. _____ inflammation of the pancreas

19. _____ erosion of the mucous membrane of the stomach or duodenum associated with increased secretion of acid from the stomach, bacterial infection (*Helicobacter pylori*), or use of nonsteroidal antiinflammatory drugs

20. _____ tumorlike growth extending outward from a mucous membrane

21. _____ hernia of the rectum

22. _____ disease characterized by inflammation of the colon with the formation of ulcers, which can cause bloody diarrhea

23. _____ chronic disease of the liver with gradual destruction of cells and formation of scar tissue; commonly caused by alcoholism and certain types of viral hepatitis

EXERCISE L   **Diagnostic Tests and Equipment**

Write the medical terms for diagnostic tests and equipment next to their definitions.

1. _____ diagnostic procedure in which a series of radiographic images is taken of the large intestine after the rectal administration of the contrast agent

2. _____ visual examination of the colon

3. CT _____ radiographic imaging of the colon (using a CT scanner and software)

4. _____ endoscopic procedure involving radiographic imaging of the biliary ducts and pancreatic ducts

5. _____ visual examination of the esophagus, stomach, and duodenum

6. _____ instrument used for visual examination of the stomach

7. _____ visual examination of the stomach

8. _____ instrument used for visual examination of the abdominal cavity

9. _____ pertaining to visual examination of the abdominal cavity

10. _____ visual examination of the abdominal cavity

11. _____ instrument used for visual examination of the rectum

12. _____ visual examination of the rectum

13. _____ visual examination of the sigmoid colon

14. _____ diagnostic procedure in which a series of radiographic images is taken of the pharynx, esophagus, stomach, and duodenum after oral administration of the contrast agent barium

EXERCISE M   **Surgical Procedures**

Write the medical terms for surgical procedures next to their definitions.

1. _____ surgical puncture to remove fluid from the abdominal cavity

2. _____ excision of the appendix

3. _____ surgical reduction of gastric capacity to treat morbid obesity, a condition that can cause serious illness

4. _____ excision of the gallbladder

5. _____ excision of the colon

6. _____ creation of an artificial opening into the colon

7. _____ excision of the stomach

8. _____ creation of an artificial opening into the stomach

9. _____ creation of an artificial opening into the ileum

10. _____ creation of an artificial opening into the jejunum

11. _____ incision into the abdominal cavity

EXERCISE N   Specialties and Professions

Write the medical terms for specialties and professions next to their definitions.

1. _____ physician who studies and treats diseases of the stomach and intestines

2. _____ study of the stomach and intestines

EXERCISE O   Medical Terms Related to the Digestive System

Write the medical terms related to the digestive system next to their definitions.

1. _____ pertaining to the anus

2. _____ pertaining to the duodenum

3. _____ pertaining to the esophagus

4. _____ pertaining to the stomach

5. _____ pertaining to the stomach and esophagus

6. _____ pertaining to the mouth

7. _____ pertaining to the pancreas

8. _____ pertaining to the rectum

9. _____ pertaining to under the tongue

10. _____ pertaining to treatment other than through the digestive system

11. _____ surgical opening between an organ and the surface of the body

OBJECTIVE 5

Use medical language in clinical statements, the case study, and a medical record.

Check responses for the following exercises in Appendix C.

EXERCISE P   Use Medical Terms in Clinical Statements

Circle the medical terms and abbreviations defined in the bolded phrases. For pronunciation practice, read the answers aloud.

1. The patient came to the hospital with epigastric pain, fat intolerance, and jaundice. The physician ordered abdominal sonography, which confirmed a diagnosis of **inflammation of the gallbladder** (cholecystitis, cholelithiasis, hepatitis). The patient was scheduled for exploratory **visual examination of the abdominal cavity** (sigmoidoscopy, laparoscopy, colonoscopy) with the understanding that **excision of the gallbladder** (gastrectomy, abdominocentesis, cholecystectomy) would be performed if necessary.

2. A(n) **creation of an artificial opening into the stomach** (jejunostomy, ileostomy, gastrostomy) was performed to feed a patient diagnosed with a cancerous **pertaining to the esophagus** (esophageal, gastroesophageal, duodenal) tumor.

3. A(n) **visual examination of the esophagus, stomach, and duodenum** (endoscopic retrograde cholangiopancreatography, esophagogastroduodenoscopy, abdominal ultrasonography) is performed by a **physician who studies and treats diseases of the stomach and intestines** (gastroenterologist, hepatologist, urologist) to diagnose **erosion of the mucous membrane of the stomach or duodenum** (ulcerative colitis, dysentery, peptic ulcer).

4. **Enlarged liver** (Hepatitis, Hepatomegaly, Hepatoma) may be associated with **inflammation of the liver** (hepatitis, hepatomegaly, hepatoma), **tumor of the liver** (hepatitis, hepatomegaly, hepatoma), **chronic disease of the liver with gradual destruction of cells and formation of scar tissue** (celiac disease, cirrhosis, Crohn disease), fatty liver, or even normal pregnancy.

5. Symptoms of chronic **disorder characterized by the abnormal backward flow of the gastrointestinal contents into the esophagus** (GERD, ERCP, EGD) are often caused by dysfunction of the **pertaining to the stomach and esophagus** (esophageal, gastroesophageal, ileocecal) sphincter. Symptoms may include condition of **difficult swallowing** (dyspepsia, dysentery, dysphagia), **inflammation of the esophagus** (gastritis, esophagitis, pancreatitis), and bleeding.

6. Dentists and dental hygienists treat disorders related to the **pertaining to the mouth** (oral, rectal, anal) cavity. They check for **inflammation of the gums** (gingivitis, gingivalgia, stomatitis) and **inflammation of the tongue** (gingivitis, glossitis, gastroenteritis), and examine the **pertaining to under the tongue** (subcostal, sublingual, subcutaneous) surface, looking for oral cancer or other abnormalities.

7. **Disease characterized by inflammation of the colon with the formation of ulcers** (Crohn disease, Peptic ulcers, Ulcerative colitis) does not affect the small intestine. For those with severe disease a **total excision of the colon** (appendectomy, colectomy, cholecystectomy), with the **creation of an artificial opening into the ileum** (ileostomy, jejunostomy, colostomy), is a permanent cure.

EXERCISE Q   **Apply Medical Terms to the Case Study**

Think back to Ruth Clifton, who was introduced in the case study at the beginning of the lesson. After working through Lesson 8 on the digestive system, consider the medical terms that might be used to describe her experience. List two terms relevant to the case study and their meanings. ■

Medical Term   Definition

1. _____   _____

2. _____   _____

EXERCISE R   **Use Medical Terms in a Document**

Ms. Clifton made an appointment with a gastroenterologist. He recommended an endoscopic procedure; the report is documented in the following medical record.

Use the definitions in numbers 1-9 to write medical terms within the document on the next page.

1. difficult digestion

2. visual examination of the esophagus, stomach, and duodenum

3. pertaining to within a vein

4. pertaining to a side

5. instrument used for visual examination of the stomach

6. pertaining to the stomach

7. pertaining to away

8. inflammation of the stomach

9. pertaining to the duodenum

Refer to the medical record to answer questions 10-12.

10. In the history section of the medical document, there are some terms that you may not have seen before. One of them is **hematemesis.** The suffix -**emesis** means **vomiting.** Use your knowledge of word parts to translate **hemat/emesis.**

    hemat/o means: _____

    -**emesis** means: _____

    Remembering that the definition usually starts with the meaning of the suffix, **hematemesis** is defined as

    _____.

```
┌─────────────────────────────────────────────────────────────────┐
│ 038721 CLIFTON, Ruth                                     _ □ ✕    │
│ File    Patient    Navigate    Custom Fields    Help              │
│  ‹  ›  👤 👥 ▯ ▮ ▤ ⬠ Rx ⏰ ⊘ ✂ ▯ ⊠ ▦ ✔ ⊙ 🔍 ?                    │
│ Chart Review │ Encounters │ Notes │ Labs │ Imaging │ Procedures │ Rx │ Documents │ Referrals │ Scheduling │ Billing │
│ Name: CLIFTON, Ruth        MR#: 038721      Sex: F    │ Allergies: None Known           │
│                            DOB: 9/15/19XX   Age: 40   │ PCP: Steinburge, Daniel DO      │
├─────────────────────────────────────────────────────────────────┤
```

Endoscopy Report:
Date: 12 December 20XX 10:15

History of Present Illness: A 40-year-old woman was referred to the endoscopy
clinic for evaluation. Patient reports nausea and vomiting with upper abdominal pain.
She complains of (1.)_____ but denies hematemesis.
She denies using alcohol or salicylates. The medications she states she is taking are not
known for ulcerogenic side effects.

Procedure: (2.)_____: The patient was
given 2 mg of (3.)_____ Versed along with lidocaine spray to
the pharynx. After the patient was placed in the left (4.)_____
position, the (5.)_____was passed into the pharynx
without difficulty. No evidence of reflux. The stomach was entered and some
(6.)_____ juices were aspirated. The esophagus, cardia, and body
of the stomach were free of abnormalities. A biopsy of the gastric mucosa was taken
for *H. pylori.* In the (7.)_____ antral area some mild
erythematous changes were noted. The pylorus had normal peristaltic activity. In the
first part of the duodenum, however, a single 1 cm ulceration of the proximal duodenum
was observed. The second part of the duodenum was free of mucosal abnormalities.
Withdrawing the scope confirmed the findings upon entry. The patient tolerated the
procedure quite well and recovered uneventfully.

Vital signs will be taken every half hour for the next 2 hours.

Postprocedural Diagnosis:

(8.) _____

(9.)_____ ulcer

Electronically signed: Garcia, Jesus MD on 12 December 20XX 11:02

```
│ Start │ Log On/Off │ Print │ Edit │                    🖨 ◁ ⌕ 🖨  │
└─────────────────────────────────────────────────────────────────┘
```

> **FYI**   -emesis can be used as a suffix, as noted above in **hematemesis**, or as in **hyperemesis** (excessive vomiting).
> **Emesis** can also be used as a stand-alone term, such as "the patient complained of nausea and emesis." In each case,
> the term **emesis** comes from the Greek **emein** meaning **to vomit**.

11. Another term in the history is ulcer/o/genic. Ulcerogenic means _____ ulcers.

12. Identify two new medical terms in the medical record you would like to investigate. Use your medical dictionary or an online resource to look up the definition.

Medical Term	Definition
1. _____	_____
2. _____	_____

EXERCISE S   Use Medical Language in Electronic Health Records Online

Select the correct medical terms to complete three medical records in one patient's electronic file.

🌐 Access online resources at evolve.elsevier.com > Evolve Resources > Practice Student Resources > Activities > Lesson 8 > Electronic Health Records

Topic: Partial Bowel Obstruction
Record 1: Office Visit
Record 2: Radiology Report
Record 3: Colonoscopy Report

❏   Check the box when complete.

OBJECTIVE 6

Recall and assess knowledge of word parts, medical terms, and abbreviations.

EXERCISE T   Online Review of Lesson Content

🌐 *Recall and assess your learning from working through the lesson by completing online learning activities at evolve. elsevier.com > Evolve Resources > Student Resources.*

❏   Check the box when complete.

EXERCISE U   Lesson Content Quiz

Test your knowledge of the terms and abbreviations introduced in this lesson. Circle the letter for the medical term or abbreviation related to the words in italics.

1. A patient diagnosed with *gallstones* has:
   a. cholelithiasis
   b. cholecystitis
   c. colitis

2. Symptoms of bloody diarrhea, abdominal pain and cramping, and fatigue may be associated with *disease characterized by inflammation of the colon with the formation of ulcers, which can cause bloody diarrhea.*
   a. UC
   b. IBS
   c. GERD

3. *Surgical reduction of gastric capacity to treat morbid obesity, a condition that can cause serious illness* may be necessary in some patients with morbid obesity, especially if it is associated with hypertension or diabetes.
   a. abdominocentesis
   b. bariatric surgery
   c. laparoscopy

4. *Difficult swallowing* may be a complication of Parkinson disease.
   a. dysphagia
   b. aphagia
   c. dyspepsia

5. Eating very spicy food may lead to *inflammation of the tongue*.
   a. gingivitis
   b. pancreatitis
   c. glossitis

6. *Inflammation of the stomach* may have some symptoms that are similar to peptic ulcers; a(n) *instrument used for visual examination of the stomach* may help differentiate between the two diseases.
   a. gastroesophageal reflux disease; laparoscope
   b. gastritis; gastroscope
   c. gastroenteritis; proctoscope

7. A *creation of an artificial opening into the colon* may be necessary if there is blockage proximal to the *pertaining to the rectum* portion of the colon.
   a. colonoscopy; oral
   b. colostomy; rectal
   c. colectomy; anal

8. *Malabsorption syndrome caused by an immune reaction to gluten* is considered a multisystem disorder with varying signs and symptoms, including abdominal bloating and pain, chronic diarrhea or constipation, steatorrhea (excessive fat in the stool), vomiting, weight loss, fatigue, and iron deficiency anemia.
   a. Crohn disease
   b. dysentery
   c. celiac disease

9. *Visual examination of the esophagus, stomach, and duodenum* may be performed to diagnose *disorder characterized by the abnormal backward flow of the gastrointestinal contents into the esophagus*.
   a. EGD; GERD
   b. ERCP; IBS
   c. BE; PEG

10. *Enlargement of the liver* may be due to hepatitis, fatty liver, or biliary disease.
    a. hemorrhoids
    b. hepatoma
    c. hepatomegaly

11. As part of the workup for her frequent heartburn, Mrs. Patel was scheduled for a(n) *diagnostic procedure in which a series of radiographic images is taken of the pharynx, esophagus, stomach, and duodenum after oral administration of the contrast agent barium*.
    a. upper GI series
    b. CT colonography
    c. barium enema

12. For *pertaining to under the tongue* administration of nitroglycerin, used to treat chest pain, the tablet is placed under the tongue to dissolve and absorb into the bloodstream through the tissue.
    a. gastric
    b. sublingual
    c. gastroesophageal

LESSON AT A GLANCE DIGESTIVE SYSTEM WORD PARTS

COMBINING FORMS			SUFFIX
abdomin/o	enter/o	lingu/o	-algia
an/o	esophag/o	or/o	
append/o	gastr/o	pancreat/o	
appendic/o	gingiv/o	peps/o	
chol/e	gloss/o	phag/o	
col/o	hepat/o	proct/o	
colon/o	ile/o	rect/o	
duoden/o	jejun/o	sigmoid/o	
	lapar/o		

LESSON AT A GLANCE   DIGESTIVE SYSTEM MEDICAL TERMS AND ABBREVIATIONS

SIGNS AND SYMPTOMS
aphagia
constipation
diarrhea
dyspepsia
dysphagia
gingivalgia
hepatomegaly

DISEASES AND DISORDERS
appendicitis
celiac disease
cholecystitis
cholelithiasis
cirrhosis
colitis
Crohn disease
dysentery
esophagitis
gastritis
gastroenteritis
gastroesophageal reflux disease
   (GERD)
gingivitis
glossitis
hemorrhoids
hepatitis
hepatoma
irritable bowel syndrome (IBS)
pancreatitis

peptic ulcer
polyp
rectocele
ulcerative colitis (UC)

DIAGNOSTIC TESTS AND EQUIPMENT
barium enema (BE)
colonoscopy
CT colonography (CTC)
endoscopic retrograde
   cholangiopancreatography (ERCP)
esophagogastroduodenoscopy (EGD)
gastroscope
gastroscopy
laparoscope
laparoscopic
laparoscopy
proctoscope
proctoscopy
sigmoidoscopy
upper GI series (UGI series)

SURGICAL PROCEDURES
abdominocentesis
appendectomy
bariatric surgery
cholecystectomy
colectomy
colostomy

gastrectomy
gastrostomy
ileostomy
jejunostomy
laparotomy

SPECIALTIES AND PROFESSIONS
gastroenterologist
gastroenterology

RELATED TERMS
anal
duodenal
esophageal
gastric
gastroesophageal
oral
pancreatic
parenteral
rectal
stoma
sublingual

ABBREVIATIONS
BE	ERCP	PEG
BM	GERD	TPN
CTC	GI	UC
EGD	IBS	UGI series

Eye and Ear

CASE STUDY **Javier Berjarano**

Javier moved into an assisted living community 6 months ago. He is doing well, but lately he notices that he can't see or hear as well as he used to. He isn't really sure when it started, but now he can't see details on the TV, even when he wears his glasses. Everything looks kind of cloudy. He also keeps trying to turn up the volume, but his neighbors get mad because it is too loud even though he can barely hear it. His right ear is really itchy, like when he was a kid with all those ear infections. He wonders if all these eye and ear problems are just from getting older. His daughter comes to visit and decides he needs to get this checked out. She schedules appointments for him with an eye doctor and an ear doctor.

■ *Consider Javier's situation as you work through the lesson on the eye and ear. We will return to this case study and identify medical terms used to describe and document his experiences.*

OBJECTIVES

1 ■ Build, translate, pronounce, and spell medical terms built from word parts (p. 275).

2 ■ Define, pronounce, and spell medical terms NOT built from word parts (p. 287).

3 ■ Write abbreviations (p. 292).

4 ■ Identify medical terms by clinical category (p. 292).

5 ■ Use medical language in clinical statements, the case study, and a medical record (p. 295).

6 ■ Recall and assess knowledge of word parts, medical terms, and abbreviations (p. 298).

INTRODUCTION TO THE EYE AND THE EAR

Anatomic Structures of the Eye	
choroid (KŌR-oid)	middle layer of the eye containing many blood vessels
cornea (KŌR-nē-a)	transparent anterior part of the sclera that lies over the iris and pupil
iris (Ī-ris)	pigmented muscular structure that regulates the amount of light entering the eye by controlling the size of the pupil
lens (lenz)	lies directly behind the pupil; focuses and bends light
optic nerve (OP-tik) (nurv)	carries visual images from the retina to the brain
pupil (PŪ-pil)	opening through which light passes in the center of the iris

Continued

Anatomic Structures of the Eye—cont'd

retina (RET-i-nah)	innermost layer of the eye; contains the vision receptors
sclera (SKLER-ah)	outer protective layer of the eye (also called **white of the eye**)

Function of the Eye

- Vision

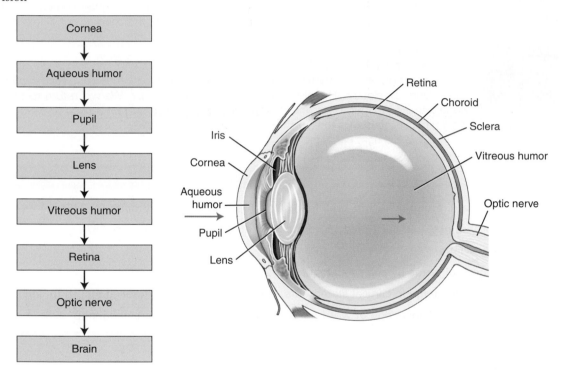

Figure 9.1 Pathway of light.

Anatomic Structures of the Ear

auricle (pinna) (AW-ri-kl), (PIN-a)	external, visible part of the ear located on both sides of the head; directs sound waves to the external auditory canal
cochlea (KŌK-lē-ah)	coiled portion of the inner ear that contains the organ for hearing
eustachian tube (yū-STĀ-shan) (toob)	passage between the middle ear and the pharynx; equalizes air pressure on both sides of the tympanic membrane
FYI **Eustachian tube** is named for Bartolomeo Eustachi, a sixteenth century Italian anatomist, who described the structure. Eustachian, an eponym, is often not capitalized because of its common usage.	
external auditory canal (ek-STER-nal) (AW-di-tor-ē) (kah-NAL)	short tube ending at the tympanic membrane (also called **external auditory meatus**)

Continued

Anatomic Structures of the Ear—cont'd

outer ear (OU-ter) (ēr)	consists of the auricle and external auditory canal (also called **external ear**)
inner ear (labyrinth) (IN-ar) (ēr), (LAB-e-rinth)	bony spaces within the temporal bone of the skull that contain the cochlea, the semicircular canals, and vestibule. The cochlea facilitates hearing. The semicircular canals and vestibule facilitate equilibrium and balance.
middle ear (MID-l) (ēr)	consists of the tympanic membrane, eustachian tube, and ossicles
ossicles (OS-i-kalz)	bones of the middle ear (stapes, incus, and malleus) that carry sound vibrations
tympanic membrane (eardrum) (tim-PAN-ik) (MEM-brān), (ĒR-drum)	semitransparent membrane that separates the external auditory canal (meatus) and the middle ear cavity; transmits sound vibrations to the ossicles

Functions of the Ear

- Hearing
- Sense of balance

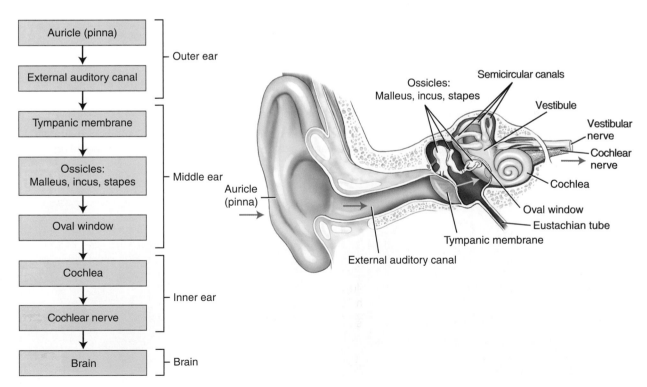

Figure 9.2 Perception of sound.

How the Eye and the Ear Work

The eye and the ear are organs of the sensory system, which communicates outside stimuli to the brain for interpretation. In addition to vision and hearing, the sensory system communicates information regarding pain, touch, pressure, taste, and other sensations.

The eye is the organ of vision. Light first passes through the **cornea.** The **iris** regulates the amount of light entering the eye by controlling **pupil** size. The **lens** lies behind the pupil and focuses the light projected onto the **retina**. The cornea and lens are the main structures responsible for refraction, which is the ability of the eye to focus images on the retina. The **optic nerve** transmits the image from the retina to the brain, where it is interpreted. The **sclera,** which appears white, forms the outer protective layer of the eye. Cavities within the eye are filled with transparent fluids, called humors, that maintain the shape of the eye. The eyebrows, eyelids, and eyelashes are accessory structures of the eye.

The ear, which is the organ of hearing and balance, is made up of three parts: the **external ear,** the **middle ear,** and the **inner ear**. The process of hearing begins as sound waves, directed by the **auricles,** enter the **external auditory canal.** As the sound waves ripple through the external ear, the **tympanic membrane** vibrates. The **ossicles** in the middle ear carry the vibration to the inner ear, where the stimulus is transmitted by the cochlear nerve to the brain where it is interpreted as sound. Balance is a function of the **inner ear** and is maintained through a series of complex processes. The vestibular nerve transmits information about motion and body position from the semicircular canals and the vestibule to the brain for interpretation.

CAREER FOCUS | Professionals Who Work with the Eye and Ear

- **Ophthalmic medical technicians** are supervised by ophthalmologists and perform a variety of clinical and administrative duties, including taking patient medical histories, providing patient instruction, performing vision and diagnostic tests, scheduling appointments, and other clerical tasks.

- **Opticians** are specialists who generally work closely with optometrists to fill prescriptions for lenses. They provide fitting for glasses and contact lenses and often have administrative duties, including answering phones, scheduling appointments, and processing payments.

- **Audiology technicians** are supervised by audiologists and perform a variety of clinical and administrative duties, including performing hearing tests, fitting hearing aids, providing patient instruction, scheduling appointments, and other clerical tasks.

Figure 9.3 An optician fitting glasses.

Figure 9.4 An audiology technician fits a hearing aid for a patient.

OBJECTIVE 1

Build, translate, pronounce, and spell medical terms built from word parts.

WORD PARTS Use the paper or online **flashcards** to familiarize yourself with the following word parts.

COMBINING FORM (WR + CV)	DEFINITION	COMBINING FORM (WR + CV)	DEFINITION
EYE		**EAR**	
blephar/o	eyelid	**audi/o**	hearing
ir/o, irid/o	iris	**myring/o**	eardrum (tympanic membrane)
kerat/o	cornea (also means hard, horny tissue)	**ot/o**	ear
		tympan/o	middle ear
ophthalm/o	eye		
opt/o	vision		
retin/o	retina		
scler/o	sclera		
SUFFIX (S)	DEFINITION	SUFFIX (S)	DEFINITION
-metry	measurement	**-ptosis**	drooping, sagging, prolapse
-plegia	paralysis		

FYI In Greek mythology, **Iris** was the special messenger of the queen of heaven. She passed from heaven to earth over the rainbow while dressed in rainbow hues. Her name was applied to the circular eye muscle because of its varied colors.

WORD PARTS PRESENTED IN PREVIOUS LESSONS		Used to Build Terms for the Eye and Ear	
COMBINING FORM (WR + CV)	DEFINITION	COMBINING FORM (WR + CV)	DEFINITION
laryng/o	larynx (voice box)		
SUFFIX (S)	DEFINITION	SUFFIX (S)	DEFINITION
-al, -ic	pertaining to	**-meter**	instrument used to measure
-ectomy	surgical removal, excision	**-plasty**	surgical repair
-itis	inflammation	**-scope**	instrument used for visual examination
-logist	one who studies and treats (specialist, physician)		
-logy	study of	**-tomy**	cut into, incision

Refer to Appendix A, Word Parts Used in *Basic Medical Language*, for alphabetical lists of word parts and their meanings.

EXERCISE A Build and Translate Terms Built from Word Parts

Use the **Word Parts Tables** to complete the following questions. Check your responses with the Answer Key in Appendix C.

1. LABEL: Write the combining forms for anatomic structures of the eye on Figure 9.5. These anatomic combining forms will be used to build and translate medical terms in Exercise A.

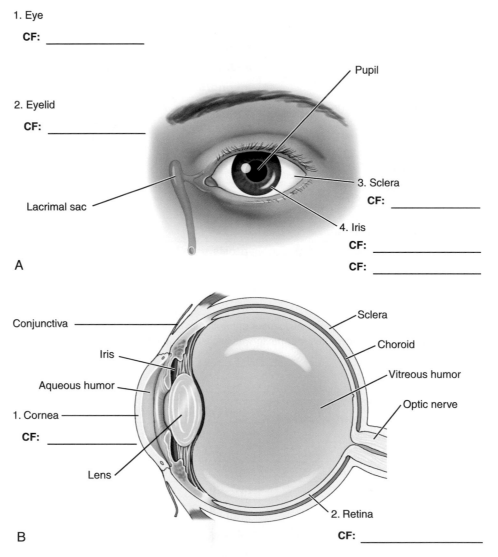

1. Eye

    CF: _____

2. Eyelid

    CF: _____

Pupil

Lacrimal sac

3. Sclera

    CF: _____

4. Iris

    CF: _____

    CF: _____

A

Conjunctiva

Iris

Aqueous humor

1. Cornea

    CF: _____

Lens

Sclera

Choroid

Vitreous humor

Optic nerve

2. Retina

    CF: _____

B

Figure 9.5 Anatomy of the eye. **A.** Anterior view. **B.** Lateral view.

2. MATCH: *Draw a line to match the suffix with its definition.*

    a. -logy   instrument used for visual examination
    b. -scope   instrument used to measure
    c. -logist   study of
    d. -meter   inflammation
    e. -itis   one who studies and treats (specialist, physician)

---

3. BUILD: *Using the combining form **ophthalm/o**, build the following terms. Remember, the definition usually starts with the meaning of the suffix.*

    a. study of the eye   _____/ o /_____
                                                   wr   cv   s

    b. physician who studies and treats diseases of the eye   _____/ o /_____
                                                     wr   cv   s

---

4. TRANSLATE: *Complete the definitions of the following diagnostic terms. Remember, the definition usually starts with the meaning of the suffix.*

    a. ophthalm/o/scope   _____ used for visual examination of the _____
    b. kerat/o/meter   instrument used to _____ (the curvature of) the _____

> **FYI** Look carefully at the spelling of **ophthalm.** Note that it is **o-ph-thalm.** Often this word is misspelled by omitting the first *h.* Think of the pronunciation of the word part beginning with **o-ph,** which sounds like the word **off,** followed by the **th** sound of **thalm.**

---

5. LABEL: *Write word parts to complete Figure 9.6.*

Figure 9.6 **A.** Visual examination of the eye. **B.** _____/o/_____.
                                               eye   instrument used for visual examination
           C. Ophthalmoscopic view of the retina.

6. READ: **Ophthalmology** (of-thal-MOL-o-jē), abbreviated **Ophth**, is the branch of medicine specializing in the study of diseases and disorders of the eye. An **ophthalmologist** (of-thal-MOL-o-jist) is a medical doctor specializing in eye and vision care. In addition to diagnosing and treating diseases and disorders of the eye, ophthalmologists provide a wide range of services, including performing eye surgery and prescribing corrective lenses. An **ophthalmoscope** (of-THAL-mō-skōp) is used to direct light into the eye and examine the retina, blood vessels, and other structures. A **keratometer** (ker-a-TOM-e-ter), also called an ophthalmometer, gives information about the curvature of the cornea and is used in the fitting of contact lenses.

7. TRANSLATE: *Complete the definitions of the following terms describing inflammation of structures of the eye.*

a. blephar/itis   _____ of the _____

b. ir/itis   inflammation of the _____

c. retin/itis   inflammation of the _____

d. scler/itis   inflammation of the _____

8. LABEL: *Write word parts to complete Figure 9.7.*

Figure 9.7 Types of inflammation. **A.** _____/_____. **B.** _____/_____.
                                          sclera   inflammation   eyelid   inflammation

9. **Blepharitis** (blef-a-RĪ-tis), often caused by bacteria, is an irritating condition accompanied by erythema (redness), crusted eyelashes, itchiness, and a burning sensation. **Iritis** (ī-RĪ-tis), **retinitis** (ret-i-NĪ-tis), and **scleritis** (skle-RĪ-tis) are more serious conditions that can lead to vision loss. Iritis has several causes, including injury, bacterial and fungal infections, and underlying autoimmune disorders. Cytomegalovirus (CMV) retinitis can lead to the destruction of the retina, resulting in blindness. Scleritis, a painful inflammatory disease, may be associated with other systemic conditions such as rheumatoid arthritis.

10. MATCH: *Draw a line to match the suffix with its definition.*

a. -ptosis   excision

b. -plegia   surgical repair

c. -ectomy   drooping, sagging, prolapse

d. -plasty   paralysis

11. **BUILD:** *Build the following terms using suffixes indicating surgical procedures.*

a. excision of (a portion of) the iris (*Hint:* Use the combining form for iris with a "d" in it.)

    _____ / _____
           wr   s

b. surgical repair of the eyelid

    _____ / o / _____
           wr   cv   s

c. surgical repair of the cornea

    _____ / o / _____
           wr   cv   s

12. **TRANSLATE:** *Complete the definitions of the following terms by using the meaning of word parts to fill in the blanks.*

a. irid/o/plegia   _____ of the _____

b. blephar/o/ptosis (*Hint:* Use the definition for the suffix that begins with a "d.")   _____ of the _____

13. **LABEL:** *Write word parts to complete Figure 9.8.*

Figure 9.8 Congenital _____ / o / _____.
                        eyelid   drooping

14. **READ:** **Blepharoptosis** (blef-ar-op-TŌ-sis), also called **ptosis,** may be unilateral, affecting one eyelid, or bilateral, affecting both eyelids. Blepharoptosis is most often seen in older adults, though it may be congenital (present at birth) and impair normal vision development in children. **Blepharoplasty** (BLEF-a-rō-plas-tē) may be performed to correct blepharoptosis and to restore vision. In **iridoplegia** (ir-i-dō-PLĒ-ja)**,** the pupil size does not change in response to a change in light. Paralysis of the iris may be due to injury, inflammation, or use of pupil-dilating drops used for an eye exam. **Iridectomy** (ir-i-DEK-to-mē) is a surgical procedure used to treat closed-angle glaucoma and melanoma of the iris. **Keratoplasty** (KER-a-tō-plas-tē) is a surgical procedure performed for several reasons, including corneal transplants, excision of corneal lesions, and repair of refraction errors such as myopia (nearsightedness) and hyperopia (farsightedness).

> **FYI** **Refraction** refers to how the anterior surface of the eye and the lens bend light to focus on the retina for visual perception. **Refraction errors,** which primarily cause blurry vision, may occur as a result of the shape of the eye, curvature of the cornea, and shape or age of the lens. Common refraction errors include **myopia, hyperopia, astigmatism,** and **presbyopia**. Corrective lenses and surgery are used to treat visual impairments.

15. MATCH: *Draw a line to match the combining form or suffix with its definition.*

    a. -al, -ic   measurement
    b. -metry   vision
    c. opt/o   pertaining to

16. BUILD: *Write word parts to build the following terms. (Hint: Use the suffix ending in "c" for pertaining to.)*

    a. measurement of vision   _____ / o / _____
                                           wr   cv   s

    b. pertaining to vision   _____ / _____
                                          wr   s

    c. pertaining to the eye   _____ / _____
                                          wr   s

17. TRANSLATE: *Complete the definitions of the following terms built with the suffix –al.*

    a. scler/al   _____ to the _____
    b. retin/al   _____ to the _____

18. READ: **Optometry** (op-TOM-e-trē) is a healthcare profession that provides primary vision care. **Optic** (OP-tik) and **ophthalmic** (of-THAL-mik) are adjectives used to describe nouns related to vision and to the eye, respectively. Examples include optic nerve and ophthalmic exam. **Scleral** (SKLE-ral) buckling is a surgical procedure used to repair **retinal** (RET-i-nal) detachment.

19. REVIEW OF EYE TERMS BUILT FROM WORD PARTS: *The following is an alphabetical list of terms built and translated in the previous exercises.*

MEDICAL TERMS BUILT FROM WORD PARTS

TERM	DEFINITION	TERM	DEFINITION
1. blepharitis (blef-a-RĪ-tis)	inflammation of the eyelid (Figure 9.7, *B*)	**4. iridectomy** (ir-i-DEK-to-mē)	excision of (a portion of) the iris
2. blepharoplasty (BLEF-a-rō-plas-tē)	surgical repair of the eyelid	**5. iridoplegia** (ir-i-dō-PLĒ-ja)	paralysis of the iris
3. blepharoptosis (blef-ar-op-TŌ-sis)	drooping of the eyelid (also called **ptosis**) (Figure 9.8)	**6. iritis** (ī-RĪ-tis)	inflammation of the iris

Continued

MEDICAL TERMS BUILT FROM WORD PARTS—cont'd

TERM	DEFINITION	TERM	DEFINITION
7. **keratometer** (ker-a-TOM-e-ter)	instrument used to measure (the curvature of) the cornea; (also called **ophthalmometer**)	13. **optic** (OP-tik)	pertaining to vision
8. **keratoplasty** (KER-a-tō-plas-tē)	surgical repair of the cornea	14. **optometry** (op-TOM-e-trē)	measurement of vision
9. **ophthalmic** (of-THAL-mik)	pertaining to the eye	15. **retinal** (RET-i-nal)	pertaining to the retina
10. **ophthalmologist** (of-thal-MOL-o-jist)	physician who studies and treats diseases of the eye	16. **retinitis** (ret-i-NĪ-tis)	inflammation of the retina
11. **ophthalmology (Ophth)** (of-thal-MOL-o-jē)	study of the eye	17. **scleral** (SKLE-ral)	pertaining to the sclera
12. **ophthalmoscope** (of-THAL-mō-skōp)	instrument used for visual examination of the eye (Figure 9.6, *B*)	18. **scleritis** (skle-RĪ-tis)	inflammation of the sclera (Figure 9.7, *A*)

EXERCISE B   Pronounce and Spell Terms Built from Word Parts

Practice pronunciation and spelling on paper and online.

1. **Practice on Paper**
   a. **Pronounce**: Read the phonetic spelling and say aloud the terms listed in the previous table, Review of Eye Terms Built from Word Parts.
   b. **Spell**: Have a study partner read the terms aloud. Write the spelling of the terms on a separate sheet of paper.

2. **Practice Online** 🌐
   a. **Access** online learning resources. Go to evolve.elsevier.com > Evolve Resources > Practice Student Resources.
   b. **Pronounce**: Select Audio Glossary > Lesson 9 > Exercise B. Select a term to hear its pronunciation and repeat aloud.
   c. **Spell**: Select Activities > Lesson 9 > Spell Terms > Exercise B. Select the audio icon and type the correct spelling of the term.

❏ Check the box when complete.

EXERCISE C   Build and Translate MORE Medical Terms Built from Word Parts

1. LABEL: *Write the combining forms for anatomic structures of the ear on Figure 9.9. These anatomic combining forms will be used to build and translate medical terms in Exercise C.*

1. Ear CF: _____

Figure 9.9 Anatomy of the ear.

2. MATCH: *Draw a line to match the suffix with its definition.*

    a. -rrhea   instrument used for visual examination
    b. -plasty   flow, discharge
    c. -scope   inflammation
    d. -itis   surgical repair

3. TRANSLATE: *Complete the definitions of the following terms built from the combining form **ot/o**, meaning ear.*

    a. ot/o/rrhea *(Hint: Use the*   _____ from the _____
        definition that starts with
        a "d" for the suffix.)

    b. ot/o/scope   _____ used for visual _____

                           of the _____

    c. ot/o/plasty   _____ _____ of the (outer) ear

4. LABEL: *Write word parts to complete Figure 9.10.*

Figure 9.10 Visual examination of the ear with

an _____ /o/ _____ .

      ear   instrument used for visual examination

5. BUILD: *Using word parts, build the following terms describing inflammation of structures of the ear.*

  a. inflammation of the ear   _____ / _____

                                            wr   s

  b. inflammation of the eardrum   _____ / _____

                                            wr   s

6. READ: **Otorrhea** (ō-tō-RĒ-a) refers to discharge from the ear as seen with **otitis** (ō-TĪ-tis) media, an infection of the middle ear. **Myringitis** (mir-in-JĪ-tis) is associated with acute otitis media and refers to the inflammation of the eardrum. An **otoscope** (Ō-tō-skōp) is useful for detecting inflammation of the eardrum and auditory canal. **Otoplasty** (Ō-tō-plas-tē) is a surgical procedure to reshape the outer ear (auricle).

7. LABEL: *Write word parts to complete Figure 9.11.*

Figure 9.11 **A.** Healthy eardrum (tympanic membrane).

           B. Eardrum with acute _____ / _____ media.

                           ear   inflammation

8. MATCH: *Draw a line to match the word part with its definition.*

a. -ic   surgical repair
b. -tomy   incision
c. -plasty   pertaining to
d. -logy   larynx (voice box)
e. -logist   study of
f. laryng/o   one who studies and treats (specialist, physician)

---

9. BUILD: *Write word parts to build the following terms using the combining form **tympan/o**, meaning middle ear.*

a. pertaining to the middle ear   _____ / _____
                                              wr   s

b. surgical repair of the middle ear   _____ /_o_/_____
                                              wr   cv   s

---

10. TRANSLATE: *Complete the definitions of the following terms built from the combining form **myring/o**, meaning eardrum.*

a. myring/o/tomy   _____ of the _____
b. myring/o/plasty   surgical _____ of the _____

---

11. READ: Tympanic (tim-PAN-ik) is an adjective used to describe a noun, as in tympanic membrane (a membrane of the middle ear called the eardrum). **Tympanoplasty** (TIM-pa-nō-plas-tē) involves surgery of the middle ear; it repairs the eardrum, but may also repair the ossicles. **Myringoplasty** (mi-RING-gō-plas-tē) is a less complicated surgical procedure to repair a perforated eardrum. Many practitioners use these terms interchangeably. **Myringotomy** (mir-ing-GOT-o-mē) is a surgical procedure that can be used to place a tube through the eardrum to help drain fluid from the middle ear with the goal of reducing ear infections.

---

12. LABEL: *Write word parts to complete Figure 9.12.*

Figure 9.12 _____ /o/_____
                eardrum   incision
is performed to release pus from the middle ear through the tympanic membrane to treat acute otitis media.

13. BUILD: *Write word parts to build the following terms using ot/o, meaning ear.*

a. study of the ear, (nose), and the larynx (throat) _____ / o / _____ / o / _____
                                                         wr   cv   wr   cv   s

b. physician who studies and treats diseases of _____ / o / _____ / o / _____
   the ear, (nose), and the larynx (throat)   wr   cv   wr   cv   s

14. Otolaryngology (ō-tō-lar-ing-GOL-o-jē) is the medical specialty dedicated to medical and surgical treatment of the head and neck, including the ear, nose, and throat **(ENT).** Surgical procedures on structures of the ear are performed by an **otolaryngologist** (ō-tō-lar-ing-GOL-o-jist). Otolaryngologists are referred to as ENT physicians or, more simply, ENTs.

> **FYI** The terms **otolaryngology** and **otolaryngologist** are shortened versions of the terms **otorhinolaryngology** and **otorhinolaryngologist**. In the longer versions, reference to the ear, nose, and throat can be more clearly seen with the inclusion of the corresponding combining forms: **ot/o** (ear), **rhin/o** (nose), and **laryng/o** (larynx/throat).

15. MATCH: *Draw a line to match the word part with its definition.*

a. audi/o   measurement
b. -logy   one who studies and treats (specialist, physician)
c. -logist   instrument used to measure
d. -meter   hearing
e. -metry   study of

16. TRANSLATE: *Complete the definitions of the following terms using the combining form **audi/o**.*

a. audi/o/logy   _____ of _____

b. audi/o/logist   specialist who _____ and _____ (impaired) _____

c. audi/o/meter   _____ used to _____ _____

d. audi/o/metry   _____ of _____

17. READ: Audiology (aw-dē-OL-o-jē) is a healthcare profession dedicated to diagnosing and treating hearing disorders. An **audiologist** (aw-dē-OL-o-jist) measures hearing using an **audiometer** (aw-dē-OM-e-ter) and other equipment. **Audiometry** (aw-dē-OM-e-trē) results are graphed, showing hearing deficits according to loudness and tonal frequency.

18. LABEL: *Write word parts to complete Figure 9.13.*

Figure 9.13 _____ /o/ _____.
            hearing   instrument used to measure

---

19. REVIEW OF EAR TERMS BUILT FROM WORD PARTS: *The following is an alphabetical list of terms built and translated in the previous exercises.*

MEDICAL TERMS BUILT FROM WORD PARTS

TERM	DEFINITION	TERM	DEFINITION
1. audiologist (aw-dē-OL-o-jist)	specialist who studies and treats (impaired) hearing	**9. otoplasty** (Ō-tō-plas-tē)	surgical repair of the (outer) ear
2. audiology (aw-dē-OL-o-jē)	study of hearing	**10. otolaryngologist (ENT)** (ō-tō-lar-ing-GOL-o-jist)	physician who studies and treats diseases of the ear, (nose), and larynx (throat)
3. audiometer (aw-dē-OM-e-ter)	instrument used to measure hearing (Figure 9.13)	**11. otolaryngology** (ō-tō-lar-ing-GOL-o-jē)	study of the ear, (nose), and larynx (throat)
4. audiometry (aw-dē-OM-e-trē)	measurement of hearing	**12. otorrhea** (ō-tō-RĒ-a)	discharge from the ear
5. myringitis (mir-in-JĪ-tis)	inflammation of the eardrum	**13. otoscope** (Ō-tō-skōp)	instrument used for visual examination of the ear (Figure 9.10)
6. myringoplasty (mi-RING-gō-plas-tē)	surgical repair of the eardrum	**14. tympanic** (tim-PAN-ik)	pertaining to the middle ear
7. myringotomy (mir-ing-GOT-o-mē)	incision into the eardrum (Figure 9.12)	**15. tympanoplasty** (TIM-pa-nō-plas-tē)	surgical repair of the middle ear
8. otitis (ō-TĪ-tis)	inflammation of the ear (Figure 9.11, *B*)		

EXERCISE D **Pronounce and Spell MORE Terms Built from Word Parts**

Practice pronunciation and spelling on paper and online.

1. **Practice on Paper**

   a. **Pronounce**: Read the phonetic spelling and say aloud the terms listed in the previous table, Review of Ear Terms Built from Word Parts.

   b. **Spell**: Have a study partner read the terms aloud. Write the spelling of the terms on a separate sheet of paper.

2. **Practice Online** 🌐

   a. **Access** online learning resources. Go to evolve.elsevier.com > Evolve Resources > Practice Student Resources.

   b. **Pronounce**: Select Audio Glossary > Lesson 9 > Exercise D. Select a term to hear its pronunciation and repeat aloud.

   c. **Spell**: Select Activities > Lesson 9 > Spell Terms > Exercise D. Select the audio icon and type the correct spelling of the term.

   ❑ Check the box when complete.

OBJECTIVE 2

Define, pronounce, and spell medical terms NOT built from word parts.

The terms listed below may contain word parts, but are difficult to translate literally.

MEDICAL TERMS NOT BUILT FROM WORD PARTS

TERM	DEFINITION
1. **astigmatism (AST)** (a-STIG-ma-tizm)	irregular curvature of the refractive surfaces of the eye (cornea or lens); causes blurry vision (Figure 9.14, *C*)
2. **cataract** (KAT-a-rakt)	clouding of the lens of the eye

FYI **Cataracts** are the gradual development of cloudiness within the lenses of the eyes, not a film over the eye, as commonly thought. They usually occur in both eyes. Most cataracts develop in persons aged 50 years or older and are caused by degenerative changes.

3. **glaucoma** (glaw-KŌ-ma)	eye disorder characterized by optic nerve damage usually caused by an abnormal increase of intraocular pressure
4. **hyperopia** (*hī*-per-Ō-pē-a)	farsightedness (Figure 9.14, *B*)
5. **LASIK** (LĀ-sik)	laser procedure that reshapes the corneal tissue beneath the surface of the cornea; LASIK is an acronym composed of the first letters of words in the term **laser-assisted in situ keratomileusis**
6. **macular degeneration** (MAC-ū-lar) (dē-gen-e-RĀ-shun)	progressive deterioration of the central portion of the retina, resulting in a loss of central vision; when caused by the aging process, it is referred to as age-related macular degeneration and is abbreviated as **AMD**

Continued

MEDICAL TERMS NOT BUILT FROM WORD PARTS—cont'd

TERM	DEFINITION
7. **myopia** (mī-Ō-pē-a)	nearsightedness (Figure 9.14, *A*)
8. **optometrist** (op-TOM-e-trist)	healthcare professional who performs eye exams, administers vision tests, and prescribes corrective lenses. Optometrists are state-licensed healthcare professionals who have earned doctorate degrees (OD).
9. **otitis media (OM)** (ō-TĪ-tis) (MĒ-dē-a)	inflammation of the middle ear
10. **presbycusis** (pres-bē-KŪ-sis)	hearing impairment occurring with age
11. **presbyopia** (pres-bē-Ō-pē-a)	vision impairment occurring with age
12. **retinal detachment** (RET-in-al) (dē-TACH-ment)	separation of the retina from the choroid in the posterior portion of the eye, resulting in a disruption of vision that may be permanent if treatment is delayed; onset may be gradual or sudden and is not painful
13. **tinnitus** (TIN-i-tus)	ringing in the ears

FYI   The pronunciation of **tinnitus** varies. While healthcare professionals pronounce it as (TIN-i-tus), often the general population uses the alternate pronunciation (tin-NĪ-tus), as though the term ends with the suffix -itis.

A. Myopia (nearsightedness).   **B.** Hyperopia (farsightedness).   **C.** Astigmatism.

Figure 9.14 Refractive errors result from an imbalance in the focusing structures of the eye. In myopia (A), distant targets are focused in front of the retina, while near objects can be seen clearly. In hyperopia (B), near objects are focused behind the retina, while distant targets are clear. In astigmatism (C), the cornea or lens has an abnormal shape, causing blurred vision at all distances.

EXERCISE E **Label**

Write the medical terms pictured and defined using the previous table of Medical Terms NOT Built from Word Parts. Check your work with the Answer Key in Appendix C.

1. _____
   clouding of the lens of the eye

2. _____
   separation of the retina from the choroid in the posterior portion of the eye

3. _____
   progressive deterioration of the central portion of the retina, resulting in loss of central vision

4. _____
   laser procedure that reshapes the corneal tissue beneath the surface of the cornea

Flap of cornea

5. _____
   healthcare professional who performs eye exams, administers vision tests, and prescribes corrective lenses

6. _____
   ringing in the ears

7. a. _____   b. _____
     vision impairment occurring with age   hearing impairment occurring with age

---

EXERCISE F   Match

Match the terms in the first column with their correct descriptions in the second column. Answers are listed in Appendix C.

_____ **1.** glaucoma
_____ **2.** hyperopia
_____ **3.** astigmatism
_____ **4.** myopia
_____ **5.** otitis media

a. irregular curvature of the refractive surfaces of the eye
b. nearsightedness
c. inflammation of the middle ear
d. farsightedness
e. usually caused by an abnormal increase of intraocular pressure

---

EXERCISE G   Learn Medical Terms NOT Built from Word Parts

Fill in the blanks with medical terms defined in bold using the Medical Terms NOT Built from Word Parts table. Check responses in Appendix C.

1. A **laser procedure that reshapes corneal tissue**, or _____, is used to correct **irregular curvature of the refractive surfaces of the eye**, or _____. **Farsightedness**, or _____, and **nearsightedness**, or _____, can also be corrected using this technique.

2. **Eye disorder usually caused by abnormally increased intraocular pressure,** or _____, leads to atrophy of the optic nerve and results in blindness. Early treatment is essential because loss of vision from this condition cannot be regained.

3. **Clouding of the lens of the eye,** or a(n) _____, is most commonly caused by the deterioration of the lens as a result of the aging process. Surgery may be advised if visual impairment is significant. A **healthcare professional who performs eye exams, administers vision tests, and prescribes corrective lenses,** or a(n) _____, may assist after surgery with a change in the prescription for eyeglasses for the patient.

4. A distortion of central vision may be an early symptom of **a progressive deterioration of the central portion of the retina, resulting in a loss of central vision,** or _____. Although there is no known cure, **AMD,** or _____ macular degeneration, may be treated with anti-VEGF injections, photodynamic therapy, and laser surgery.

5. **Separation of the retina from the choroid,** or _____, is a medical emergency that can result in permanent vision loss if not treated quickly. Usually, a tear in the retina causes fluid to leak, pulling it away from supporting tissue.

6. A myringotomy may be performed in a severe case of **inflammation of the middle ear,** or _____ _____, to release pus accumulated behind the tympanic membrane.

7. A common symptom of diseases and conditions of the ear is **ringing in the ears,** or _____, and warrants further examination by a healthcare professional.

8. **Vision impairment occurring with age**, or _____, usually becomes noticeable as a person reaches the mid to late 40s. **Hearing impairment occurring with age**, or _____ _____, usually presents as bilateral hearing loss after the age of 50.

EXERCISE H   **Pronounce and Spell Terms NOT Built from Word Parts**

Practice pronunciation and spelling on paper and online.

1. **Practice on Paper**
   a. **Pronounce**: Read the phonetic spelling and say aloud the terms listed in the previous table, Medical Terms NOT Built from Word Parts.
   b. **Spell**: Have a study partner read the terms aloud. Write the spelling of the terms on a separate sheet of paper.

2. **Practice Online** ⊕
   a. **Access** online learning resources. Go to evolve.elsevier.com > Evolve Resources > Practice Student Resources.
   b. **Pronounce**: Select Audio Glossary > Lesson 9 > Exercise H. Select a term to hear its pronunciation and repeat aloud.
   c. **Spell**: Select Activities > Lesson 9 > Spell Terms > Exercise H. Select the audio icon and type the correct spelling of the term.

❏   Check the box when complete.

OBJECTIVE 3

Write abbreviations.

ABBREVIATIONS RELATED TO THE EYE AND EAR

Use the online **flashcards** to familiarize yourself with the following abbreviations.

ABBREVIATION	TERM	ABBREVIATION	TERM
AMD	age-related macular degeneration	**IOP**	intraocular pressure
AST	astigmatism	**OM**	otitis media
ENT	ear, nose, and throat; otolaryngologist	**Ophth**	ophthalmology
HOH	hard of hearing	**VA**	visual acuity

EXERCISE I   Abbreviate Medical Terms

Write the correct abbreviation next to its medical term. Abbreviations may be used twice.

1. Signs and Symptoms:

   a. _____ intraocular pressure

   b. _____ hard of hearing

2. Diseases and Disorders:

   a. _____ otitis media

   b. _____ astigmatism

   c. _____ age-related macular degeneration

3. Diagnostic Test:

   _____ visual acuity

4. Specialties and Professions:

   a. _____ ophthalmology

   b. _____ otolaryngologist

5. Related:

   _____ ears, nose, and throat

 OBJECTIVE 4

Identify medical terms by clinical category.

Now that you have worked through the lesson on the eye and the ear, review and practice medical terms grouped by clinical category. Categories include signs and symptoms, diseases and disorders, diagnostic tests and equipment, surgical procedures, specialties and professions, and other terms related to the eye and ear. Check your responses with the Answer Key in Appendix C.

EXERCISE J   Signs and Symptoms

Write the medical terms for signs and symptoms next to their definitions.

1. _____ discharge from the ear

2. _____ ringing in the ears

Diseases and Disorders

Write the medical terms for diseases and disorders next to their definitions.

1. _____ irregular curvature of the refractive surfaces of the eye (cornea or lens)

2. _____ inflammation of the middle ear

3. _____ nearsightedness

4. _____ farsightedness

5. _____ clouding of the lens of the eye

6. _____ progressive deterioration of the central portion of the retina, resulting in loss of central vision

7. _____ separation of the retina from the choroid in the posterior portion of the eye, resulting in a disruption of vision

8. _____ eye disorder characterized by optic nerve damage usually caused by an increase of intraocular pressure

9. _____ hearing impairment occurring with age

10. _____ vision impairment occurring with age

11. _____ inflammation of the eyelid

12. _____ drooping of the eyelid

13. _____ paralysis of the iris

14. _____ inflammation of the iris

15. _____ inflammation of the sclera

16. _____ inflammation of the retina

17. _____ inflammation of the eardrum

18. _____ inflammation of the ear

Diagnostic Tests and Equipment

Write the medical terms for diagnostic tests and equipment next to their definitions.

1. _____ instrument used for visual examination of the eye

2. _____ instrument used to measure (the curvature of) the cornea

3. _____ instrument used to measure hearing

4. _____ instrument used for visual examination of the ear

5. _____ measurement of hearing

EXERCISE M   Surgical Procedures

Write the medical terms for surgical procedures next to their definitions.

1. _____   surgical repair of the eyelid

2. _____   excision of (a portion of) the iris

3. _____   surgical repair of the cornea

4. _____   laser procedure that reshapes the corneal tissue beneath the surface of the cornea

5. _____   surgical repair of the eardrum

6. _____   incision into the eardrum

7. _____   surgical repair of the (outer) ear

8. _____   surgical repair of the middle ear

EXERCISE N   Specialties and Professions

Write the medical terms for specialties and professions next to their definitions.

1. _____   physician who studies and treats diseases of the eye

2. _____   study of the eye

3. _____   measurement of vision

4. _____   healthcare professional who performs eye exams, administers vision tests, and prescribes corrective lenses

5. _____   specialist who studies and treats impaired hearing

6. _____   study of hearing

7. _____   physician who studies and treats diseases of the ear, (nose), and the larynx (throat)

8. _____   study of the ear, (nose), and larynx (throat)

EXERCISE O   Medical Terms Related to the Eye and Ear

Write the medical terms related to the eye and ear sensory systems to their definitions.

1. _____   pertaining to the eye

2. _____   pertaining to vision

3. _____   pertaining to the retina

4. _____   pertaining to the sclera

5. _____   pertaining to the middle ear

OBJECTIVE 5

Use medical language in clinical statements, the case study, and a medical record.

Check responses for the following exercises in Appendix C.

EXERCISE P **Use Medical Terms in Clinical Statements**

Circle the medical terms defined in the bolded phrases. For pronunciation practice, read the answers aloud.

1. The **physician who studies and treats diseases of the eye** (ophthalmologist, optometrist, optician) is trained in surgery and specializes in eye and vision care, including the diagnosis and treatment of diseases and disorders of the eye, performing eye surgery, and prescribing lenses.

2. **A procedure using a laser to reshape corneal tissue** (iridectomy, LASIK, blepharoplasty) was performed to correct **farsightedness** (astigmatism, hyperopia, myopia).

3. **Excision of a portion of the iris**, called an (iritis, iridectomy, iridoplegia), may be performed to treat some forms of an **eye disorder characterized by optic nerve damage, usually caused by an abnormal increase of intraocular pressure** (glaucoma, cataracts, macular degeneration).

4. The goal of **surgical repair of the eyelids** (blepharoptosis, blepharoplasty, blepharitis) is to correct impaired peripheral vision caused by **drooping eyelids** (blepharoptosis, blepharoplasty, blepharitis).

5. The optometrist used a(n) **instrument used to measure (the curvature) of the cornea** (keratoplasty, keratometer, ophthalmoscope) to collect data for the fitting of the patient's contact lenses.

6. **Vision loss occurring with age** (AMD, Presbyopia, Presbycusis) may be diagnosed and treated by a(n) **healthcare professional who performs eye exams, administers vision tests, and prescribes corrective lenses** (ophthalmologist, optometrist, audiologist).

7. The patient presented with a painful redness in both eyes, photophobia, and diminished vision, which suggested the diagnosis of **inflammation of the pigmented muscular structure (colored portion) of the eye** (retinitis, scleritis, iritis).

8. The **instrument used to visually examine the ear** is called an (otoscope, ophthalmoscope, audiometer). The **instrument used to measure hearing** is called an (otoscope, ophthalmoscope, audiometer).

9. The pediatric **ENT** (audiologist, otolaryngologist, ophthalmologist) is planning to release pus from a child's middle ear by performing a(n) **incision into the eardrum** (tympanoplasty, myringoplasty, myringotomy).

10. **Surgical repair of the eardrum** (Myringotomy, Myringitis, Myringoplasty) is one form of **surgical repair of the middle ear** (keratoplasty, tympanoplasty, otoplasty).

11. **Hearing loss occurring with age** (Tinnitus, Presbyopia, Presbycusis) may be diagnosed and treated by a(n) **specialist who studies and treats impaired hearing** (otolaryngologist, optometrist, audiologist).

EXERCISE Q   **Apply Medical Terms to the Case Study**

Think back to Javier, introduced in the case study at the beginning of the lesson. After working through Lesson 9 on the eye and the ear, consider the medical terms that might be used to describe his experiences. List three terms relevant to the case study and their meanings. ■

Medical Term   **Definition**

1. _____   _____

2. _____   _____

3. _____   _____

EXERCISE R   **Use Medical Terms in a Document**

With the help of his daughter, Javier is able to visit the ophthalmologist and otolaryngologist. His experiences are documented in the following consultation report.

Use the definitions in numbers 1-14 to write abbreviations and medical terms within the consultation report.

1. abbreviation for ear, nose, and throat

2. ringing in the ears

3. inflammation of the middle ear

4. surgical repair of the middle ear

5. eye disorder characterized by optic nerve damage usually caused by an abnormal increase of intraocular pressure

6. physician who studies and treats diseases of the eye

7. healthcare professional who performs eye exams, administers vision tests, and prescribes corrective lenses

8. instrument used for visual examination of the ear

9. pertaining to the middle ear

10. discharge from the ear

11. specialist who studies and treats impaired hearing

12. inflammation of the ear

13. study of hearing

14. physician who studies and treats diseases of the ear, (nose), and the larynx (throat)

118003 BERJARANO, Javier

File　Patient　Navigate　Custom Fields　Help

Chart Review | Encounters | Notes | Labs | Imaging | Procedures | Rx | Documents | Referrals | Scheduling | Billing

Name: **Berjarano, Javier**　　MR#: 118003　　Gender: M　　**Allergies:** None known
　　　　　　　　　　　DOB: 11/03/19XX　　Age: 81　　**PCP:** Rose Duarte MD

(1.) _____ **Consultation**
Date of Consultation: 05/22/20XX
Requesting Physician: Rose Duarte, MD
Reason for Consultation: Hearing Loss

History: This 81-year-old male is brought to the office by his daughter with complaints of gradual hearing loss. It has probably been occurring for months, but seems to have worsened recently. He also notes some itching in his right ear. He denies any
(2.) _____ or dizziness. Past medical history is significant for recurrent
(3.) _____ as a child with right **(4.)** _____ at that time. During the review of symptoms, his daughter reported that he has been having trouble with his vision. He was recently diagnosed with **(5.)**_____ by an
(6.) _____. He is now on medication for this. He also has an appointment with an **(7.)** _____ to get new glasses.

Physical Examination: Vital signs are normal. He is an elderly male in no acute distress. Examination of the head and face reveals no scars, lesions or masses. Sinuses are palpated and normal. Salivary gland examination is normal with no masses noted. Eyes show normal extraocular movement. The left exterior ear is normal, and examination of the ear canal using an **(8.)** _____ shows some cerumen but otherwise no abnormalities. The **(9.)** _____ membrane is intact. The right exterior ear is normal, but there is inflammation in the canal and **(10.)** _____ is present, in addition to heavy cerumen. The tympanic membrane is scarred but intact.

Diagnostic Studies:
Audiology Report: Mr. Berjarano saw the **(11.)** _____ and the testing revealed moderate to severe sensorineural hearing loss on the left and profound sensoineural hearing loss on the right. Speech understanding was 40% for the left ear and 24% for the right. Based on these results, Mr. Berjarano has great difficulty hearing all speech sounds without amplification.

Impression and Plan:
1. Right **(12.)** _____ externa: apparent infection of the right ear canal. We will treat with topical antibiotics. He was also given a medication for treating wax buildup in the ear canals.
2. Bilateral sensorineural hearing loss. Mr. Berjarano appears to be a good candidate for hearing aid amplification; however, I would like to see his right ear infection resolve and then repeat the **(13.)** _____ testing in about 2 weeks, at which time he can be fitted for hearing aids.
3. He will follow up as above or call our office if symptoms worsen or do not improve.

Thank you for this consultation. Please do not hesitate to contact me with any questions.
Electronically signed: James Cohen, MD, **(14.)** _____

Start | Log On/Off | Print | Edit

Refer to the ENT Consultation to answer questions 15-17.

15. The term **ocular**, used in the medical record to describe the movement observed, is built from word parts. Use your medical dictionary or a reliable online source to define the word parts, and then use your skills to build the term.

ocul/o means _____

-ar means _____

Remember, most definitions begin with the suffix.

ocul/ar means _____

16. The term **lesion** was presented in the integumentary system lesson. Can you recall its meaning?

lesion _____

17. Identify two new medical terms in the medical record you would like to investigate. Use your medical dictionary or an online reference to look up the definition.

Medical Term	Definition
1. _____	_____
2. _____	_____

EXERCISE S   **Use Medical Language in Electronic Health Records Online**

Select the correct medical terms to complete three medical records in one patient's electronic file.

⊕ Access online resources at evolve.elsevier.com > Evolve Resources > Practice Student Resources > Activities > Lesson 9 > Electronic Health Records

Topic: Glaucoma
Record 1: New Patient Evaluation
Record 2: Consultation Letter to PCP
Record 3: Operative Note

❏   Check the box when complete.

OBJECTIVE 6

Recall and assess knowledge of word parts, medical terms, and abbreviations.

EXERCISE T   **Online Review of Lesson Content**

⊕ *Recall and assess your learning from working through the lesson by completing online learning activities at evolve. elsevier.com > Evolve Resources > Student Resources.*

❏   Check the box when complete.

EXERCISE U Lesson Content Quiz

Test your knowledge of the terms and abbreviations introduced in this lesson. Circle the letter for the medical term or abbreviation related to the words in italics.

1. *Separation of the retina from the choroid in the posterior portion of the eye, resulting in a disruption of vision,* may cause a sudden increase in floaters, flashes of light, and worsening vision.
   a. retinal detachment
   b. glaucoma
   c. cataract

2. *Irregular curvature of the refractive surfaces of the eye* can produce blurred or distorted vision.
   a. myopia
   b. macular degeneration
   c. astigmatism

3. Presbycusis is an age-related condition which may cause one to be *hard of hearing.*
   a. HH
   b. HOH
   c. IOP

4. The patient was scheduled for ophthalmic surgery with an intraocular lens implant to treat the *cataract* in her left eye.
   a. eye disorder caused by optic nerve damage
   b. farsightedness
   c. clouding of the lens of the eye

5. *Progressive deterioration of the central portion of the retina resulting in a loss of central vision* is more common after age 60 and in those with a history of smoking.
   a. retinal detachment
   b. macular degeneration
   c. iridoplegia

6. The child said he could read the book but had difficulty reading road signs. The ophthalmologist said he had *nearsightedness.*
   a. astigmatism
   b. hyperopia
   c. myopia

7. *Surgical repair of the eyelid* may be performed for functional or cosmetic reasons. In patients with ptosis, the procedure can significantly improve visual fields.
   a. keratoplasty
   b. blepharoplasty
   c. tympanoplasty

8. The nurse practitioner used *the instrument for visual examination of the eye* to check on the health of the patient's eyes during her annual physical exam.
   a. ophthalmoscope
   b. opthalmoscope
   c. ophthaloscope

9. The child's right outer ear became misshapen following a dog bite to the right side of his face. *Surgical repair of the (outer) ear* was performed by the plastic surgeon.
   a. otoplasty
   b. blepharoplasty
   c. tympanoplasty

10. The baby was tugging at her ears, crying more than normal, and was not sleeping. The pediatrician used an otoscope to examine her ears and noted *inflammation of the eardrum* on the right.
    a. tinnitus
    b. iritis
    c. myringitis

11. The patient reported *ringing in the ears* after working at the airport for many years.
    a. presbycusis
    b. tinnitus
    c. otorrhea

12. A(n) *instrument used to measure hearing* is used to determine whether a patient needs hearing aids.
    a. otoscope
    b. audiometer
    c. keratometer

LESSON AT A GLANCE — EYE AND EAR WORD PARTS

COMBINING FORMS

Eye	**Ear**
blephar/o	audi/o
ir/o	myring/o
irid/o	ot/o
kerat/o	tympan/o
ophthalm/o	
opt/o	
retin/o	
scler/o	

SUFFIXES
-metry
-plegia
-ptosis

LESSON AT A GLANCE — EYE AND EAR MEDICAL TERMS AND ABBREVIATIONS

SIGNS AND SYMPTOMS
otorrhea
tinnitus

DISEASES AND DISORDERS
astigmatism (AST)
blepharitis
blepharoptosis
cataract
glaucoma
hyperopia
iridoplegia
iritis
macular degeneration
myopia
myringitis
otitis
otitis media (OM)
presbycusis
presbyopia
retinal detachment
retinitis
scleritis

DIAGNOSTIC TESTS AND EQUIPMENT
audiometer
audiometry
keratometer
ophthalmoscope
otoscope

SURGICAL PROCEDURES
blepharoplasty
iridectomy
keratoplasty
LASIK
myringoplasty
myringotomy
otoplasty
tympanoplasty

SPECIALTIES AND PROFESSIONS
audiologist
audiology
ophthalmologist
ophthalmology (Ophth)
optometrist
optometry
otolaryngologist (ENT)
otolaryngology

RELATED TERMS
ophthalmic
optic
retinal
scleral
tympanic

ABBREVIATIONS

AMD	HOH	Ophth
AST	IOP	VA
ENT	OM	

Musculoskeletal System

Shanti was walking to the store to buy more cigarettes. It was cold and icy and the sidewalks were slippery. She saw a pile of slush on the sidewalk in front of her and tried to scoot around it. Unfortunately, she slipped on some ice on the pavement. She tried to use her hand to brace her fall, but her hand and wrist buckled under her when she fell. Now her wrist is really swollen and very painful. She also has muscle pain all over and thinks she may have bruised her hip bone.

■ *Consider Shanti's situation as you work through the lesson on the musculoskeletal system. At the end of the lesson, we will return to this case study and identify medical terms used to document Shanti's experience and the care she receives.*

OBJECTIVES

1   ■ Build, translate, pronounce, and spell medical terms built from word parts (p. 303).

2   ■ Define, pronounce, and spell medical terms NOT built from word parts (p. 326).

3   ■ Write abbreviations (p. 331).

4   ■ Identify medical terms by clinical category (p. 332).

5   ■ Use medical language in clinical statements, the case study, and a medical record (p. 336).

6   ■ Recall and assess knowledge of word parts, medical terms, and abbreviations (p. 340).

INTRODUCTION TO THE MUSCULOSKELETAL SYSTEM

Anatomic Structures of the Musculoskeletal System	
bone (bōn)	organ made up of hard connective tissue with a dense outer layer and spongy inner layer
bone marrow (bōn) (MAR-ō)	material found in the cavities of bones; red marrow is responsible for blood cell formation, and yellow marrow serves as a storehouse for fat
bursa (*pl.* bursae) (BER-sa), (BER-sē)	fluid-filled sac that allows for easy movement of one part of a joint over another
cartilage (KAR-ti-lej)	firm connective tissue primarily found in joints; covers the contacting surfaces of bones
ilium (IL-ē-um)	upper wing-shaped part on each side of the pelvis
ischium (IS-kē-um)	lower posterior portion of the pelvis on which one sits
joint (joint)	structure forming the union between bones and often allowing for movement

Continued

Anatomic Structures of the Musculoskeletal System—cont'd

ligament (LIG-a-ment)	flexible, tough bands of fibrous connective tissue that attach one bone to another at a joint
muscle (MUS-el)	tissue composed of specialized cells with the ability to contract to produce movement
pubis (PŪ-bis)	anterior portion of the pelvis
sternum (STUR-num)	long, flat bone attached to the collarbone and first seven ribs, forming the center front of the chest wall (also called **breastbone**)
tendon (TEN-den)	band of fibrous connective tissue that attaches muscle to bone
vertebral column (ver-TĒ-brel) (KOL-em)	made up of bones called vertebrae (pl.) or vertebra (s.) through which the spinal cord runs. The vertebral column protects the spinal cord, supports the head, and provides points of attachment for ribs and muscles. It has five sections, including the cervical spine, thoracic spine, lumbar spine, sacrum, and coccyx (see Figure 10.4).

Functions of the Musculoskeletal System

- Provides body framework, support, and movement
- Protects internal organs
- Stores calcium
- Produces blood cells

How the Musculoskeletal System Works

Muscles, bones, and joints, along with other associated structures, provide the body with a flexible and protective framework. More than 600 **muscles** cover the bones, maintain posture, and move the body through a process of contracting and relaxing. Two hundred and six **bones** form the adult human skeleton and provide structure for the body as a whole (Figure 10.2). There are several types of bones performing various functions, such as bearing weight and protecting organs. Although bones are hard and seem lifeless, they are complete organs with living cells integrated into a mineral framework, which stores calcium. Bones have a dense outer layer and a spongy inner layer. Red **bone marrow,** found in some bones, generates blood cells. **Joints** form the union between bones and often allow for movement, although some do not. Most of the joints in the skeleton are freely moving and contain **cartilage** and **bursae. Cartilage** provides smooth surfaces within the joint and supports weight-bearing activities. **Bursae,** resting between the joint and tendon, allow **tendons** to slide over bones as they move. The organs and structures of the musculoskeletal system work together to protect, support, and move the body.

CAREER FOCUS **Professionals Who Work with the Musculoskeletal System**

- **Surgical technologists**, also called operating room technicians or scrub techs, work under the supervision of surgeons and are in charge of the instruments, supplies, and maintaining a sterile environment during surgical procedures. They assist surgeons with gowns and gloves, pass instruments, apply dressings, and prepare the operating room between procedures.

- **Occupational therapy assistants (OTAs)** work under the direction of occupational therapists to implement treatment plans that help restore or maintain a patient's ability to function independently. Their duties include teaching mobility techniques, monitoring patient progress, and alerting the therapists if changes in the prescribed regimen are needed.

- **Physical therapist assistants (PTAs)** work directly with patients to regain movement and manage pain. Under the direction of licensed physical therapists, PTAs implement treatment plans, which may include massage, exercises, training for the use of medical equipment (such as a walker), and other therapies, such as electrical stimulation.

Figure 10.1 Physical therapist assistant conducting strength training with a patient.

OBJECTIVE 1

Build, translate, pronounce, and spell medical terms built from word parts.

WORD PARTS Use the paper or online **flashcards** to familiarize yourself with the following word parts.

COMBINING FORM (WR + CV)	DEFINITION	COMBINING FORM (WR + CV)	DEFINITION
arthr/o	joint(s)	**lord/o**	bent forward (lumbar spine)
burs/o	bursa	**necr/o**	death
carp/o	carpals, wrist (bone)	**oste/o**	bone
chondr/o	cartilage	**phalang/o**	phalanx (*pl.* phalanges) (any bone of the fingers or toes)
cost/o	rib(s)		
crani/o	skull (cranium)	**pub/o**	pubis (anterior portion of the pelvis)
femor/o	femur (upper leg bone)		
ili/o	ilium (upper wing-shaped part on each side of the pelvis)	**rachi/o**	vertebra, spine, vertebral column
		scoli/o	crooked, curved (spine)
		spondyl/o	vertebra, spine, vertebral column
ischi/o	ischium (lower posterior portion of the pelvis on which one sits)	**stern/o**	sternum (breastbone)
		ten/o, tendin/o	tendon
		troph/o	development
kinesi/o	movement, motion	**vertebr/o**	vertebra, spine, vertebral column
kyph/o	hump (thoracic spine)		

Continued

WORD PARTS	Use the paper or online **flashcards** to familiarize yourself with the following word parts.—cont'd

SUFFIX (S)	DEFINITION	SUFFIX (S)	DEFINITION
-asthenia	weakness	-malacia	softening
-desis	binding, fusion	-schisis	split, fissure
PREFIX	**DEFINITION**		
inter-	between		

WORD PARTS PRESENTED IN PREVIOUS LESSONS	Used to Build Terms for the Musculoskeletal System

COMBINING FORM (WR + CV)	DEFINITION	COMBINING FORM (WR + CV)	DEFINITION
my/o	muscle(s), muscle tissue	path/o	disease
electr/o	electrical activity	sarc/o	flesh, connective tissue
SUFFIX (S)	**DEFINITION**	**SUFFIX (S)**	**DEFINITION**
-a, -y	no meaning	-itis	inflammation
-ac, -al, -eal, -ic	pertaining to	-logy	study of
-algia	pain	-oma	tumor
-centesis	surgical puncture to remove fluid	-osis	abnormal condition
		-penia	abnormal reduction (in number)
-ectomy	surgical removal, excision	-plasty	surgical repair
-gram	record, radiographic image	-scopic	pertaining to visual examination
-ia	diseased state, condition of	-scopy	visual examination
-iasis	condition	-tomy	cut into, incision
PREFIX (P)	**DEFINITION**	**PREFIX (P)**	**DEFINITION**
a-, an-	absence of, without	hyper-	above, excessive
brady-	slow	intra-	within
dys-	difficult, painful, abnormal	sub-	below, under

Refer to Appendix A, Word Parts Used in *Basic Medical Language*, for alphabetical lists of word parts and their meanings.

EXERCISE A **Build and Translate Medical Terms Built from Word Parts**

Use the **Word Parts Tables** to complete the following questions. Check your responses with the Answer Key in Appendix C.

1. LABEL: Write the combining forms for anatomic structures of the musculoskeletal system on Figure 10.2. These anatomic combining forms will be used to build and translate medical terms in Exercise A.

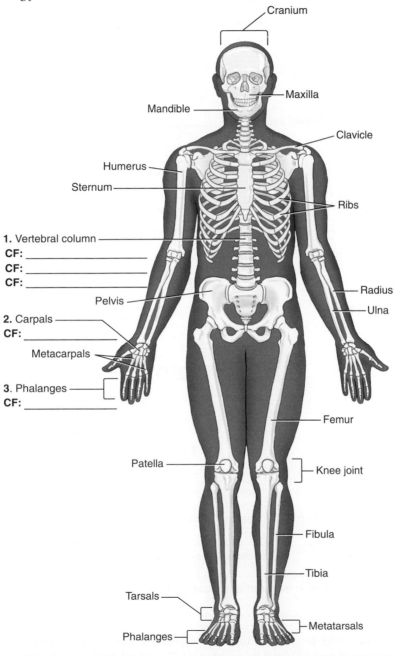

Cranium

Maxilla

Mandible

Clavicle

Humerus

Sternum

Ribs

1. Vertebral column
CF: _____
CF: _____
CF: _____

Pelvis

Radius

Ulna

2. Carpals
CF: _____

Metacarpals

3. Phalanges
CF: _____

Femur

Patella

Knee joint

Fibula

Tibia

Tarsals

Metatarsals

Phalanges

Figure 10.2 Skeletal system, anterior view, with combining forms.

2. MATCH: *Draw a line to match the word part with its definition.*

a. -al   surgical repair
b. -ectomy   between
c. -plasty   pertaining to
d. inter-   excision

3. BUILD: *Using the combining form **vertebr/o** and the word parts reviewed in the previous exercise, build the following terms related to the vertebra and spine. Remember, the definition usually starts with the meaning of the suffix.*

a. pertaining to the vertebra(e)   _____ / _____
                                              wr   s

b. pertaining to between the vertebrae _____ / _____ / _____
                                              p   wr   s

c. excision of a vertebra   _____ / _____
                                              wr   s

d. surgical repair of a vertebra   _____ / o / _____
                                              wr   cv   s

4. LABEL: *Write word parts to complete Figure 10.3.*

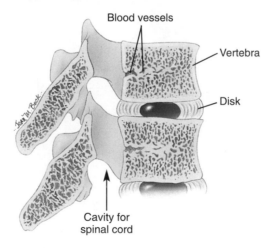

Blood vessels

Vertebra

Disk

Cavity for
spinal cord

Figure 10.3 Vertebrae. Sagittal section of vertebrae showing normal
_____ / _____ / _____ disks.
  between   vertebrae   pertaining to

FYI Disk is sometimes spelled **disc** in names of bony structures.

5. READ: The **vertebral** (VER-te-bral) column is composed of three main sets of bones, called vertebrae (Figure 10.4). The cervical vertebrae are abbreviated C1-C7 and referred to as the cervical spine. The thoracic vertebrae are T1-T12, called the thoracic spine. The lumbar vertebrae are L1-L5, called the lumbar spine. The sacrum and coccyx complete the column. The **intervertebral** (in-ter-VER-te-bral) disks fill the spaces between vertebrae and are composed of a fibrous, cartilage-type tissue. A **vertebroplasty** (VER-te-brō-plas-tē) may be performed in cases where a vertebra has collapsed due to osteoporosis, while a **vertebrectomy** (ver-te-BREK-to-mē) might be performed if the vertebra cannot be repaired and must be replaced.

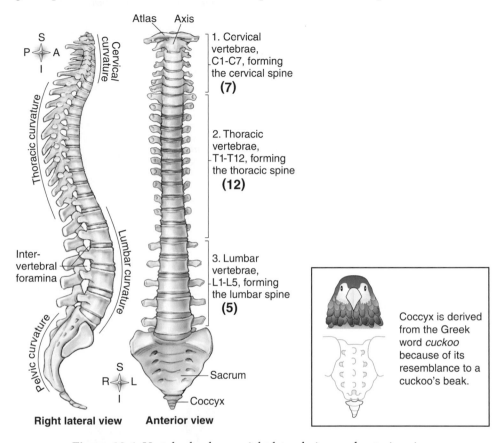

Atlas   Axis

1. Cervical vertebrae, C1-C7, forming the cervical spine
(7)

2. Thoracic vertebrae, T1-T12, forming the thoracic spine
(12)

3. Lumbar vertebrae, L1-L5, forming the lumbar spine
(5)

Intervertebral foramina

Sacrum

Coccyx

Coccyx is derived from the Greek word *cuckoo* because of its resemblance to a cuckoo's beak.

Right lateral view   **Anterior view**

Figure 10.4 Vertebral column, right lateral view and anterior view.

6. MATCH: *Draw a line to match the word part with its definition.*

a. -schisis   joint(s)
b. -tomy   inflammation
c. -itis   split, fissure
d. arthr/o   incision

7. TRANSLATE: *Complete the definitions of the following terms built from the combining form **rachi/o**, meaning vertebral column. Remember, the definition usually starts with the meaning of the suffix.*

a. rachi/schisis   _____ of the _____ column
b. rachi/o/tomy   _____ into the vertebral _____

8. **BUILD**: *Using the combining form* **spondyl/o,** *meaning vertebra, spine, vertebral column, and the word parts reviewed in the matching exercise, build the following term:*

inflammation of the spinal joints

_____/_____/_____
          wr   wr   s

9. **READ**: **Rachischisis** (rā-KIS-kis-sis) refers to a split in a vertebra, and is commonly seen in spina bifida. **Spondylarthritis** (spon-dil-ar-THRĪ-tis) may present with back pain, stiffness, and inflammation of the tendons that attach to the spine. A **rachiotomy** (rā-kē-OT-o-mē) is a surgical procedure that allows access to the spinal column through a vertebra.

10. **MATCH**: *Draw a line to match the word part with its definition.*

   a. -osis   crooked, curved (spine)
   b. kyph/o   hump (thoracic spine)
   c. lord/o   abnormal condition
   d. scoli/o   bent forward (lumbar spine)

11. **TRANSLATE**: *Complete the definitions of the following terms:*

   a. scoli/osis   _____ _____ of crooked, curved (spine)
   b. kyph/osis   abnormal condition of a _____ (thoracic spine)
   c. lord/osis   _____ _____ of bent _____ (lumbar spine)

12. **LABEL**: *Write word parts to complete Figure 10.5.*

Figure 10.5 Abnormal curvatures of the vertebral column.

A. _____/_____.
     bent forward (lumbar spine)   abnormal condition

B. _____/_____.
     hump (thoracic spine)   abnormal condition

C. _____/_____.
     crooked, curved   abnormal condition

13. **MATCH**: *Draw a line to match the word part with its definition.*

   a. -al, -eal   excision
   b. -ectomy   pertaining to

14. **BUILD:** *Using the combining form **carp/o**, meaning wrist, and the word parts reviewed in the previous exercise, build the following terms:*

   a. pertaining to the wrist   _____ / _____
                                          wr   s

   b. excision of a wrist (bone)   _____ / _____
                                          wr   s

15. **READ: Carpal** (KAR-pal) means pertaining to the wrist bones (Figure 10.6). "Meta-" is a prefix meaning "beyond." Metacarpal refers to the bones beyond (distal to) the carpals, between the wrist bones and the fingers. A **carpectomy** (kar-PEK-to-mē) refers to removal of a wrist bone, which may be performed in cases of severe arthritis.

Figure 10.6 The carpal, metacarpal, and phalangeal bones.

16. **TRANSLATE:** *Complete the definitions of the following terms using the word root **phalang/o**, meaning phalanx (any bone of the fingers or toes).*

   a. phalang/eal   _____ to a _____ (any bone of the fingers or toes)
   b. phalang/ectomy   _____ of a _____ (any bone of the fingers or toes)

17. **READ:** When **phalangeal** (fa-LAN-jē-al) terms are used, they are accompanied by descriptive words to designate a specific finger or toe bone. For example, a physician would say "The patient had a **phalangectomy** (fal-an-JEK-to-mē) of the distal phalanx of the fifth finger, right hand." The thumb is counted as the first finger, the index finger is second, and thus the pinky is the fifth finger.

18. **MATCH:** *Draw a line to match the word part with its definition.*

   a. a-   above, excessive
   b. dys-   no meaning
   c. hyper-   absence of, without
   d. -y   pertaining to
   e. -ic   difficult, painful, abnormal

19. BUILD: *Using the combining form **troph/o** and the word parts reviewed in the previous exercise, build the following terms related to growth.*

a. abnormal development

_____/_____/_y_____
p   wr   s

b. without development (process of wasting away)

_____/_____/_y_____
p   wr   s

c. excessive development

_____/_____/_y_____
p   wr   s

d. pertaining to excessive development

_____/_____/_____
p   wr   s

20. READ: Hypertrophy (hī-PER-tro-fē) occurs when muscles are overdeveloped, which may result from weight lifting. Almost any muscle can become **hypertrophic** (hī-per-TRŌF-ik); when the heart muscle is overdeveloped, it is called hypertrophic cardiomyopathy. Loss of muscle mass, or **atrophy** (AT-rō-fē), occurs when muscles are not used, which may result from disability or a sedentary lifestyle. Muscular **dystrophy** (DIS-tro-fē), or **MD**, is a group of hereditary diseases characterized by abnormal muscles and weakness.

21. LABEL: *Write word parts to complete Figure 10.7.*

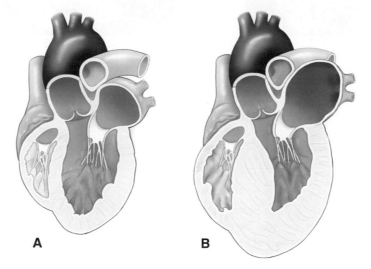

A   B

Figure 10.7 **A.** Normal heart muscle.

B. _____/_____/_____ heart muscle in cardiomyopathy.
        excessive   development   pertaining to

22. **LABEL:** *Write the combining forms for anatomic structures of a joint in Figure 10.8.*

Bone

Tendon

Femur

Patella

Cartilage

Joint

1. Bursa
CF: _____

Tibia

Figure 10.8 Knee joint and related combining form for bursa.

---

23. **MATCH:** *Draw a line to match the word part with its definition.*

 a. -itis   excision
 b. -ectomy   incision
 c. -tomy   inflammation

---

24. **TRANSLATE:** *Complete the definitions of the following terms using the combining form **burs/o**, meaning bursa.*

 a. burs/ectomy   excision of a _____

 b. burs/itis   _____ of the _____

 c. burs/o/tomy   _____ into a bursa

---

25. **READ:** **Bursitis** (ber-SĪ-tis) refers to inflammation of the fluid-filled sac around a joint. Over time, this fluid can increase and the bursa may thicken. Sometimes a **bursotomy** (ber-SOT-o-mē) is performed and a drain is placed if the swelling becomes severe. In chronic bursitis, the bursa may become thickened or even infected and a **bursectomy** (ber-SEK-to-mē) may be performed.

---

26. **LABEL:** *Write word parts to complete Figure 10.9.*

Figure 10.9 Olecranon (elbow) _____/_____.
                    bursa   inflammation

27. LABEL: *Write the combining forms for anatomic structures of the pelvis on Figure 10.10.*

1. Ilium
   CF: _____

2. Pubis
   CF: _____

3. Ischium
   CF: _____

Sacrum

Coccyx

Pubic symphysis

> **FYI** Compare the combining form for ilium, **ili/o,** the portion of the pelvis, with the combining form for ileum, **ile/o,** the distal portion of the small intestine. The pronunciation is the same. Think of i**l**ium with an **i** and int**e**stine with an **e** to help distinguish the word roots.

Figure 10.10 Pelvis, anterior view, with combining forms.

---

28. MATCH: *Draw a line to match the word part with its definition.*

a. -al, -ac, -ic   pertaining to
b. femor/o   femur (see Figure 10.2)

---

29. TRANSLATE: *Complete the definitions of the following terms.*

a. ili/ac   pertaining to the _____

b. femor/al   _____ to the femur

c. ili/o/femor/al pertaining to the _____ and the _____

d. ischi/al   _____ to the ischium

e. ischi/o/pub/ic pertaining to the _____ and the pubis

---

30. READ: The **ischial** (IS-kē-al) bones are referred to as the "sitting bones." The **iliofemoral** (il-lē-ō-FEM-or-al) ligament is one of the strongest in the body; it connects the pelvis to the thighbone. At birth, the three bones of the pelvis are separate and distinct, but in childhood they fuse together. The first fusion results in the **ischiopubic** (is-kē-ō-PŪ-bik) ramus (a projection of the bones where they meet).

---

31. MATCH: *Draw a line to match the word part with its definition.*

a. -algia   electrical activity
b. -asthenia   pain
c. -gram   record, radiographic image
d. electr/o   muscle(s), muscle tissue
e. my/o   weakness

32. BUILD: *Using the combining form* **my/o** *and the word parts reviewed in the previous exercise, build the following terms related to muscle. Hint: For a. and b. the definition of the term starts with the meaning of the combining form.*

a. muscle pain

_____/_____
  wr   s

b. muscle weakness

_____/_____
  wr   s

c. record of the electrical activity of a muscle

_____/_o_/_____/_o_/_____
  wr   cv   wr   cv   s

33. READ: Myalgia (mī-AL-ja) is a symptom of many disorders. Fibromyalgia is a disorder characterized by widespread musculoskeletal pain accompanied by fatigue, sleep, memory, and mood issues. **Myasthenia** (mī-as-THĒ-nē-a) gravis, abbreviated MG, is an autoimmune neuromuscular disease leading to fluctuating muscle loss and fatigue. Symptoms may include drooping eyelids, blurred vision, or slurred speech. An **electromyogram** (ē-lek-trō-MĪ-ō-gram) may show patterns that are specific to MG.

34. LABEL: *Write word parts to complete Figure 10.11.*

Figure 10.11 Diagram of an _____/o/_____/o/_____ (EMG) of the forearm.
                           electrical activity   muscle   record

35. MATCH: *Draw a line to match the word part with its definition.*

    a. brady-   no meaning

    b. dys-   slow

    c. -a   difficult, painful, abnormal

36. BUILD: *Using the combining form **kinesi/o** and the word parts reviewed in the previous exercise, build the following terms related to movement.*

    a. slow movement   _____ / _____ / _____a_____

                                            p   wr   s

    b. painful movement   _____ / _____ / _____a_____

                                            p   wr   s

37. READ: Bradykinesia (brad-ē-ki-NĒ-zha) and **dyskinesia** (dis-ki-NĒ-zha) refer to abnormalities in muscle movement caused by neurological irregularities and are usually associated with Parkinson disease. Shuffling when walking and having little or no facial expressions are types of unusually slow movement seen in bradykinesia. Dyskinesias are involuntary movements, such as swaying of the body, twitching, and bobbing of the head.

38. REVIEW OF MUSCULOSKELETAL SYSTEM TERMS BUILT FROM WORD PARTS: *The following is an alphabetical list of terms built and translated in the previous exercises.*

MEDICAL TERMS BUILT FROM WORD PARTS

TERM	DEFINTION	TERM	DEFINTION
1. atrophy (AT-rō-fē)	without development (process of wasting away)	**8. dyskinesia** (dis-ki-NĒ-zha)	painful movement
2. bradykinesia (brad-ē-ki-NĒ-zha)	slow movement	**9. dystrophy** (DIS-tro-fē)	abnormal development
3. bursectomy (ber-SEK-to-mē)	excision of the bursa	**10. electromyogram (EMG)** (ē-lek-trō-MĪ-ō-gram)	record of the electrical activity of the muscle (Figure 10.11)
4. bursitis (ber-SĪ-tis)	inflammation of the bursa (Figure 10.9)	**11. femoral** (FEM-or-al)	pertaining to the femur
5. bursotomy (ber-SOT-o-mē)	incision into the bursa	**12. hypertrophic** (hī-per-TRŌF-ik)	pertaining to excessive development (Figure 10.7, *B*)
6. carpal (KAR-pal)	pertaining to the wrist (Figure 10.6)	**13. hypertrophy** (hī-PER-tro-fē)	excessive development
7. carpectomy (kar-PEK-to-mē)	excision of a wrist (bone)	**14. iliac** (IL-ē-ak)	pertaining to the ilium

Continued

MEDICAL TERMS BUILT FROM WORD PARTS—cont'd

TERM	DEFINTION	TERM	DEFINTION
15. **iliofemoral** (il-lē-ō-FEM-or-al)	pertaining to the ilium and femur	24. **phalangectomy** (fal-an-JEK-to-mē)	excision of a phalanx (any bone of the fingers or toes)
16. **intervertebral** (in-ter-VER-te-bral)	pertaining to between the vertebrae (Figure 10.3)	25. **rachiotomy** (rā-kē-OT-o-mē)	incision into the vertebral column
17. **ischial** (IS-kē-al)	pertaining to the ischium	26. **rachischisis** (rā-KIS-kis-sis)	fissure of the vertebral column
18. **ischiopubic** (is-kē-ō-PŪ-bik)	pertaining to the ischium and pubis	27. **scoliosis** (skō-lē-Ō-sis)	abnormal condition of crooked, curved (spine) (Figure 10.5, *C*)
19. **kyphosis** (kī-FŌ-sis)	abnormal condition of a hump (thoracic spine) (Figure 10.5, *B*)	28. **spondylarthritis** (spon-dil-ar-THRĪ-tis)	inflammation of the vertebral joints
20. **lordosis** (lōr-DŌ-sis)	abnormal condition of bent forward (lumbar spine) (Figure 10.5, *A*)	39. **vertebral** (VER-te-bral)	pertaining to the vertebra(e)
21. **myalgia** (mī-AL-ja)	muscle pain	30. **vertebrectomy** (ver-te-BREK-to-mē)	excision of the vertebra
22. **myasthenia** (mī-as-THĒ-nē-a)	muscle weakness	31. **vertebroplasty** (VER-te-brō-plas-tē)	surgical repair of the vertebra
23. **phalangeal** (fa-LAN-jē-al)	pertaining to a phalanx (any bone of the fingers or toes) (Figure 10.6)		

EXERCISE B   Pronounce and Spell Terms Built from Word Parts

Practice pronunciation and spelling on paper and online.

1. **Practice on Paper**

   a. **Pronounce**: Read the phonetic spelling and say aloud the terms listed in the previous table, Review of Terms Built from Word Parts.

   b. **Spell**: Have a study partner read the terms aloud. Write the spelling of the terms on a separate sheet of paper.

2. **Practice Online** ⊕

   a. **Access** online learning resources. Go to evolve.elsevier.com > Evolve Resources > Practice Student Resources.

   b. **Pronounce**: Select Audio Glossary > Lesson 10 > Exercise B. Select a term to hear its pronunciation and repeat aloud.

   c. **Spell**: Select Activities > Lesson 10 > Spell Terms > Exercise B. Select the audio icon and type the correct spelling of the term.

❑ Check the box when complete.

EXERCISE C Build and Translate MORE Medical Terms Built from Word Parts

*Use the **Word Parts Tables** to complete the following questions. Check your responses with the Answer Key in Appendix C.*

1. **LABEL:** *Write the combining forms for anatomic structures of the musculoskeletal system on Figure 10.12. These anatomic combining forms will be used to build and translate medical terms in Exercise C.*

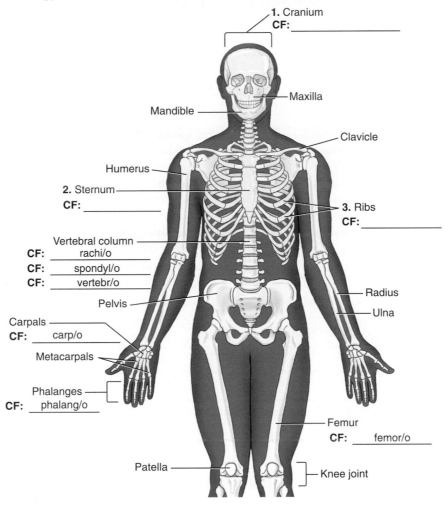

1. Cranium
CF: _____

Maxilla

Mandible

Clavicle

Humerus

2. Sternum
CF: _____

3. Ribs
CF: _____

Vertebral column
CF: _____rachi/o_____
CF: _____spondyl/o_____
CF: _____vertebr/o_____

Pelvis

Radius

Ulna

Carpals
CF: _____carp/o_____

Metacarpals

Phalanges
CF: _____phalang/o_____

Femur
CF: _____femor/o_____

Patella

Knee joint

Figure 10.12 Skeletal system, anterior view, with combining forms.

2. **MATCH:** *Draw a line to match the word part with its definition.*

a. -tomy   pertaining to
b. intra-   incision
c. -schisis   within
d. -malacia   split, fissure
e. -al   diseased state, condition of
f. -ia   softening

3. BUILD: *Using the combining form* **crani/o** *and the word parts reviewed in the previous exercise, build the following terms related to the skull (cranium). Remember, the definition usually starts with the meaning of the suffix.*

a. pertaining to within the skull
_____/_____/_____
                       p   **wr**   **s**

b. fissure of the skull
_____/ o /_____
                   wr   **cv**   **s**

c. incision into the skull
_____/ o /_____
                   wr   **cv**   **s**

d. softening of the skull
_____/ o /_____
                   wr   **cv**   **s**

4. READ: An **intracranial** (in-tra-KRĀ-nē-al) hemorrhage may be caused by extremely high blood pressure, an aneurysm, a stroke, or by various traumatic injuries. If it is severe, a **craniotomy** (krā-nē-OT-o-mē) may be required to access the brain and evacuate the blood. **Cranioschisis** (krā-nē-OS-ki-sis) usually occurs along the midsagittal plane of the skull and may be accompanied by protrusion of the brain and its meninges (linings). **Craniomalacia** (krā-nē-ō-ma-LĀ-sha) may be discovered during examination of the newborn, in which gentle pressure on the skull produces a sudden collapse.

5. LABEL: *Write the word parts to complete Figure 10.13.*

Blood appears white on this MRI

Figure 10.13 Magnetic resonance imaging (MRI) of a subdural hematoma,

a type of _____/_____/_____ bleeding.
              within   **skull**   **pertaining to**

6. MATCH: *Draw a line to match the word part with its definition.*

a. -al   between
b. inter-   pertaining to
c. sub-   below, under

7. TRANSLATE: *Complete the definitions of the following terms by using the meaning of the word parts to fill in the blanks.*

a. stern/al   pertaining to the _____
b. stern/o/cost/al   pertaining to the sternum and the _____

8. READ: The sternum is a bony plate at the anterior wall of the chest. It is divided into three parts, called the manubrium, the body, and the xiphoid process. The **sternal** (STER-nal) angle divides the manubrium from the sternal body. The xiphoid process is at the bottom of the sternum and can usually be felt on exam. The **sternocostal** (ster-nō-KOS-tal) joints connect the sternum to the ribs.

---

9. LABEL: *Write the word parts to complete Figure 10.14.*

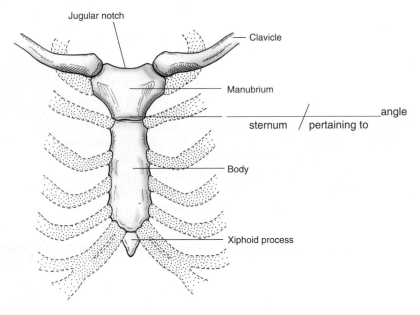

Jugular notch

Clavicle

Manubrium

_____/_____angle
sternum / pertaining to

Body

Xiphoid process

Figure 10.14 Sternum and rib joints.

---

10. BUILD: *Using the combining form **cost/o** and the word parts reviewed in the previous matching exercise, build the following terms related to the ribs.*

a. pertaining to between the ribs   _____/_____/_____
                                                    p   wr   s

b. pertaining to below the ribs   _____/_____/_____
                                                    p   wr   s

---

11. READ: The **intercostal** (in-ter-KOS-tal) muscles are responsible for forced (voluntary) respiratory inspiration and expiration. **Subcostal** (sub-KOS-tal) retractions appear as the sucking in of the skin and muscles beneath the sternum (breastbone) and ribs and can be a sign of respiratory difficulty.

---

12. LABEL: *Write the combining forms for anatomic structures of the musculoskeletal system on Figure 10.15.*

1. Tendon
   CF: _____
   CF: _____

2. Cartilage
   CF: _____

Bursa
CF: _____ burs/o _____

Patella

3. Bone
   CF: _____

Femur

4. Joint
   CF: _____

Tibia

Figure 10.15 Knee joint and related combining forms

13. MATCH: *Draw a line to match the word part with its definition.*

a. -itis   pertaining to
b. -ectomy   excision
c. -malacia   softening
d. -al   inflammation

14. TRANSLATE: *Complete the definitions of the following terms built from the combining form **chondr/o**, meaning cartilage. Use the meaning of word parts to fill in the blanks.*

a. cost/o/chondr/al   pertaining to _____ and cartilage
b. chondr/itis   inflammation of _____
c. chondr/ectomy   _____ of _____
d. chondr/o/malacia   _____ of cartilage

> **FYI** **Cartilage** is made up of connective tissue and covers the ends of two adjoining bones. It is also found in other semirigid structures such as the nose, ear, and trachea.

15. READ: Chondromalacia (kon-drō-ma-LĀ-sha) patella is a general term meaning damage to the cartilage under the kneecap. It is also called "runner's knee." **Chondritis** (kon-DRĪ-tis) can occur in the ear cartilage after piercing and often indicates an infection. A **chondrectomy** (kon-DREK-to-mē) may be necessary, and plastic surgery may be required to restore the appearance of the ear. Another common form of chondritis occurs at the **costochondral** (kos-tō-KON-dral) joints and can cause pain with breathing or coughing; it is referred to as costochondritis.

16. LABEL: *Write the word parts to complete Figure 10.16.*

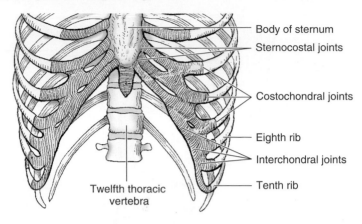

Body of sternum
Sternocostal joints
Costochondral joints
Eighth rib
Interchondral joints
Tenth rib
Twelfth thoracic vertebra

Figure 10.16 Lower sternum and ribs, showing sternocostal,

_____/o/_____/_____, and interchondral joints.

    ribs   cartilage   pertaining to

---

17. MATCH: *Draw a line to match the word part with its definition.*

a. -osis   death
b. -itis   abnormal condition
c. necr/o   inflammation

---

18. BUILD: *Use the combining form* **oste/o**, *along with the word parts reviewed in the previous exercise, to build terms related to bone.*

a. abnormal condition of death

                                        _____/_____
                                               wr   s

b. abnormal condition of death of the bone (tissue)

                                        _____/_o_/_____/_____
                                               wr   cv   wr   s

c. inflammation of the bone and cartilage

                                        _____/_o_/_____/_____
                                               wr   cv   wr   s

---

19. READ: Osteonecrosis (os-tē-ō-ne-KRŌ-sis) is the death of bone cells due to lack of blood flow. **Avascular necrosis** (ne-KRŌ-sis) is another term for this. **Osteochondritis** (os-tē-ō-kon-DRĪ-tis) dissecans is actually a type of osteonecrosis because small pieces of cartilage and bone become separated from the end of a bone and lose their blood supply.

20. MATCH: *Draw a line to match the word part with its definition.*

a. path/o   no meaning
b. -malacia   abnormal reduction
c. -penia   softening
d. -y   disease

21. TRANSLATE: *Complete the definitions of the following terms by using the meaning of the word parts to fill in the blanks.*

a. oste/o/path/y   _____ of the bone
b. oste/o/penia   abnormal _____ of _____ mass
c. oste/o/malacia   _____ of the bone

> **FYI**   The suffix **-penia** comes from the Greek word meaning **poverty** or **need**. In Lesson 7, the suffix -penia was used to describe an **abnormal reduction in number**, such as with **leukocytopenia** (abnormal reduction in the number of white cells). Here, -penia refers to an **abnormal reduction**, not in the number of bone cells, but of the bone mass itself.

22. READ: Osteomalacia (os-tē-ō-ma-LĀ-sha) is often caused by vitamin D deficiency and is a defect in the bone building process. **Osteopenia** (os-tē-ō-PĒ-ne-a) is any reduction of the bone mass below normal, and means that existing bone cells are being reabsorbed by the body faster than new ones can be made. While **osteopathy** (os-tē-OP-a-thē) refers to disease of the bone, it also refers to a practice of medicine.

> **FYI**   **Osteopathy** practice uses the same forms of treatment and diagnosis as conventional medicine but places greater emphasis on the relationship between body organs and the musculoskeletal system. A physician who practices osteopathy is called a doctor of osteopathy, or DO (most commonly referred to as an "osteopath"). A physician who practices conventional (allopathic) medicine is a doctor of medicine, or MD.

23. MATCH: *Draw a line to match the word part with its definition.*

a. sarc/o   tumor
b. -oma   inflammation
c. -itis   flesh, connective tissue

24. BUILD: *Use the combining form **oste/o**, along with the word parts reviewed in the previous exercise, to build terms related to bone.*

a. inflammation of the bone(s) and the joint(s)   _____/ o /_____/_____
                                                    wr   cv   wr   s

b. tumor of the bone and connective tissue   _____/ o /_____/_____
                                                    wr   cv   wr   s

25. READ: **Osteoarthritis** (os-tē-ō-ar-THRĪ-tis) is the most common form of arthritis and is the result of degeneration and loss of bone cartilage, especially of the knees and hips. **Osteosarcoma** (os-tē-ō-sar-KŌ-ma) is a malignant tumor that arises from connective tissues and most frequently involves the long bones.

26. LABEL: *Write the word parts to complete Figure 10.17.*

Figure 10.17 Lateral radiograph (A) and pathology specimen (B) of _____/o/_____/_____.
                                                                            bone   connective tissue   tumor

27. MATCH: *Draw a line to match the word part with its definition.*

    a. -algia   surgical repair
    b. -desis   inflammation
    c. -plasty   binding, fusion
    d. -itis   pain

28. TRANSLATE: *Complete the definitions of the following terms built from the combining form **arthr/o,** meaning joint(s). Use the meaning of word parts to fill in the blanks.*

    a. arthr/algia   pain in the _____

    b. arthr/itis   _____ of the joint(s)

    c. arthr/o/desis   _____ of a joint

    d. arthr/o/plasty   surgical _____ of a _____

29. READ: Osteoarthritis, rheumatoid arthritis, and gout are three forms of **arthritis** (ar-THRĪ-tis). While **arthralgia** (ar-THRAL-ja) is associated with all three forms, they differ in terms of other symptoms, such as swelling, redness, and stiffness. In **arthrodesis** (ar-thrō-DĒ-sis), two bones on the end of a joint are fused or "welded" together, eliminating the joint itself. The joint becomes immobile to reduce pain. In **arthroplasty** (AR-thrō-plas-tē), the joint space is preserved, and the joint is restored to its full range of motion.

30. MATCH: *Draw a line to match the word part with its definition.*

a. -centesis   visual examination
b. -gram   record, radiographic image
c. -scopy   pertaining to visual examination
d. -scopic   surgical puncture to remove fluid

31. BUILD: *Continue using the combining form* **arthr/o,** *along with the word parts reviewed in the previous exercise, to build terms related to joints.*

a. surgical puncture of a joint to remove fluid   _____/ o /_____
                                                      wr   cv   s

b. radiographic image of a joint   _____/ o /_____
                                                      wr   cv   s

c. visual examination of a joint   _____/ o /_____
                                                      wr   cv   s

d. pertaining to visual examination of a joint   _____/ o /_____
                                                      wr   cv   s

32. LABEL: *Write the word parts to complete Figure 10.18.*

Figure 10.18 An arthroscope is used to perform a(n) _____/o/_____
                                                          joint   visual examination

for diagnostic purposes or for _____/o/_____
                                 joint   pertaining to visual examination

surgery to repair ligaments or to remove cartilage.

33. MATCH: *Draw a line to match the word part with its definition.*

a. -desis   inflammation
b. -itis   surgical repair
c. -plasty   binding, fusion

34. TRANSLATE: *Complete the definitions of the following terms built from the combining forms **ten/o** and **tendin/o**, meaning tendon. Use the meaning of word parts to fill in the blanks. Note that the combining form **tendin/o** contains an i compared with the term itself, **tendon**, which is spelled with an o.*

a. tendin/itis   _____ of the tendon(s)

b. ten/o/plasty   surgical _____ of a _____

c. ten/o/desis   _____ of a tendon (to a bone or ligament)

35. READ: In some patients with biceps **tendinitis** (ten-di-NĪ-tis), **tenodesis** (ten-ō-DĒ-sis) may be needed to remove the biceps at its attachment to the shoulder and to reinsert it in a different area. In cases of Achilles tendon rupture, **tenoplasty** (TEN-ō-plas-tē) may be needed to restore function of the ankle.

> **FYI**   The **Achilles tendon**, located between the calf muscle and the heel, is the thickest and strongest tendon in the body. Its name is derived from the classical tale of Achilles. To make him invulnerable, Achilles' mother dipped him into the river Styx. She held him by this tendon, which was not immersed, and later a mortal wound was inflicted on Achilles' heel.

36. REVIEW OF MORE MUSCULOSKELETAL SYSTEM TERMS BUILT FROM WORD PARTS: *The following is an alphabetical list of terms built and translated in the previous exercises.*

MEDICAL TERMS BUILT FROM WORD PARTS

TERM	DEFINITION	TERM	DEFINITION
1. arthralgia (ar-THRAL-ja)	pain in the joint	11. chondromalacia (kon-drō-ma-LĀ-sha)	softening of cartilage
2. arthritis (ar-THRĪ-tis)	inflammation of the joint(s)	12. costochondral (kos-tō-KON-dral)	pertaining to the ribs and cartilage (Figure 10.16)
3. arthrocentesis (ar-thrō-sen-TĒ-sis)	surgical puncture of a joint to remove fluid	13. craniomalacia (krā-nē-ō-ma-LĀ-sha)	softening of the skull
4. arthrodesis (ar-thrō-DĒ-sis)	fusion of a joint	14. cranioschisis (krā-nē-OS-ki-sis)	fissure of the skull
5. arthrogram (AR-thrō-gram)	radiographic image of a joint	15. craniotomy (krā-nē-OT-o-mē)	incision into the skull
6. arthroplasty (AR-thrō-plas-tē)	surgical repair of a joint	16. intercostal (in-ter-KOS-tal)	pertaining to between the ribs
7. arthroscopic (ar-thrō-SKOP-ik)	pertaining to visual examination of a joint (Figure 10.18)	17. intracranial (in-tra-KRĀ-nē-al)	pertaining to within the skull (Figure 10.13)
8. arthroscopy (ar-THROS-ko-pē)	visual examination of a joint (Figure 10.18)	18. necrosis (ne-KRŌ-sis)	abnormal condition of death
9. chondrectomy (kon-DREK-to-mē)	excision of cartilage	19. osteoarthritis (OA) (os-tē-ō-ar-THRĪ-tis)	inflammation of the bone(s) and the joint(s)
10. chondritis (kon-DRĪ-tis)	inflammation of cartilage	20. osteochondritis (os-tē-ō-kon-DRĪ-tis)	inflammation of the bone and cartilage

Continued

MEDICAL TERMS BUILT FROM WORD PARTS—cont'd

TERM	DEFINITION	TERM	DEFINITION
21. **osteomalacia** (os-tē-ō-ma-LĀ-sha)	softening of the bone	27. **sternocostal** (ster-nō-KOS-tal)	pertaining to the sternum and the ribs (Figure 10.16)
22. **osteonecrosis** (os-tē-ō-ne-KRŌ-sis)	abnormal condition of death of bone (tissue)	28. **subcostal** (sub-KOS-tal)	pertaining to below the ribs
23. **osteopathy** (os-tē-OP-a-thē)	disease of the bone	29. **tendinitis** (ten-di-NĪ-tis)	inflammation of the tendon(s)
24. **osteopenia** (os-tē-ō-PĒ-ne-a)	abnormal reduction of bone mass	30. **tenodesis** (ten-ō-DĒ-sis)	binding of a tendon (to a bone or ligament)
25. **osteosarcoma** (os-tē-ō-sar-KŌ-ma)	tumor of the bone and the connective tissue (Figure 10.17)	31. **tenoplasty** (TEN-ō-plas-tē)	surgical repair of a tendon
26. **sternal** (STER-nal)	pertaining to the sternum (Figure 10.14)		

EXERCISE D   Pronounce and Spell MORE Terms Built from Word Parts

Practice pronunciation and spelling on paper and online.

1. **Practice on Paper**
   a. **Pronounce**: Read the phonetic spelling and say aloud the terms listed in the previous table, Review of MORE Terms Built from Word Parts.
   b. **Spell**: Have a study partner read the terms aloud. Write the spelling of the terms on a separate sheet of paper.

2. **Practice Online** 🌐
   a. **Access** online learning resources. Go to evolve.elsevier.com > Evolve Resources > Practice Student Resources.
   b. **Pronounce**: Select Audio Glossary > Lesson 10 > Exercise D. Select a term to hear its pronunciation and repeat aloud.
   c. **Spell**: Select Activities > Lesson 10 > Spell Terms > Exercise D. Select the audio icon and type the correct spelling of the term.

❏ Check the box when complete.

OBJECTIVE 2

Define, pronounce, and spell medical terms NOT built from word parts

The terms listed below may contain word parts, but are difficult to translate literally.

MEDICAL TERMS NOT BUILT FROM WORD PARTS

TERM	DEFINITION
1. **carpal tunnel syndrome (CTS)** (KAR-pl)(TUN-el) (SIN-drōm)	common nerve entrapment disorder of the wrist caused by compression of the median nerve. Symptoms include pain, tingling, and numbness in portions of the hand and fingers.
2. **chiropractic** (kī-rō-PRAK-tik)	system of treatment that consists of manipulation of the vertebral column
3. **dual x-ray absorptiometry (DXA)** (du-al) (EKS-rā) (ab-sorp-shē-OM-e-trē)	radiographic imaging, usually of the lumbar spine and hips, to measure bone loss and bone mineral density; the procedure utilizes low doses of radiation and is used in the diagnosis of osteoporosis and monitoring of treatment (also called **dual-energy x-ray absorptiometry [DEXA], bone densitometry**, and **bone density test)**
4. **fracture (Fx)** (FRAK-chūr)	broken bone
5. **gout** (gowt)	disease in which an excessive amount of uric acid in the blood causes sodium urate crystals to be deposited in the joints, especially that of the great toe, producing arthritis
6. **hernia** (HUR-nē-ah)	protrusion of an organ or structure through an abnormal opening. Hernias often occur due to weakness of the mucsles or ligaments in the surrounding area.
7. **herniated disk** (HER-nē-āt-ed) (disk)	rupture of the intervertebral disk cartilage, which allows the contents to protrude through it, putting pressure on the spinal nerve roots
8. **Lyme disease** (līm) (di-ZĒZ)	immune response caused by a bite from a deer tick infected with *Borrelia burgdorferi*; causes symptoms including fever, headache, and joint pain, and mimics other musculoskeletal diseases. A rash (target lesion) may initially arise at the site of the tick bite.
9. **muscular dystrophy (MD)** (MUS-kū-lar) (DIS-tro-fē)	group of hereditary diseases characterized by degeneration of muscle and weakness
10. **orthopedics (ortho)** (or-thō-PĒ-diks)	study and treatment of diseases and abnormalities of the musculoskeletal system
11. **orthopedist** (or-thō-PĒ-dist)	physician who specializes in the study and treatment of diseases and abnormalities of the musculoskeletal system
12. **osteoporosis** (os-tē-ō-po-RŌ-sis)	disease caused by abnormal loss of bone density occurring predominantly in postmenopausal women, which can lead to an increase in fractures of the ribs, thoracic and lumbar vertebrae, hips, and wrists
13. **plantar fasciitis** (PLAN-tar) (fas-ē-Ī-tis)	inflammation of the connective tissue of the sole of the foot; common cause of heel pain
14. **rheumatoid arthritis (RA)** (RŪ-ma-toyd) (ar-THRĪ-tis)	chronic systemic disease characterized by autoimmune inflammatory changes in the connective tissue throughout the body
15. **spinal stenosis** (SPĪ-nal) (ste-NŌ-sis)	narrowing of the spinal canal with compression of nerve roots. Symptoms include pain, numbness, and tingling in the thigh that radiates to lower extremities.

EXERCISE E Label

Write the medical terms pictured and defined using the previous table of Medical Terms NOT Built from Word Parts. Check your work with the Answer Key in Appendix C.

1. _____

immune response caused by a bite from an infected deer tick; a rash (target lesion) may initially arise at the site of the tick bite

2. _____

common nerve entrapment disorder of the wrist caused by compression of the median nerve

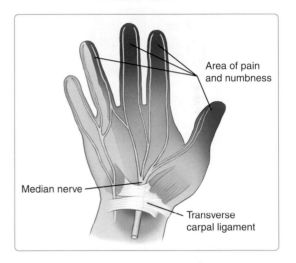

Area of pain and numbness

Median nerve

Transverse carpal ligament

3. _____

broken bone

4. _____

disease in which an excessive amount of uric acid in the blood causes sodium urate crystals to be deposited in the joints

5. _____

disease caused by abnormal loss of bone density that may lead to an increase in fractures

6. _____

rupture of the intervertebral disk cartilage, which allows the contents to protrude through it, putting pressure on the spinal nerve roots

7. _____

narrowing of the spinal canal with compression of nerve roots.

8. _____

inflammation of the connective tissue of the sole of the foot; common cause of heel pain

9. _____

radiographic imaging, usually of the lumbar spine and hips, to measure bone loss and bone mineral density

10. _____

physician who specializes in the study and treatment of diseases and abnormalities of the musculoskeletal system

11. _____

chronic systemic disease characterized by autoimmune inflammatory changes in the connective tissue throughout the body

---

EXERCISE F **Match**

Match the terms in the first column with their correct descriptions in the second column. Answers are listed in Appendix C.

_____ **1.** muscular dystrophy

_____ **2.** orthopedics

_____ **3.** hernia

_____ **4.** chiropractic

a. system of treatment that consists of manipulation of the vertebral column

b. group of hereditary diseases characterized by degeneration of muscle and weakness

c. protrusion of an organ or structure through an abnormal opening

d. the study and treatment of diseases and abnormalities of the musculoskeletal system

---

EXERCISE G **Learn Medical Terms NOT Built from Word Parts**

Fill in the blanks with medical terms, defined in bold, using the Medical Terms NOT Built from Word Parts table. Answers are listed in Appendix C.

1. _____ is the branch of medicine dealing with the **study and treatment of diseases and abnormalities of the musculoskeletal system**. A **physician who specializes in the study and treatment of diseases and abnormalities of the musculoskeletal system** is called a(n) _____. This term was devised in 1740 and comes from *orthos*, meaning straight, and *ped*, meaning children; it literally means to straighten children. At that time rickets, osteomyelitis, tuberculosis, and poliomyelitis were the main orthopedic problems, often resulting in deformities. Correcting these deformities by straightening or aligning bones was common. Today, an orthopedist may be required to repair a **broken bone,** or _____, fix a **rupture of the intervertebral disk cartilage,** or _____, or treat a patient with **narrowing of the spinal canal with compression of nerve roots**, or

_____.

2. A rheumatologist may see a person with swelling, pain, and stiffness in a joint and request a blood test to diagnose a **chronic systemic disease characterized by autoimmune inflammatory changes in the connective tissue**, or _____.

3. _____, a **disease in which an excessive amount of uric acid in the blood causes sodium urate crystals to be deposited in the joints**, generally affects the great toe, but may also affect joints in the feet, ankles, wrists, and hands. The sharp sodium urate crystals cause inflammation and pain as they collect in the joints. Risk factors include diets high in red meat or seafood, excessive alcohol use, certain medications, and genetic predisposition.

4. Usually diagnosed in children by the age of 5 years, a **group of hereditary diseases characterized by degeneration of muscle and weakness**, or _____, is characterized by the replacement of muscle tissue with fat and scar tissue.

5. **Common nerve entrapment disorder of the wrist caused by compression of the median nerve**, or _____, can be caused by many factors, including repetitive work stress, traumatic injuries such as fractures or sprains, or arthritis in the wrist joint. Another condition that may be caused by repetitive stress, **inflammation of the connective tissue of the sole of the foot**, or _____, may occur in runners due to repeated stretching and small tears. Treatment may involve rest, ice packs, therapeutic exercises, massage, antiinflammatory or steroidal medications, or surgery.

6. The **disease caused by abnormal loss of bone density occurring predominantly in postmenopausal women**, or _____, can cause kyphosis of the spine and increased risk for fractures. **Radiographic imaging to measure bone loss and bone mineral density**, or _____, is used in diagnosis, assessment of fracture risk, and to monitor treatment. Diets high in calcium and vitamin D and use of weight-bearing exercise over a lifetime can help prevent this debilitating chronic disease.

7. **A protrusion of an organ or structure through an abnormal opening**, or _____, often occurs within the abdominal cavity. Common types include inguinal, which occur near the groin, umbilical, which are around the umbilicus (belly button), and hiatal, in which a portion of the stomach pushes up through the diaphragm.

8. **System of treatment that consists of manipulation of the vertebral column**, or _____, is a healthcare profession that focuses on the relationship between the body's structure and its functioning. In North America, it is often considered a complementary health approach.

9. **Immune response caused by a bite from a deer tick infected with *Borrelia burgdorferi***, or _____, may have symptoms similar to a number of other musculoskeletal diseases, including rheumatoid arthritis, gout, and ankylosing spondylitis. A two-step process for diagnosing this disease is currently recommended to prevent misdiagnosis and improper treatment.

EXERCISE H **Pronounce and Spell Terms NOT Built from Word Parts**

Practice pronunciation and spelling on paper and online.

1. **Practice on Paper**
   a. **Pronounce**: Read the phonetic spelling and say aloud the terms listed in the previous table, Medical Terms NOT Built from Word Parts.
   b. **Spell**: Have a study partner read the terms aloud. Write the spelling of the terms on a separate sheet of paper.

2. **Practice Online** 🌐
   a. **Access** online learning resources. Go to evolve.elsevier.com > Evolve Resources > Practice Student Resources.
   b. **Pronounce**: Select Audio Glossary > Lesson 10 > Exercise H. Select a term to hear its pronunciation and repeat aloud.
   c. **Spell**: Select Activities > Lesson 10 > Spell Terms > Exercise H. Select the audio icon and type the correct spelling of the term.

   ❏ Check the box when complete.

OBJECTIVE 3

Write abbreviations.

ABBREVIATIONS RELATED TO THE MUSCULOSKELETAL SYSTEM

Use the online **flashcards** to familiarize yourself with the following abbreviations.

ABBREVIATION	TERM	ABBREVIATION	TERM
C1-C7	cervical vertebrae	OA	osteoarthritis
CTS	carpal tunnel syndrome	ortho	orthopedics
DC	doctor of chiropractic	OT	occupational therapy
DEXA	dual-energy x-ray absorptiometry	PT	physical therapy
DO	doctor of osteopathy	RA	rheumatoid arthritis
DXA	dual x-ray absorptiometry	ROM	range of motion
FYI DXA and DEXA are spoken as a whole word (deh-XA).			
EMG	electromyogram	T1-T12	thoracic vertebrae
Fx	fracture	THA	total hip arthroplasty
L1-L5	lumbar vertebrae	TKA	total knee arthroplasty
MD	muscular dystrophy		

EXERCISE I   Abbreviate Medical Terms

Write the correct abbreviation next to its medical term.

1. Diseases and Disorders:

   a. _____ carpal tunnel syndrome

   b. _____ fracture

   c. _____ muscular dystrophy

   d. _____ osteoarthritis

   e. _____ rheumatoid arthritis

2. Diagnostic Tests and Equipment:

   a. _____ electromyogram

   b. _____ dual x-ray absorptiometry

   c. _____ dual-energy x-ray
   absorptiometry

3. Surgical Procedures:

   a. _____ total knee arthroplasty

   b. _____ total hip arthroplasty

4. Specialties and Professions:

   a. _____ orthopedics

   b. _____ physical therapy

   c. _____ doctor of osteopathy

   d. _____ occupational therapy

   e. _____ doctor of chiropractic

5. Related Terms:

   a. _____ cervical vertebrae

   b. _____ lumbar vertebrae

   c. _____ thoracic vertebrae

   d. _____ range of motion

OBJECTIVE 4

Identify medical terms by clinical category.

Now that you have worked through the musculoskeletal system lesson, review and practice medical terms grouped by clinical category. Categories include signs and symptoms, diseases and disorders, diagnostic tests and equipment, surgical procedures, specialties and professions, and other terms related to the musculoskeletal system. Check your responses with the Answer Key in Appendix C.

EXERCISE J   Signs and Symptoms

Write the medical terms for signs and symptoms next to their definitions.

1. _____ pain in the joint

2. _____ without development (process of wasting away)

3. _____ slow movement

4. _____ painful movement

5. _____ abnormal development

6. _____ excessive development

7. _____ muscle pain

8. _____ muscle weakness

EXERCISE K **Diseases and Disorders**

Write the medical terms for diseases and disorders next to their definitions.

1. _____ inflammation of the joint(s)

2. _____ inflammation of the connective tissue of the sole of the foot

3. _____ inflammation of the bursa

4. _____ common nerve entrapment disorder of the wrist caused by compression of the median nerve

5. _____ inflammation of cartilage

6. _____ softening of cartilage

7. _____ softening of the skull

8. _____ fissure of the skull

9. _____ broken bone

10. _____ disease in which an excessive amount of uric acid in the blood causes sodium urate crystals to be deposited in the joints, especially that of the great toe, producing arthritis

11. _____ rupture of the intervertebral disk cartilage, which allows the contents to protrude through it, putting pressure on the spinal nerve roots

12. _____ abnormal condition of a hump (thoracic spine)

13. _____ abnormal condition of bent forward (lumbar spine)

14. _____ group of hereditary diseases characterized by degeneration of muscle and weakness

15. _____ abnormal condition of death

16. _____ inflammation of the bone(s) and the joint(s)

17. _____ inflammation of the bone and cartilage

18. _____ softening of the bone

19. _____ abnormal condition of death of the bone (tissue)

20. _____ disease of the bone

21. _____ abnormal reduction of bone mass

22. _____ disease caused by abnormal loss of bone density occurring predominantly in postmenopausal women, which can lead to an increase in fractures of the ribs, thoracic and lumbar vertebrae, hips, and wrists

23. _____ tumor of the bone and the connective tissue

24. _____ fissure of the vertebral column

25. _____ chronic systemic disease characterized by autoimmune inflammatory changes in the connective tissue throughout the body

26. _____ abnormal condition of crooked, curved (spine)

27. _____ inflammation of the vertebral joints

28. _____ inflammation of the tendon(s)

29. _____ narrowing of the spinal canal with compression of nerve roots

30. _____ immune response caused by a bite from a deer tick infected with *Borrelia burgdorferi*; causes symptoms including fever, headache, and joint pain, and mimics other musculoskeletal diseases

31. _____ protrusion of an organ or structure through an abnormal opening

EXERCISE L   Diagnostic Tests and Equipment

Write the medical terms for diagnostic tests and equipment next to their definitions.

1. _____ radiographic image of a joint

2. _____ pertaining to visual examination of a joint

3. _____ visual examination of a joint

4. _____ record of the electrical activity of a muscle

5. _____ radiographic imaging, usually of the lumbar spine and hips, to measure bone loss and bone mineral density; the procedure utilizes low doses of radiation and is used in the diagnosis of osteoporosis and monitoring of treatment

EXERCISE M   Surgical Procedures

Write the medical terms for surgical procedures next to their definitions.

1. _____ surgical puncture of a joint to remove fluid

2. _____ fusion of a joint

3. _____ surgical repair of a joint

4. _____ excision of a bursa

5. _____ incision into a bursa

6. _____ excision of a wrist (bone)

7. _____ excision of cartilage

8. _____ incision into the skull

9. _____ excision of a phalanx (any bone of the fingers or toes)

10. _____ incision into the vertebral column

11. _____ binding of a tendon (to a bone or ligament)

12. _____ surgical repair of a tendon

13. _____ excision of a vertebra

14. _____ surgical repair of a vertebra

EXERCISE N   Specialties and Professions

Write the medical terms for specialties and professions next to their definitions.

1. _____ study and treatment of diseases and abnormalities of the musculoskeletal system

2. _____ physician who specializes in the study and treatment of diseases and abnormalities of the musculoskeletal system

3. _____ system of treatment that consists of manipulation of the vertebral column

---

EXERCISE O   Medical Terms Related to the Musculoskeletal System

Write the medical terms related to the musculoskeletal system next to their definitions.

1. _____ pertaining to the wrist

2. _____ pertaining to the ribs and cartilage

3. _____ pertaining to the femur

4. _____ pertaining to excessive development

5. _____ pertaining to the ilium

6. _____ pertaining to the ilium and the femur

7. _____ pertaining to between the ribs

8. _____ pertaining to between the vertebra(e)

9. _____ pertaining to within the skull

10. _____ pertaining to the ischium

11. _____   pertaining to the ischium and the pubis

12. _____   pertaining to a phalanx (any bone of the fingers or toes)

13. _____   pertaining to the sternum

14. _____   pertaining to the sternum and the ribs

15. _____   pertaining to below the ribs

16. _____   pertaining to the vertebrae

OBJECTIVE 5

Use medical language in clinical statements, the case study, and a medical record.

Check responses for the following exercises in Appendix C.

EXERCISE P   Use Medical Terms in Clinical Statements

Circle the medical terms and abbreviations defined in the bolded phrases. For pronunciation practice, read the answers aloud.

1. Carmen McCroskey is experiencing pain in her ankle caused by traumatic **inflammation of the joint(s)** (arthralgia, arthritis, osteoarthritis) resulting from a **broken bone** (herniated disk, gout, fracture) several years ago. Her orthopedic surgeon will perform a triple **fusion of a joint** (arthrodesis, arthrogram, arthrocentesis) in an attempt to reduce the pain in the area.

2. If **radiographic image of a joint** (arthroscopy, arthrocentesis, arthrogram) findings indicate that surgery is needed, a(n) **visual examination of a joint** (arthroscopy, arthrocentesis, arthrodesis) may be performed to repair ligaments, fix a torn meniscus, or address other minor injuries. Common types of **pertaining to visual examination of a joint** (arthroplasty, arthroscopic, arthralgia) surgery include rotator cuff repair of the shoulder and meniscus repair of the knee.

3. Total hip replacement and total knee **surgical repair of a joint** (arthroscopy, arthrodesis, arthroplasty) are common orthopedic procedures. Various prostheses are used to rebuild joints that have been damaged by trauma or, more commonly, **inflammation of the bone(s) and the joint(s)** (osteochondritis, osteoarthritis, osteopathy).

4. During her lifetime, Abigail Carpenter experienced multiple changes to the curvature of her vertebral column. During elementary school, she was diagnosed with mild **abnormal condition of crooked, curved spine** (scoliosis, spondylarthritis, muscular dystrophy). While pregnant with twins, as her spine adjusted to the extra weight, she had prominent **abnormal condition of bent forward (lumbar spine)** (lordosis, rachischisis, scoliosis). After menopause, she lost 2 inches of height as she developed **abnormal condition of a hump (thoracic spine)** (scoliosis, kyphosis, hernia) due to **disease caused by abnormal loss of bone density** (muscular dystrophy, osteosarcoma, osteoporosis).

5. To assist in determining the patient's diagnosis of **a group of hereditary diseases characterized by degeneration of muscle and weakness** (myasthenia, rheumatoid arthritis, muscular dystrophy), the physician ordered a(n) **record of the electrical activity of a muscle** (arthroscopy, electromyogram, rachiotomy).

6. While playing soccer, Eli Kleinman experienced pain above the posterior aspect of his heel and could not continue playing. The **physician who specializes in the study and treatment of diseases and abnormalities of the musculoskeletal system** (chiropractic, orthopedist, pulmonologist) told Eli's mother that he strained his Achilles tendon, causing **inflammation of his tendon** (tendinitis, bursitis, chondritis). The orthopedist prescribed analgesics and cautioned against physical activity to avoid the risk of a tendon rupture, which might require **surgical repair of a tendon** (arthroplasty, vertebroplasty, tenoplasty).

7. **Inflammation of a bursa** (Osteoarthritis, Chondritis, Bursitis) may be precipitated by **inflammation of the joint(s)** (bursitis, tendinitis, arthritis). The chief symptom is severe pain. In chronic cases a(n) **incision into a bursa** (rachiotomy, bursotomy, vertebrectomy) to remove calcium deposits may be required.

8. **Softening of cartilage** (Craniomalacia, Osteomalacia, Chondromalacia) of the patella (kneecap) may occur after a knee injury. It is characterized by swelling, pain, and degenerative changes. **Softening of the bone** (Craniomalacia, Osteomalacia, Chondromalacia) results from many diseases. It is caused by an inadequate amount of phosphorus and calcium in the blood, resulting in impaired mineralization of the bone.

9. **Excessive development** (Atrophy, Dystrophy, Hypertrophy) occurs when muscles are overdeveloped, which may result from weight lifting. Loss of muscle mass, **without development** (atrophy, dystrophy, hypertrophy), occurs when muscles are not used, which may result from disability or a sedentary lifestyle.

10. George Robenowski was seen in the **system of treatment that consists of manipulation of the vertebral column** (chiropractic, orthopedic, physical therapy) clinic for chronic back pain; he was later referred to an orthopedist for his **narrowing of the spinal canal with compression of nerve roots** (plantar fasciitis, Lyme disease, spinal stenosis).

11. Some medical terms are used to indicate areas of the body when noting pain and other observations in medical records. Examples include:
    - **pertaining to within the skull** (intracranial, intervertebral, intravascular) bleeding
    - **pertaining to between the ribs** (costochondral, sternocostal, intercostal) muscles
    - discomfort in the **pertaining to below the ribs** (subcostal, subdural, subxiphoid) region
    - **pertaining to the ischium and the pubis** (ischial, iliofemoral, ischiopubic) bruising
    - a lesion noted over the left **pertaining to the ilium** (iliac, ileal, ischial) region
    - pain in the left **pertaining to the sternum and the ribs** (costochondral, sternocostal, intercostal) region
    - stiffness in the **pertaining to the vertebra(e)** (vertebral, intervertebral, phalangeal) column
    - **pertaining to the femur** (femoral, carpal, ischial) artery occlusion
    - **pertaining to the sternum** (vertebral, sternal, intercostal) incision

---

EXERCISE Q **Apply Medical Terms to the Case Study**

Think back to Shanti Mehra, who was introduced in the case study at the beginning of the lesson. After working through Lesson 10 on the musculoskeletal system, consider the medical terms that might be used to describe her experience. List two terms relevant to the case study and their meanings. ■

Medical Term   **Definition**

1. _____

2. _____

EXERCISE R   Use Medical Terms in a Document

Mrs. Mehra went to the Emergency Department. After a nurse took her vital signs, an emergency physician examined her and ordered an x-ray [radiograph]. A radiologist reviewed the results. She was then given medication for pain and referred to an orthopedist. This visit is documented in the following medical record.

Use the definitions in numbers 1-9 to write medical terms within the document.

1. study and treatment of diseases and abnormalities of the musculoskeletal system

2. broken bone

3. muscle pain

4. abnormal condition of hump (thoracic spine)

5. pertaining to the vertebra(e)

6. pertaining to the ilium

7. pertaining to the wrist

8. pertaining to a phalanx

9. disease caused by abnormal loss of bone density, occurring predominantly in postmenopausal women

Refer to the medical record to answer questions 10-13

10. In the physical examination section of the medical document, there are many anatomic terms that identify parts of the body. For example, **iliac** means "pertaining to the ilium" and **carpal** means "pertaining to the wrist bones." Write the terms referring to the bones in the forearm that mean "pertaining to the radius" and "pertaining to the ulna." (Hint: The suffix "**-ar**" is another word part meaning "pertaining to.")

    a. _____/_____
       wr   s
    b. _____/_____
       wr   s

11. The iliac crests are the curved superior portions of the ilium. When you put your hands on your hips, they are on the tops of the iliac crests. Try to find the iliac crests on yourself and on the diagram on Figure 10.10.

12. A contusion is an injury with no break in the skin, characterized by pain, swelling, and discoloration. Name a more common term for contusion: _____.

13. Identify two new medical terms in the medical record you would like to investigate. Use your medical dictionary or an online resource to look up the definition.

    Medical Term   **Definition**

    1. _____   _____

    2. _____   _____

```
011107 MEHRA, Shanti                                                    _□X
 File      Patient     Navigate    Custom Fields    Help
 ‹  ›  👤 👥 ▯ ▤ ▤ 🖴 Rx 🕐 ⓘ ✂ ▯ 🗒 ▦ ✔ ⊘ 🔍 ?
 Chart Review  Encounters   Notes    Labs    Imaging   Procedures   Rx   Documents   Referrals   Scheduling   Billing
 Name: MEHRA, Shanti        MR#: 011107        Gender: F        Allergies: Codeine
                            DOB: 10/17/19XX     Age: 67          PCP: Kimbrell, Howard DO
```

Clinical Note
Encounter Date: 04/02/20XX

History: This 67-year-old woman is seen for a follow-up visit in (1.) _____.
She presented 1 week ago in the emergency department for treatment of a
(2.)_____ of the right wrist, with an accompanying right ulnar fracture.
She also experienced (3.) _____ and pain in her right hip. The patient
is postmenopausal with a history of cigarette smoking.

Physical Examination: The patient is 5'5" tall and weighs 137 lbs. She has prominent
dorsal (4.) _____ in the thoracic (5.) _____ column.
The examination of the right forearm and hand reveals normal color with minimal swelling.
She has contusions over the right (6.) _____ crest. AP and lateral
radiographs of the right wrist and hand reveal healing distal radial and ulnar fractures.
There are no (7.) _____, metacarpal, or (8.) _____
abnormalities noted.

Diagnostic Studies: A DEXA scan assessing bone-mineral density shows evidence of
(9.) _____.

Impression: Healing right distal radial and ulnar fractures and osteoporosis.

Recommendation: The patient was advised to continue immobilization of the right forearm
for another 3 weeks. Calcium and vitamin D therapy were recommended. Smoking
cessation was strongly encouraged. Alendronate was prescribed as treatment for her
osteoporosis. A follow-up visit is scheduled in 3 weeks.

Electronically signed: Maxwell S. Kline, MD 04/02/20XX 16:30

```
 ◄                                                                        ►
 Start   Log On/Off   Print    Edit                              🖨 ◄) ✗ 🖥
```

EXERCISE S   **Use Medical Language in Electronic Health Records Online**

Select the correct medical terms to complete three medical records in one patient's electronic file.

🌐 Access online resources at evolve.elsevier.com > Evolve Resources > Practice Student Resources > Activities >
Lesson 10 > Electronic Health Records.

Topic: Fracture Right Arm
Record 1: Admission Note
Record 2: Radiology Report
Record 3: Neurology Consultation

❏   Check the box when complete.

OBJECTIVE 6

Recall and assess knowledge of word parts, medical terms, and abbreviations.

EXERCISE T   Online Review of Lesson Content

🌐 *Recall and assess your learning from working through the lesson by completing online learning activities at evolve.elsevier.com > Evolve Resources > Student Resources.*

❏   Check the box when complete.

EXERCISE U   Lesson Content Quiz

Test your knowledge of the terms and abbreviations introduced in this lesson. Circle the letter for the medical term or abbreviation related to the words in italics.

1. Sometimes, people with *immune response caused by a bite from a deer tick infected with Borrelia burgdorferi* do not have any memory of a tick bite or rash.
   a. rheumatoid arthritis
   b. Lyme disease
   c. chondritis

2. Orthopedists may perform *visual examination of a joint* to diagnose and sometimes treat problems in the knee, shoulder, or elbow.
   a. arthroscopy
   b. arthrogram
   c. arthrocentesis

3. A total hip *surgical repair of a joint* may be necessary in patients with severe osteoarthritis if other measures are no longer effective.
   a. arthrodesis
   b. arthroplasty
   c. chondroplasty

4. The causes of *abnormal condition of bone death* are not always clear, but some known factors include steroid medications, alcohol use, previous injury, and increased pressure inside the bone.
   a. osteomalacia
   b. osteosarcoma
   c. osteonecrosis

5. Injuries from an automobile accident may result in *pertaining to the ribs and cartilage* pain.
   a. costochondral

   b. subcostal
   c. intercostal

6. Symptoms of Parkinson disease may include tremors, *slow movement*, and dementia.
   a. dyskinesia
   b. bradykinesia
   c. hypertrophy

7. *Abnormal condition of crooked, curved (spine)* is more common in girls and is usually graded in terms of mild, moderate, or severe; braces or surgery may be recommended in some cases.
   a. lordosis
   b. kyphosis
   c. scoliosis

8. In patients with long-standing diabetes mellitus, poor circulation may result in osteonecrosis of the toe, and may require *excision of any bone of the fingers or toes*.
   a. bursectomy
   b. phalangectomy
   c. chondrectomy

9. Mrs. Lipai, who had been experiencing ongoing pain, radiating numbness, and weakness in her left leg, was scheduled for an MRI to determine if a *rupture of the intervertebral disk cartilage* had occurred.
   a. herniated disk
   b. fracture
   c. chondritis

10. In mild to moderate cases of *common nerve entrapment disorder of the wrist caused by compression of the median nerve*, the use of wrist splints at night can be very helpful.
    a. rachischisis
    b. rheumatoid arthritis
    c. carpal tunnel syndrome

11. Symptoms of ocular *muscle weakness* associated with an autoimmune condition can include diplopia and ptosis.
    a. myalgia
    b. myasthenia
    c. atrophy

12. Mr. Rodriguez awoke in the middle of the night with intense pain in the big toe of his right foot. In the morning he noticed the toe was red and swollen. A joint fluid test revealed the presence of urate crystals, and he was diagnosed with *disease in which an excessive amount of uric acid in the blood causes sodium urate crystals to be deposited in the joints*.
    a. arthralgia
    b. plantar fasciitis
    c. gout

LESSON AT A GLANCE   MUSCULOSKELETAL SYSTEM WORD PARTS

COMBINING FORMS

arthr/o	necr/o
burs/o	oste/o
carp/o	phalang/o
chondr/o	pub/o
cost/o	rachi/o
crani/o	scoli/o
femor/o	spondyl/o
ili/o	stern/o
ischi/o	ten/o, tendin/o
kinesi/o	troph/o
kyph/o	vertebr/o
lord/o	

SUFFIXES
-asthenia
-desis
-malacia
-schisis

PREFIX
inter-

SIGNS AND SYMPTOMS
arthralgia
atrophy
bradykinesia
dyskinesia
dystrophy
hypertrophy
myalgia
myasthenia

DISEASES AND DISORDERS
arthritis
bursitis
carpal tunnel syndrome (CTS)
chondritis
chondromalacia
craniomalacia
cranioschisis
fracture (Fx)
gout
hernia
herniated disk
kyphosis
lordosis
Lyme disease
muscular dystrophy (MD)
necrosis
osteoarthritis (OA)
osteochondritis
osteomalacia
osteonecrosis
osteopathy
osteopenia

osteoporosis
osteosarcoma
plantar fasciitis
rachischisis
rheumatoid arthritis (RA)
scoliosis
spinal stenosis
spondylarthritis
tendinitis

**DIAGNOSTIC TESTS
AND EQUIPMENT**
arthrogram
arthroscopic
arthroscopy
dual x-ray absorptiometry (DXA)
electromyogram (EMG)

SURGICAL PROCEDURES
arthrocentesis
arthrodesis
arthroplasty
bursectomy
bursotomy
carpectomy
chondrectomy
craniotomy
phalangectomy
rachiotomy
tenodesis
tenoplasty
vertebrectomy
vertebroplasty

RELATED TERMS
carpal
costochondral
femoral
hypertrophic
iliac
iliofemoral
intercostal
intervertebral
intracranial
ischial
ischiopubic
phalangeal
sternal
sternocostal
subcostal
vertebral

SPECIALTIES AND PROFESSIONS
chiropractic
orthopedics (ortho)
orthopedist

ABBREVIATIONS

C1–C7	Fx	RA
CTS	L1–L5	ROM
DC	MD	T1–T12
DEXA	OA	THA
DO	ortho	TKA
DXA	OT	
EMG	PT	

Nervous System and Behavioral Health

CASE STUDY

Koji Kaneshiro

Kazuno Kaneshiro is worried about her husband, Koji. He was eating breakfast with her when he suddenly stopped speaking and dropped his spoon onto the table. "He never does that!" she thought. He wasn't making any sense, though he was definitely trying to say something. Also, his right arm was hanging limply by his side. She noticed that the left side of his face was also droopy. She had seen a billboard about strokes and was afraid he might be having one. She remembered the billboard saying that every minute counts, so she called 911 immediately.

■ *Consider Koji's situation as you work through the lesson on the nervous system and behavioral health. At the end of the lesson, we will return to this case study and identify medical terms used to document Koji's experience and the care he receives.*

OBJECTIVES

1 ■ Build, translate, pronounce, and spell medical terms built from word parts (p. 346).

2 ■ Define, pronounce, and spell medical terms NOT built from word parts (p. 359).

3 ■ Write abbreviations (p. 367).

4 ■ Identify medical terms by clinical category (p. 368).

5 ■ Use medical language in clinical statements, the case study, and a medical record (p. 371).

6 ■ Recall and assess knowledge of word parts, medical terms, and abbreviations (p. 375).

INTRODUCTION TO THE NERVOUS SYSTEM

Anatomic Structures of the Nervous System	
brain (brān)	central organ of the nervous system contained within the cranium that coordinates body activities and processes sensory information transmitted through nerves. Sections of the brain include the cerebellum, the cerebrum, and the brainstem.
brainstem (BRĀN-stem)	stemlike portion of the brain that connects with the spinal cord; contains centers that control respiration and heart rate. Three structures comprise the brainstem: midbrain, pons, and medulla oblongata.
central nervous system (CNS) (SEN-trel) (NUR-vus) (SIS-tum)	brain and spinal cord (Figures 11.1 and 11.3)
cerebellum (ser-a-BEL-um)	located under the posterior portion of the cerebrum; assists in the coordination of skeletal muscles to maintain balance
cerebrospinal fluid (CSF) (ser-ē-brō-SPĪ-nel) (FLOO-id)	clear, colorless fluid contained in ventricles; cushions brain and spinal cord from shock, transports nutrients, and clears metabolic waste

Continued

Anatomic Structures of the Nervous System—cont'd

cerebrum (se-RĒ-brum)	largest portion of the brain; divided into left and right hemispheres
meninges (me-NIN-jēz)	three layers of membranes that cover the brain and spinal cord. The dura mater is the tough outer layer, the arachnoid is the delicate, weblike middle layer, and the pia mater is the thin inner layer of the meninges.
nerve (nurv)	cordlike structure made up of fibers that carries impulses from one part of the body to another
peripheral nervous system (PNS) (puh-RIF-er-ul) (NUR-vus) (SIS-tum)	system of nerves extending from the brain and spinal cord (Figure 11.1)
spinal cord (SPĪ-nel) (kord)	tubelike bundle of nerve tissue extending from the brainstem to the lower portion of the spine; conducts nerve impulses to and from the brain
ventricles (VEN-tri-kuls)	spaces within the brain that contain cerebrospinal fluid

Functions of the Nervous System

- Control and integration of body functions
- Communication
- Mental activity, thought, and memory

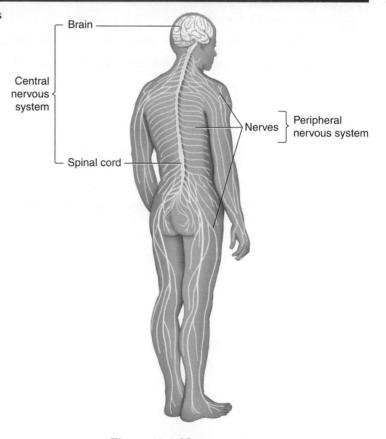

Figure 11.1 Nervous system.

How the Nervous System Works

The **brain, spinal cord,** and **nerves** form a complex communication system allowing for the coordination of body functions and activities. As a whole, the nervous system is designed to detect changes inside and outside the body, to evaluate this sensory information, and to send directions to muscles or glands in response. The nervous system may be divided into two parts: the **central nervous system** (CNS) and the **peripheral nervous system** (PNS) (Figure 11.1). The central nervous system, the **brain** and **spinal cord,** receives and processes sensory information and formulates outgoing responses. The largest portion of the brain, the **cerebrum,** controls skeletal muscles, contains centers for sight and hearing, and provides for mental activities such as thought, memory, and emotional reactions. The brain and spinal cord are covered by a three-layered membrane called the **meninges.** Further protection is provided by bone, the skull, and the spine. The peripheral nervous system forms a complex network of nerves extending from the brain and spinal cord. It carries sensory messages to the central nervous system and delivers responding messages to muscles and glands.

> **FYI** The **meninges** are made up of three layers, called the **dura mater,** the **arachnoid,** and the **pia mater.** Dura mater and pia mater were first named by a Persian physician in the tenth century. Dura mater, the outer tough layer, means tough mother. Pia mater, the delicate inner layer, means soft mother. The arachnoid resembles a spider web. Arachnida is the scientific name for spiders and is derived from Greek mythology.

Aspects of Behavioral Health

The terms "behavioral health" and "mental health" are closely related. Generally, these terms refer to our emotional, psychological, and social well-being. It reflects how we think, feel, and act. It has an impact on how we handle stress, make choices, and relate to the world around us. Behavioral health is part of an integrated approach to care of the patient as a whole. This lesson will serve as an introduction to a few common behavioral health terms.

CAREER FOCUS | Professionals Who Work with the Nervous System and in Behavioral Health

- **Speech-language pathology aides** assist with screening exams and implementation of treatment plans addressing communication and swallowing disorders. They work closely with patients and are supervised by speech-language pathologists.

- **Neurodiagnostic technicians** use special equipment to monitor how well a patient's nervous system is working (Figure 11.2). These include electroencephalograms (EEGs), polysomnograms (sleep studies), and nerve conduction studies.

- **Psychiatric aides** work under the direction of nurses and doctors to help mentally impaired or emotionally disturbed patients. They may assist with daily living activities, lead patients in educational and recreational activities, or accompany them to and from examinations and treatments.

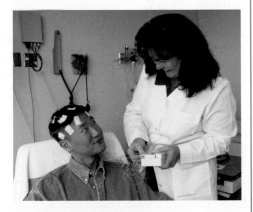

Figure 11.2 A neurodiagnostic technician performs an EEG on a patient.

OBJECTIVE 1

Build, translate, pronounce, and spell medical terms built from word parts.

WORD PARTS Use the paper or online **flashcards** to familiarize yourself with the following word parts.

COMBINING FORM (WR + CV)	DEFINITION	COMBINING FORM (WR + CV)	DEFINITION
cerebr/o	cerebrum, brain	pleg/o	paralysis
encephal/o	brain	poli/o	gray matter
mening/o, meningi/o	meninges	psych/o	mind
myel/o	spinal cord	quadr/i	four (*Note: The combining vowel is an **i**.*)
phas/o	speech		
SUFFIX (S)	**DEFINITION**		
-us	no meaning		
PREFIX	**DEFINITION**	**PREFIX (P)**	**DEFINITION**
hemi-	half	micro-	small

WORD PARTS PRESENTED IN PREVIOUS LESSONS Used to Build Nervous System and Behavioral Health Terms

COMBINING FORM (WR + CV)	DEFINITION	COMBINING FORM (WR + CV)	DEFINITION
angi/o	blood vessel(s)	my/o	muscle(s), muscle tissue
arthr/o	joint(s)	neur/o	nerve(s), nerve tissue
cephal/o	head (upward)	path/o	disease
electr/o	electrical activity	thromb/o	blood clot
hydr/o	water		
SUFFIX (S)	**DEFINITION**	**SUFFIX (S)**	**DEFINITION**
-al, -ic	pertaining to	-ia	diseased state, condition of
-algia	pain	-itis	inflammation
-cele	hernia, protrusion	-logist	one who studies and treats (specialist, physician)
-genic	producing, originating, causing	-logy	study of
-gram	record, radiographic image	-oma	tumor
-graph	instrument used to record	-osis	abnormal condition
-graphy	process of recording, radiographic imaging	-y	no meaning
PREFIX (P)	**DEFINITION**	**PREFIX (P)**	**DEFINITION**
a-	absence of, without	poly-	many, much
dys-	difficult, painful, abnormal		

Refer to Appendix A, Word Parts Used in *Basic Medical Language*, for alphabetical lists of word parts and their meanings.

EXERCISE A **Build and Translate Medical Terms Built from Word Parts**

*Use the **Word Parts Tables** to complete the following questions. Check your responses with the Answer Key in Appendix C.*

1. **LABEL:** *Write the combining forms for anatomic structures of the nervous system on Figure 11.3. These anatomic combining forms will be used to build and translate medical terms in Exercise A.*

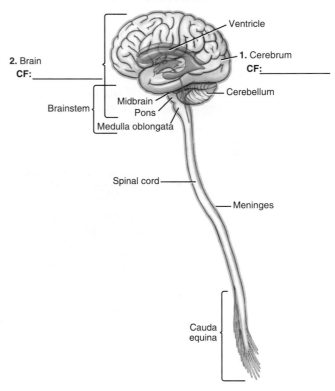

2. Brain
CF:_____

Ventricle

1. Cerebrum
CF:_____

Cerebellum

Brainstem {
Midbrain
Pons
Medulla oblongata

Spinal cord

Meninges

FYI **Cauda equina**, horse's tail in Latin, refers to the bundle of nerves extending from the spinal cord near the end of the vertebral column.

Cauda equina

Figure 11.3 The brain and spinal cord.

2. **MATCH:** *Draw a line to match the word part with its definition.*

    a. -al   blood clot
    b. angi/o   pertaining to
    c. -graphy   blood vessel(s)
    d. thromb/o   abnormal condition
    e. -osis   process of recording, radiographic imaging

3. **BUILD**: *Using the combining form **cerebr/o** and the word parts reviewed in the previous exercise, build the following terms related to the cerebrum. Remember, the definition usually starts with the meaning of the suffix.*

    a. pertaining to the cerebrum

                                         _____/_____
                                                    wr   s

    b. radiographic imaging of the blood vessels of   cerebral _____/ o /_____
       the cerebrum   wr   cv   s

    c. abnormal condition of a blood clot in the   cerebral _____/_____
       cerebrum   wr   s

4. **READ**: **Cerebral thrombosis** (se-RĒ-bral) (throm-BŌ-sis) is frequently caused by plaque formation or by an embolus (a blood clot or foreign material that enters the bloodstream and moves until it lodges at another point in the circulation). **Cerebral angiography** (se-RĒ-bral) (an-jē-OG-ra-fē) is an excellent test for diagnosing thrombosis and may also be used as therapy to break down the clot.

5. **LABEL**: *Write word parts to complete Figure 11.4.*

Figure 11.4 _____/_____ _____/o/_____ uses CT
               cerebrum   pertaining to   blood vessel   radiographic imaging

imaging to obtain images of the arterial and venous circulation.

6. **MATCH**: *Draw a line to match the word part with its definition.*

    a. -itis   disease
    b. -y   inflammation
    c. path/o   no meaning

7. **BUILD**: *Using the combining form **encephal/o**, meaning brain, and the word parts reviewed in the matching exercise, build the following terms:*

    a. disease of the brain

                                        _____/ o /_____/____y____
                                         wr   cv   wr   s

    b. inflammation of the brain

                                        _____/_____
                                         wr   s

8. READ: Viral infections are the most common causes of **encephalitis** (en-sef-a-LĪ-tis), which can sometimes be life-threatening. Fever, severe headache, or loss of consciousness are reasons to seek immediate medical care. The major symptom of **encephalopathy** (en-sef-a-LOP-a-thē) is an altered mental state. Frequent causes include infections, alcohol-related liver disease, kidney disease, trauma, and toxins.

---

9. MATCH: *Draw a line to match the word part with its definition.*

a. electr/o   instrument used to record
b. -graphy   electrical activity
c. -graph   record, radiographic image
d. -gram   process of recording, radiographic imaging

---

10. TRANSLATE: *Continue using the combining form **encephal/o** to complete the definitions of the following terms.*

a. electr/o/encephal/o/gram   _____ of _____ activity of the brain
b. electr/o/encephal/o/graph   _____used to record _____ _____of the brain
c. electr/o/encephal/o/graphy   process of _____ the electrical activity of the _____

---

11. READ: An **electroencephalogram** (ē-lek-trō-en-SEF-a-lō-gram), abbreviated EEG, is a test that detects electrical activity in the brain using flat metal discs attached to the scalp (see Figure 11.2). The **electroencephalograph** (ē-lek-trō-en-SEF-a-lō-graf) detects electrical impulses that provide information about the activity of the brain cells. **Electroencephalography** (ē-lek-trō-en-sef-a-LOG-ra-fē) is very useful in diagnosing epilepsy (seizure disorder) and is also helpful in diagnosing sleep disorders.

> **FYI** Compare **electroencephalogram** with **electromyogram** and **electrocardiogram**. Note that the combining form for the body part is the only difference between the words and therefore the meanings of each medical term.

---

12. LABEL: *Write word parts to complete Figure 11.5.*

Figure 11.5 Sample of recordings of different mental states obtained by

_____/o/_____/o/_____.
    electrical activity   brain   process of recording

13. MATCH: *Draw a line to match the word part with its definition.*

    a. -al   pain

    b. -algia   pertaining to

---

14. BUILD: *Using the combining form **neur/o**, meaning nerve(s), and the word parts reviewed in the previous exercise, build the following terms.*

    a. pertaining to the nerve(s)   _____ / _____

                                                   wr   **s**

    b. pain in the nerve(s)   _____ / _____

                                                   wr   **s**

---

15. READ: The **neural** (NŪ-ral) foramen is an opening between the vertebrae; nerves leave the spine through these openings and extend to other parts of the body. Postherpetic **neuralgia** (nū-RAL-ja) can occur after shingles. This burning, stabbing, and sometimes very severe pain can occur anywhere on the body.

---

16. LABEL: *Write word parts to complete Figure 11.6.*

Figure 11.6 Postherpetic _____ / _____

                               nerve(s)   pain

occurring on the right side of a patient's back.

---

17. MATCH: *Draw a line to match the word part with its definition.*

    a. -logist   no meaning

    b. -logy   one who studies and treats (specialist, physician)

    c. path/o   study of

    d. -y   disease

18. TRANSLATE: *Complete the definitions of the following terms using the combining form **neur/o**.*

    a. neur/o/logist   _____ who studies and treats diseases of the nervous system

    b. neur/o/logy   study of the _____ (nervous system)

    c. neur/o/path/y   _____ of the _____(nervous system)

---

19. READ: Diabetic peripheral **neuropathy** (nū-ROP-a-thē) usually occurs in patients who have had diabetes for at least 2 years. It causes decreased sensation in the feet and hands, and is often accompanied by pain. A **neurologist** (nū-ROL-o-jist) may perform special tests to determine the extent of the nerve damage. A **neurology** (nū-ROL-o-jē) consultation is especially important if the patient has developed sores or ulcers due to lack of sensation in the feet.

---

20. MATCH: *Draw a line to match the word part with its definition.*

    a. -itis   joint(s)

    b. -algia   nerve(s)

    c. arthr/o   inflammation

    d. my/o   muscle(s)

    e. neur/o   pain

---

21. BUILD: *Use the prefix **poly-**, meaning many or much, and the word parts reviewed in the previous exercise to build the following terms.*

    a. pain in many muscles   _____ / _____ / _____

                                                    p   wr   s

    b. inflammation of many joints   _____ / _____ / _____

                                                    p   wr   s

    c. inflammation of many nerves   _____ / _____ / _____

                                                     p   wr   s

---

22. READ: Polymyalgia (pol-ē-mī-AL-ja) rheumatica, abbreviated PMR, is an inflammatory disorder that mainly affects adults over the age of 65. Patients complain of muscle pain and stiffness in the shoulders, neck, upper arms, and hips. Many types of **polyarthritis** (pol-ē-ar-THRĪ-tis) exist, including rheumatoid arthritis, lupus, viral arthritis, and gout. Guillain-Barré syndrome is a type of **polyneuritis** (pol-ē-nū-RĪ-tis), which causes rapid onset of numbness, weakness, and sometimes even paralysis of the legs, arms, breathing muscles, and face.

23. REVIEW OF NERVOUS SYSTEM AND BEHAVIORAL HEALTH TERMS BUILT FROM WORD PARTS: *The following is an alphabetical list of terms built and translated in the previous exercises.*

MEDICAL TERMS BUILT FROM WORD PARTS

TERM	DEFINITION	TERM	DEFINITION
1. **cerebral** (se-RĒ-bral)	pertaining to the cerebrum	9. **neural** (NŪ-ral)	pertaining to the nerve(s)
2. **cerebral angiography** (se-RĒ-bral) (an-jē-OG-ra-fē)	radiographic imaging of the blood vessels of the cerebrum (Figure 11.4)	10. **neuralgia** (nū-RAL-ja)	pain in the nerve(s) (Figure 11.6)
3. **cerebral thrombosis** (se-RĒ-bral) (throm-BŌ-sis)	abnormal condition of a blood clot in the cerebrum (Figure 11.11, *B*)	11. **neurologist** (nū-ROL-o-jist)	physician who studies and treats diseases of the nervous system
4. **electroencephalogram (EEG)** (ē-lek-trō-en-SEF-a-lō-gram)	record of electrical activity of the brain	12. **neurology** (nū-ROL-o-jē)	study of the nerves
5. **electroencephalograph** (ē-lek-trō-en-SEF-a-lō-graf)	instrument used to record electrical activity of the brain	13. **neuropathy** (nū-ROP-a-thē)	disease of the nerves
6. **electroencephalography** (ē-lek-trō-en-sef-a-LOG-ra-fē)	process of recording the electrical activity of the brain	14. **polyarthritis** (pol-ē-ar-THRĪ-tis)	inflammation of many joints
7. **encephalitis** (en-sef-a-LĪ-tis)	inflammation of the brain	15. **polymyalgia** (pol-ē-mī-AL-ja)	pain in many muscles
8. **encephalopathy** (en-sef-a-LOP-a-thē)	disease of the brain	16. **polyneuritis** (pol-ē-nū-RĪ-tis)	inflammation of many nerves

---

EXERCISE B   Pronounce and Spell Terms Built from Word Parts

Practice pronunciation and spelling on paper and online.

1. **Practice on Paper**
   a. **Pronounce:** Read the phonetic spelling and say aloud the terms listed in the previous table, Review Terms Built from Word Parts.
   b. **Spell:** Have a study partner read the terms aloud. Write the spelling of the terms on a separate sheet of paper.

2. **Practice Online** ⊕
   a. **Access** online learning resources. Go to evolve.elsevier.com > Evolve Resources > Practice Student Resources.
   b. **Pronounce:** Select Audio Glossary > Lesson 11 > Exercise B. Select a term to hear its pronunciation and repeat aloud.
   c. **Spell:** Select Activities > Lesson 11 > Spell Terms > Exercise B. Select the audio icon and type the correct spelling of the term.

❑ Check the box when complete.

EXERCISE C **Build and Translate MORE Medical Terms Built from Word Parts**

*Use the **Word Parts Tables** to complete the following questions. Check your responses with the Answer Key in Appendix C.*

1. **LABEL:** *Write the combining forms for ana-tomic structures of the nervous system on Figure 11.7. These anatomic combining forms will be used to build and translate medical terms in Exercise C.*

Ventricle

Cerebrum
CF: <u>cerebr/o</u>

Brain
CF: <u>encephal/o</u>

Cerebellum

Midbrain
Brainstem
Pons
Medulla oblongata

1. Spinal cord
   CF:_____

2. Meninges
   CF:_____
   CF:_____

Cauda equina

Figure 11.7 The brain and spinal cord.

2. **MATCH:** *Draw a line to match the word part with its definition.*

   a. -oma   hernia, protrusion
   b. -itis   tumor
   c. -cele   inflammation

3. **BUILD:** *Use the combining forms for meninges and the word parts reviewed in the previous exercise to build the following terms. Remember, the definition usually starts with the meaning of the suffix. Hint: Use **mening/o** for a and b and **meningi/o** for c.*

   a. hernia of the meninges   _____ / o / _____
                                        wr   cv   s

   b. inflammation of the meninges   _____ / _____
                                        wr   s

   c. tumor of the meninges   _____ / _____
                                        wr   s

4. **READ:** Spina bifida occurs when the vertebral column doesn't close completely during development; this may result in a **meningocele** (me-NING-gō-sēl). A **meningioma** (me-nin-je-Ō-ma) is usually benign and slow growing, and occurs most often in the brains of older women. **Meningitis** (men-in-JĪ-tis) is usually caused by a bacterial or viral infection of the fluid surrounding the brain and spinal cord.

5. **LABEL:** *Write word parts to complete Figure 11.8.*

Figure 11.8 A large _____/_____ in a female patient.
　　　　　　　　　　　　　 meninges　　　　　tumor

6. **MATCH:** *Draw a line to match the word part with its definition.*

a. -itis　　　　gray matter
b. poli/o　　　inflammation

7. **TRANSLATE:** *Complete the definitions of the following terms using the combining form **myel/o**, meaning spinal cord. Use the meaning of the word parts to fill in the blanks. Remember, the definition usually starts with the meaning of the suffix.*

a. mening/o/myel/itis　　　_____ of the meninges and spinal cord
b. poli/o/myel/itis　　　　inflammation of the _____ matter of the _____ cord

8. **READ:** **Meningomyelitis** (me-ning-gō-mī-e-LĪ-tis) is a rare condition that is usually caused by a virus. **Poliomyelitis** (pō-lē-ō-mī-e-LĪ-tis) is often referred to as polio or infantile paralysis. It is a viral disease that has been eradicated from most countries in the world, thanks to the development of vaccines in 1952 and 1962 and mass vaccination campaigns.

9. **MATCH:** *Draw a line to match the word part with its definition.*

a. -graphy　　　　record, radiographic image
b. -gram　　　　　process of recording, radiographic imaging

10. BUILD: *Continue using* **myel/o**, *along with the word parts reviewed in the previous exercise, to build the following terms related to the spinal cord.*

a. radiographic image of the spinal cord   _____ / o / _____
                                            wr   cv   s

b. radiographic imaging of the spinal cord   _____ / o / _____
                                             wr   cv   s

11. READ: Myelography (mī-e-LOG-ra-fē) is an invasive procedure that has been largely replaced by magnetic resonance imaging (MRI). For those who cannot have an MRI, such as a patient with a pacemaker, a CT **myelogram** (MĪ-e-lō-gram) is performed by injecting a contrast medium into the cerebrospinal fluid (CSF) that surrounds the spinal cord and obtaining images of the area in question.

12. LABEL: *Write word parts to complete Figure 11.9.*

Spinal cord

Figure 11.9 Image obtained by CT _____ /o/ _____.
                                  spinal cord   radiographic imaging

13. MATCH: *Draw a line to match the word part with its definition.*

a. -algia   small
b. -us   pain
c. hydr/o   no meaning
d. micro-   water

14. TRANSLATE: *Complete the definitions of the following terms built from the combining form* **cephal/o**, *meaning head. Use the meaning of word parts to fill in the blanks.*

a. micro/cephal/us   small _____
b. hydr/o/cephal/us   _____ (cerebrospinal fluid) in the _____ (brain)
c. ceph/algia   _____ in the head (headache)

NOTE: the **al** *is dropped from the combining form cephal/o in the term cephalgia.*

15. READ: Cephalgia (sef-AL-ja) refers to a headache and is used to describe cluster headaches associated with migraines and headaches accompanied by facial pain. **Microcephalus** (mī-krō-SEF-a-lus), also called microcephaly (mī-krō-SEF-a-lē), refers to an abnormally small circumference of a baby's head. It may be present at birth (congenital) or occur in the first few years of life (acquired). **Hydrocephalus** (hī-drō-SEF-a-lus) may be congenital or acquired and is caused by increased amounts of cerebrospinal fluid in the brain. Congenital hydrocephalus may result in an enlargement of the infant's cranium.

16. MATCH: *Draw a line to match the word part with its definition.*

a. a-   diseased state, condition of
b. dys-   half
c. hemi-   four
d. quadr/i   difficult, painful, abnormal
e. -ia   absence of, without

17. BUILD: *Use the combining form **phas/o**, meaning speech, along with the word parts reviewed in the previous exercise to build the following terms.*

a. condition of without speech   _____/_____/_____
                                                            p   wr   s

b. condition of difficulty with speech   _____/_____/_____
                                                            p   wr   s

18. READ: Aphasia (a-FĀ-zha) describes a condition in which a person cannot communicate; it affects the ability to express oneself through both spoken and written language. **Dysphasia** (dis-FĀ-zha) is a less severe condition in which some speech and language abilities are preserved. Either may be the result of a stroke or head injury.

19. TRANSLATE: *Complete the definitions of the following terms built from the combining form **pleg/o**, meaning paralysis.*

a. hemi/pleg/ia   condition of _____ of half (right or left side of the body)
b. quadr/i/pleg/ia   condition of paralysis of _____ (limbs)

20. READ: Hemiplegia (hem-ē-PLĒ-ja) can affect either the left or right side of the body and is most commonly caused by a stroke. **Quadriplegia** (kwod-ri-PLĒ-ja) is usually a result of vertebral fractures that cause injury to the spinal cord.

21. LABEL: *Write word parts to complete Figure 11.10.*

Figure 11.10 A. _____/_____/_____.
                           half   paralysis   condition of

                    B. Paraplegia.

                    C. _____/i/_____/_____.
                           four   paralysis   condition of

A   B   C

22. **MATCH:** *Draw a line to match the word part with its definition.*

    a. -genic   no meaning
    b. path/o   producing, originating, causing
    c. -y   abnormal condition
    d. -osis   disease

23. **BUILD:** *Use the combining form **psych/o**, meaning mind, along with the word parts reviewed in the previous exercise, to build terms related to the mind.*

    a. originating in the mind   _____/ o /_____
                                                   wr   cv   s

    b. (any) disease of the mind   _____/ o /_____/___y___
                                                   wr   cv   wr   s

    c. abnormal condition of the mind _____/_____
                                                   wr   s

24. **READ:** **Psychogenic** (sī-kō-JEN-ik) disorders arise from mental or emotional sources. While **psychopathy** (sī-KOP-a-thē) refers to any disease of the mind and may be mild or severe, **psychosis** (si-KŌ-sis) implies a severe impairment in perception of reality with hallucinations, incoherent speech or behavior, and a lack of awareness of this behavior on the part of the patient.

25. **MATCH:** *Draw a line to match the word part with its definition.*

    a. -logist   study of
    b. -logy   one who studies and treats (specialist, physician)

26. **TRANSLATE:** *Complete the definitions of the following terms. Use the meaning of word parts to fill in the blanks.*

    a. psych/o/logist   specialist who studies and treats the _____
    b. psych/o/logy   _____ of the mind

27. **READ:** The American Psychological Association describes **psychology** (sī-KOL-o-jē) as the study of the mind and behavior, which ranges from the functions of the brain to the actions of nations. A **psychologist** (sī-KOL-o-jist) may work in a private or group practice, or may work in schools, hospitals, nursing homes, mental health clinics, prisons, businesses, or places of worship.

28. REVIEW OF MORE NERVOUS SYSTEM AND BEHAVIORAL HEALTH TERMS BUILT FROM WORD PARTS: *The following is an alphabetical list of terms built and translated in the previous exercises.*

MEDICAL TERMS BUILT FROM WORD PARTS

TERM	DEFINITION	TERM	DEFINITION
1. **aphasia** (a-FĀ-zha)	condition of without speech (or loss of the ability to speak)	11. **myelogram** (MĪ-e-lō-gram)	radiographic image of the spinal cord
2. **cephalgia** (sef-AL-ja)	pain in the head (also called **headache**). *Note: The* **al** *is dropped from the combining form cephal/o.*	12. **myelography** (mī-e-LOG-ra-fē)	radiographic imaging of the spinal cord (Figure 11.9)
3. **dysphasia** (dis-FĀ-zha)	condition of difficulty with speech	13. **poliomyelitis** (pō-lē-ō-mī-e-LĪ-tis)	inflammation of the gray matter of the spinal cord
4. **hemiplegia** (hem-ē-PLĒ-ja)	condition of paralysis of half (of the body) (Figure 11.10, A)	14. **psychogenic** (sī-kō-JEN-ik)	originating in the mind
5. **hydrocephalus** (hī-drō-SEF-a-lus)	water in the head (increased amount of cerebrospinal fluid in the brain)	15. **psychologist** (sī-KOL-o-jist)	specialist who studies and treats the mind
6. **meningioma** (me-nin-je-Ō-ma)	tumor of the meninges (Figure 11.8)	16. **psychology** (sī-KOL-o-jē)	study of the mind
7. **meningitis** (men-in-JĪ-tis)	inflammation of the meninges	17. **psychopathy** (sī-KOP-a-thē)	(any) disease of the mind
8. **meningocele** (me-NING-gō-sēl)	hernia of the meninges	18. **psychosis** (si-KŌ-sis)	abnormal condition of the mind (major mental disorder characterized by extreme derangement, often with delusions and hallucinations)
9. **meningomyelitis** (me-ning-gō-mī-e-LĪ-tis)	inflammation of the meninges and the spinal cord		
10. **microcephalus** (mī-krō-SEF-a-lus)	small head (also called **microcephaly**)	19. **quadriplegia** (kwod-ri-PLĒ-ja)	condition of paralysis of four (limbs) (Figure 11.10, C)

EXERCISE D   Pronounce and Spell MORE Terms Built from Word Parts

Practice pronunciation and spelling on paper and online.

1. **Practice on Paper**
   a. **Pronounce**: Read the phonetic spelling and say aloud the terms listed in the previous table, Review of MORE Terms Built from Word Parts.
   b. **Spell**: Have a study partner read the terms aloud. Write the spelling of the terms on a separate sheet of paper.

2. **Practice Online** 🌐

   a. **Access** online learning resources. Go to evolve.elsevier.com > Evolve Resources > Practice Student Resources.

   b. **Pronounce**: Select Audio Glossary > Lesson 11 > Exercise D. Select a term to hear its pronunciation and repeat aloud.

   c. **Spell**: Select Activities > Lesson 11 > Spell Terms > Exercise D. Select the audio icon and type the correct spelling of the term.

❏ Check the box when complete.

OBJECTIVE 2

Define, pronounce, and spell medical terms NOT built from word parts.

The terms listed below may contain word parts, but are difficult to translate literally.

MEDICAL TERMS NOT BUILT FROM WORD PARTS

TERM	DEFINITION
1. Alzheimer disease (AD) (AWLTZ-hī-mer) (di-ZĒZ)	type of dementia caused by degeneration of brain tissue and occurring more frequently after age 65. The brain shrinks dramatically as nerve cells die and tissues atrophy. The disease is slowly progressive and usually results in profound dementia in 5 to 10 years. A prominent feature of AD is the inability to remember the recent past, while memories of the distant past remain intact.
2. anxiety disorder (ang-ZĪ-e-tē) (dis-OR-der)	disorder characterized by feelings of apprehension, tension, or uneasiness arising typically from the anticipation of unreal or imagined danger
3. bipolar disorder (bī-PŌ-lar) (dis-OR-der)	major psychological disorder typified by a disturbance in mood. The disorder is manifested by manic (elevated or irritated mood, excessive energy, impulsiveness) and depressive episodes that may alternate, or elements of both may occur simultaneously.
4. concussion (kon-KUSH-un)	injury to the brain caused by major or minor head trauma; symptoms include vertigo, headache, and possible loss of consciousness
5. dementia (de-MEN-sha)	cognitive impairment characterized by loss of intellectual brain function, including difficulty in performing complex tasks, reasoning, learning and retaining new information, orientation, word finding, and behavior. Dementia has several causes and is not considered part of normal aging.
6. depression (dē-PRESH-un)	mood disturbance characterized by feelings of sadness, despair, discouragement, hopelessness, lack of joy, altered sleep patterns, and difficulty with decision making and daily function. Depression ranges from normal feelings of sadness through dysthymia (mild depression), to major depression.
7. epidural nerve block (ep-i-DŪ-ral) (nurv) (blok)	procedure performed for spine-related pain, or for pain from other causes such as childbirth and labor, by injection of anesthetic agent into the epidural space. Injection may be between the vertebral spines, in the cervical, thoracic, or lumbar region.
8. lumbar puncture (LP) (LUM-bar) (PUNK-chur)	diagnostic procedure performed by insertion of a needle into the subarachnoid space, usually between the third and fourth lumbar vertebrae; performed for many reasons, including the removal of cerebrospinal fluid (also called **spinal tap**)

Continued

MEDICAL TERMS NOT BUILT FROM WORD PARTS—cont'd

TERM	DEFINITION
9. **migraine** (MĪ-grān)	an intense, throbbing headache, usually one-sided, and often associated with irritability, nausea, vomiting, and extreme sensitivity to light or sound. Migraines may occur with or without aura (sensory warning symptoms such as flashes of light, blind spots, or tingling in the arms or legs).
10. **multiple sclerosis (MS)** (MUL-ti-pul) (skle-RŌ-sis)	chronic degenerative disease characterized by sclerotic patches along the brain and spinal cord; signs and symptoms fluctuate over the course of the disease; more common symptoms include fatigue, balance and coordination impairments, numbness, and vision problems
11. **paraplegia** (par-a-PLĒ-ja)	paralysis from the waist down caused by damage to the lower level of the spinal cord

FYI   The term **paraplegia** is composed of the Greek words **para**, meaning beside, and **pleg**, meaning paralysis. Paraplegia has been used since Hippocrates' time and originally meant paralysis of any limb or side of the body. It has been used to mean paralysis from the waist down since the nineteenth century.

12. **Parkinson disease (PD)** (PAR-kin-sun) (di-ZĒZ)	chronic degenerative disease of the central nervous system; symptoms include resting tremors of the hands and feet, rigidity, expressionless face, shuffling gait, and eventually dementia. It usually occurs after the age of 50 years.

FYI   **Parkinson disease** is also called **parkinsonism**, **paralysis agitans**, and **shaking palsy**. It was described by James Parkinson, an English professor, in 1817 in his **Essay on the Shaking Palsy**.

13. **psychiatrist** (sī-KĪ-a-trist)	physician with additional training and experience in the diagnosis, prevention, and treatment of mental disorders; can prescribe medications and direct therapy
14. **sciatica** (sī-AT-i-ka)	inflammation of the sciatic nerve, causing pain that travels from the buttock through the leg to the foot and toes; can be caused by injury, infection, arthritis, herniated disk, or from prolonged pressure on the nerve from sitting for long periods

FYI   The **sciatic nerve**, the longest in the body, travels through the hip from the spine to the thigh and continues with branches throughout the lower leg and foot. **Sciatica** is inflammation of the nerve along its course.

15. **seizure (Sz)** (SĒ-zher)	sudden, abnormal surge of electrical activity in the brain, resulting in involuntary body movements or behaviors
16. **stroke** (strōk)	interruption of blood supply to a region of the brain, depriving nerve cells in the affected area of oxygen and nutrients (also called **cerebrovascular accident [CVA]**) (Figure 11.11)
17. **subarachnoid hemorrhage (SAH)** (sub-e-RAK-noyd) (HEM-o-rij)	bleeding between the pia mater and arachnoid layers of the meninges (subarachnoid space) caused by a ruptured blood vessel (usually a ruptured cerebral aneurysm). The patient may experience an intense, sudden headache accompanied by nausea, vomiting, and neck pain. SAH is a critical condition that must be recognized and treated immediately to prevent permanent brain damage or death. (Figure 11.11, *A*)
18. **syncope** (SINK-o-pē)	fainting or sudden loss of consciousness caused by lack of blood supply to the cerebrum
19. **transient ischemic attack (TIA)** (TRAN-sē-ent) (is-KĒ-mik) (a-TAK)	sudden deficient supply of blood to the brain lasting a short time. The symptoms may be similar to those of stroke, but are temporary, and the usual outcome is complete recovery. TIAs are often warning signs for eventual occurrence of a stroke

EXERCISE E **Label**

Write the medical terms pictured and defined using the previous table of Medical Terms NOT Built from Word Parts. Check your work with the Answer Key in Appendix C.

1. _____

sudden deficient supply of blood to the brain lasting a short time

2. _____

interruption of blood supply to a region of the brain, depriving nerve cells in the affected area of oxygen and nutrients

3. _____

bleeding between the pia mater and arachnoid layers of the meninges caused by a ruptured blood vessel

4. _____

cognitive impairment characterized by loss of intellectual brain function, including difficulty in performing complex tasks, reasoning, learning and retaining new information, orientation, word finding, and behavior.

5. _____

type of dementia caused by degeneration of brain tissue and occurring more frequently after age 65

Normal brain

Reduced mass associated with this disease

Sulci   Gyri

6. _____

diagnostic procedure performed for the removal of cerebrospinal fluid (for testing)

End of spinal cord

Needle insertion site (L3-L4)

Cauda equina

Intervertebral disc

Vertebra (spinous process)

Dura mater

Arachnoid

Subarachnoid space

7. _____

paralysis from the waist down

8. _____

inflammation of the sciatic nerve, causing pain that travels from the thigh through the leg to the foot and toes

9. _____

an intense, throbbing headache, usually one-sided, and often associated with irritability, nausea, vomiting, and extreme sensitivity to light or sound

10. _____

physician with additional training and experience in the diagnosis, prevention, and treatment of mental disorders; can prescribe medications and direct therapy

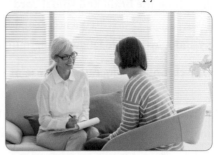

EXERCISE F Match

Match the terms in the first column with their correct descriptions in the second column. Answers are listed in Appendix C.

_____ **1.** syncope

_____ **2.** multiple sclerosis

_____ **3.** anxiety disorder

_____ **4.** depression

_____ **5.** epidural nerve block

a. mood disturbance characterized by feelings of sadness, despair, and discouragement

b. chronic degenerative disease characterized by sclerotic patches along the brain and spinal cord

c. fainting or sudden loss of consciousness

d. injection of anesthetic agent between the vertebrae; performed for spine-related pain

e. disorder characterized by feelings of apprehension, tension, or uneasiness

EXERCISE G Match

Match the terms in the first column with their correct descriptions in the second column. Answers are listed in Appendix C.

_____ **1.** bipolar disorder

_____ **2.** Parkinson disease

_____ **3.** concussion

_____ **4.** seizure

a. injury to the brain caused by major or minor head trauma

b. sudden, abnormal surge of electrical activity in the brain, resulting in involuntary body movements or behaviors

c. symptoms include resting tremors of the hands and feet, rigidity, expressionless face, and shuffling gait

d. disorder manifested by manic and depressive episodes that may alternate or may occur simultaneously

EXERCISE H   Learn Medical Terms NOT Built from Word Parts

Fill in the blanks with medical terms defined in bold using the Medical Terms NOT Built from Word Parts table. Answers are listed in Appendix C.

1. More than twice as likely to affect women than men, **chronic degenerative disease characterized by sclerotic patches along the brain and spinal cord**, or _____, abbreviated as _____, is frequently diagnosed between the ages of 20 and 40 years. Symptoms of MS vary widely and may include fatigue, pain, numbness, or problems with vision or coordination.

2. Another **chronic degenerative disease of the central nervous system**, or _____ _____, abbreviated as _____, is usually diagnosed after the age of 50 years. A hallmark symptom of PD is a resting tremor, or uncontrolled movement of a limb when at rest, that stops during purposeful, voluntary movement. Other symptoms include rigidity, expressionless face, shuffling gait, and eventually dementia.

3. **Cognitive impairment characterized by loss of intellectual brain function**, or _____, has several causes and is not considered a part of normal aging. The **type of dementia caused by degeneration of brain tissue and occurring more frequently after age 65**, or _____ (AD), is the most common type of dementia, making up 60% to 80% of all cases. It causes death of nerve cells throughout the brain, leading to tissue loss and shrinkage.

4. Vertigo and loss of consciousness can be symptoms of **injury to the brain caused by major or minor head trauma**, or _____. Major head trauma can result in **sudden, abnormal surge of electrical activity in the brain, resulting in involuntary body movements or behaviors**, or _____. In some cases, patients may develop epilepsy years after a severe concussion.

5. **Inflammation of the sciatic nerve, causing pain that travels from the buttock through the leg to the foot and toes**, or _____, may be caused by arthritis in the vertebrae or by a herniated disk. **Procedure performed for spine-related pain by injection of anesthetic agent into the epidural space**, or _____ may be needed in severe cases and usually incorporates a steroid like cortisone for long-term relief.

6. **An intense, throbbing headache, usually one-sided, and often associated with irritability, nausea, vomiting, and extreme sensitivity to light or sound**, or _____, may be triggered by hormonal changes in women, or by certain foods, food additives (like aspartame or MSG), alcohol, stress, or changes in sleep patterns.

7. A **diagnostic procedure performed by insertion of a needle into the subarachnoid space, usually between the third and fourth lumbar vertebrae**, or _____, abbreviated _____, is also called a spinal tap. It may be used to diagnose normal pressure hydrocephalus, which is a form of hydrocephalus with a gradual onset, usually affecting those 60 years of age and older.

8. **Interruption of blood supply to a region of the brain, depriving nerve cells in the affected area of oxygen and nutrients**, or _____ (also called **cerebrovascular accident** and abbreviated as _____), can be best understood by categorizing the underlying cause of the interruption of blood flow (Figure 11.11). One type of stroke is caused by bleeding within the brain or cranial space, known as hemorrhagic stroke. Another type is an ischemic stroke, which is due to a blocked vessel caused by a cerebral thrombosis or a cerebral embolus.

9. **Bleeding between the pia mater and arachnoid layers of the meninges (subarachnoid space) caused by a ruptured blood vessel**, or _____, is usually the result of a ruptured brain aneurysm, and can result in a hemorrhagic stroke.

10. **A sudden deficient supply of blood to the brain lasting a short time**, or _____ _____, abbreviated _____, usually lasts only a few minutes and causes no permanent damage. It is considered a warning sign for an ischemic stroke. Symptoms may include hemiplegia, dysphasia, loss of vision, and **fainting or sudden loss of consciousness caused by lack of blood supply to the cerebrum**, or _____.

11. **Paralysis from the waist down caused by damage to the lower level of the spinal cord**, or _____ _____, may be caused by vertebral fracture or dislocation (Figure 11.10, *B*).

Figure 11.11 Causes of stroke. **A.** Hemorrhagic stroke is the result of bleeding caused by an intracerebral hemorrhage or a subarachnoid hemorrhage, usually a result of a ruptured cerebral aneurysm. **B.** Ischemic stroke is the result of a blocked blood vessel caused by a cerebral thrombosis or cerebral embolus.

12. **Disorder characterized by feelings of apprehension, tension, or uneasiness**, or _____
_____, may be treated with psychotherapy (talk therapy) and/or medications. Making lifestyle
changes, learning coping mechanisms, and relaxation therapy can also help.

13. **Mood disturbance characterized by feelings of sadness, despair, and discouragement**, or _____
_____, may range from normal feelings of sadness (resulting from personal
loss or tragedy), through dysthymia (mild depressive symptoms that come and go), to major depressive disorder (persistent depressed feelings that impact everyday life). Both dysthymia and major depression can be
treated with psychotherapy and/or medications.

14. **Major psychological disorder typified by a disturbance in mood, manifested by manic or depressive episodes**, or _____, has symptoms that range from feelings of
hopelessness and despair (depression) to elevated or irritated mood, excessive energy, and impulsiveness
(mania). Mood shifts may occur only a few times a year, or as often as several times a day. Sometimes bipolar
disorder causes symptoms of depression and mania at the same time. Medication is the main treatment for
bipolar disorder, although psychotherapy is also very important.

15. **A physician with additional training and experience in the diagnosis, prevention, and treatment of mental
disorders**, or a _____, is trained to assess mental and physical aspects of
psychological problems. Physicians in this specialty can order and perform a variety of laboratory and psychological tests to make diagnoses and formulate treatment plans.

16. **Sudden loss of consciousness caused by lack of blood supply to the cerebrum**, or _____,
may be due to less serious causes, such as changes in body position, emotional stress, or pain. It may also be
due to more serious causes, such as atrial fibrillation, heart failure, and some medications.

EXERCISE I   **Pronounce and Spell Terms NOT Built from Word Parts**

Practice pronunciation and spelling on paper and online.

1. **Practice on Paper**
   a. **Pronounce**: Read the phonetic spelling and say aloud the terms listed in the previous table, Terms NOT
   Built from Word Parts.
   b. **Spell**: Have a study partner read the terms aloud. Write the spelling of the terms on a separate sheet of paper.

2. **Practice Online** 🌐
   a. **Access** online learning resources. Go to evolve.elsevier.com > Evolve Resources > Practice Student Resources.
   b. **Pronounce**: Select Audio Glossary > Lesson 11 > Exercise I. Select a term to hear its pronunciation and
   repeat aloud.
   c. **Spell**: Select Activities > Lesson 11 > Spell Terms > Exercise I. Select the audio icon and type the correct
   spelling of the term.

❑   Check the box when complete.

OBJECTIVE 3

Write abbreviations.

ABBREVIATIONS RELATED TO THE NERVOUS SYSTEM AND BEHAVIORAL HEALTH

Use the online **flashcards** to familiarize yourself with the following abbreviations.

ABBREVIATION	TERM	ABBREVIATION	TERM
AD	Alzheimer disease	MS	multiple sclerosis
ADHD	attention deficit/hyperactivity disorder	OCD	obsessive-compulsive disorder
ADL, ADLs	activities of daily living (such as personal hygiene, dressing, eating, ability to use the restroom, and transferring to and from a standing position)	PD	Parkinson disease
CNS	central nervous system	PNS	peripheral nervous system
CP	cerebral palsy	PTSD	posttraumatic stress disorder
CSF	cerebrospinal fluid	SAH	subarachnoid hemorrhage
CVA	cerebrovascular accident	Sz	seizure
EEG	electroencephalogram	TIA	transient ischemic attack
LP	lumbar puncture		

EXERCISE J   Abbreviate Medical Terms

Write the correct abbreviation next to its medical term.

1. Signs and Symptoms:

   a. _____ seizure

2. Diseases and Disorders:

   a. _____ Alzheimer disease

   b. _____ cerebrovascular accident

   c. _____ multiple sclerosis

   d. _____ Parkinson disease

   e. _____ subarachnoid hemorrhage

   f. _____ transient ischemic attack

   g. _____ obsessive-compulsive disorder

   h. _____ cerebral palsy

   i. _____ posttraumatic stress disorder

3. Diagnostic Tests and Equipment:

    a. _____ electroencephalogram

    b. _____ lumbar puncture

4. Related Terms:

    a. _____ central nervous system

    b. _____ cerebrospinal fluid

    c. _____ peripheral nervous system

    d. _____, _____ activities of daily living

 OBJECTIVE 4

Identify medical terms by clinical category.

Now that you have worked through the nervous system and behavioral health lesson, review and practice medical terms grouped by clinical category. Categories include signs and symptoms, diseases and disorders, diagnostic tests and equipment, surgical procedures, specialties and professions, and other terms related to the nervous system and behavioral health. Check your responses with the Answer Key in Appendix C.

EXERCISE K   **Signs and Symptoms**

Write the medical terms for signs and symptoms next to their definitions.

1. _____ condition of without speech (or loss of the ability to speak)

2. _____ pain in the head (also called headache)

3. _____ condition of difficulty with speech

4. _____ pain in the nerve(s)

5. _____ inflammation of many joints

6. _____ pain in many muscles

7. _____ inflammation of many nerves

8. _____ sudden, abnormal surge of electrical activity in the brain, resulting in involuntary body movements or behaviors

9. _____ fainting or sudden loss of consciousness caused by lack of blood supply to the cerebrum

EXERCISE L   **Diseases and Disorders**

Write the medical terms for diseases and disorders next to their definitions.

1. _____ type of dementia caused by degeneration of brain tissue and occurring more frequently after age 65

2. _____ disorder characterized by feelings of apprehension, tension or uneasiness, arising typically from the anticipation of unreal or imagined danger

3. _____ major psychological disorder typified by a disturbance in mood

4. _____ abnormal condition of a blood clot in the cerebrum

5. _____ injury to the brain caused by major or minor head trauma

6. _____ cognitive impairment characterized by loss of intellectual brain function

7. _____ mood disturbance characterized by feelings of sadness, despair, discouragement, hopelessness, lack of joy, altered sleep patterns, and difficulty with decision making and daily function

8. _____ inflammation of the brain

9. _____ disease of the brain

10. _____ condition of paralysis of half (of the body)

11. _____ water in the head (increased amount of cerebrospinal fluid in the brain)

12. _____ tumor of the meninges

13. _____ inflammation of the meninges

14. _____ hernia of the meninges

15. _____ inflammation of the meninges and the spinal cord

16. _____ an intense, throbbing headache, usually one-sided, and often associated with irritability, nausea, vomiting, and extreme sensitivity to light or sound

17. _____ chronic degenerative disease characterized by sclerotic patches along the brain and spinal cord

18. _____ disease of the nerves

19. _____ paralysis from the waist down caused by damage to the lower level of the spinal cord

20. _____ chronic degenerative disease of the central nervous system; symptoms include resting tremors of the hands and feet, rigidity, expressionless face, shuffling gait, and eventually dementia

21. _____ inflammation of the gray matter of the spinal cord
22. _____ (any) disease of the mind
23. _____ abnormal condition of the mind (major mental disorder characterized by extreme derangement, often with delusions and hallucinations)
24. _____ condition of paralysis of four (limbs)
25. _____ inflammation of the sciatic nerve, causing pain that travels from the buttock through the leg to the foot and toes
26. _____ interruption of blood supply to a region of the brain, depriving nerve cells in the affected area of oxygen and nutrients
27. _____ bleeding between the pia mater and arachnoid layers of the meninges caused by a ruptured blood vessel
28. _____ sudden deficient supply of blood to the brain lasting a short time
29. _____ small head

EXERCISE M   Diagnostic Tests and Equipment

Write the medical terms for diagnostic tests and equipment next to their definitions.

1. _____ radiographic imaging of the blood vessels of the cerebrum
2. _____ record of electrical activity of the brain
3. _____ instrument used to record electrical activity of the brain
4. _____ process of recording the electrical activity of the brain
5. _____ diagnostic procedure performed by insertion of a needle into the subarachnoid space, usually between the third and fourth lumbar vertebrae (also called a spinal tap)
6. _____ radiographic image of the spinal cord
7. _____ radiographic imaging of the spinal cord

EXERCISE N   Surgical Procedure

Write the medical term for the surgical procedure next to its definition.

_____ procedure performed for spine-related pain by injection of anesthetic agent into the epidural space

EXERCISE O **Specialties and Professions**

Write the medical terms for specialties and professions next to their definitions.

1. _____ physician who studies and treats diseases of the nervous system

2. _____ study of the nerves (nervous system)

3. _____ specialist who studies and treats the mind

4. _____ study of the mind

5. _____ physician with additional training and experience in the diagnosis, prevention, and treatment of mental disorders; can prescribe medications and direct therapy

EXERCISE P **Medical Terms Related to the Nervous System and Behavioral Health**

Write the medical terms related to the nervous system and behavioral health next to their definitions.

1. _____ pertaining to the cerebrum

2. _____ pertaining to a nerve

3. _____ originating in the mind

 OBJECTIVE 5

Use medical language in clinical statements, the case study, and a medical record.

Check responses for the following exercises in Appendix C.

EXERCISE Q **Use Medical Terms in Clinical Statements**

Circle the medical terms and abbreviations defined in the bolded phrases. For pronunciation practice, read the answers aloud.

1. **Mood disturbance characterized by feelings of sadness, despair, and hopelessness** (Anxiety disorder, Depression, Psychosis) is a diagnosis frequently encountered in the field of **study of the mind** (psychology, neurology, endocrinology). It may be accompanied by **disorder characterized by feelings of apprehension, tension, or uneasiness** (bipolar disorder, dementia, anxiety disorder). Fortunately, there are medications, which may be prescribed by a **physician with additional training and experience in the diagnosis, prevention, and treatment of mental disorders who can prescribe medications and direct therapy** (psychiatrist, psychologist, psych tech), that are helpful in treating both conditions. Psychotherapy performed by a **specialist who studies and treats the mind** (psychologist, physiologist, neurologist) can also be very helpful.

2. The manic phase of **major psychological disorder typified by a disturbance in mood** (anxiety disorder, somatoform disorder, bipolar disorder) can be very dangerous to the patient. In addition to euphoria and recklessness, some patients experience **major mental disorder characterized by extreme derangement**

(psychosis, neurosis, thrombosis), in which they may hear voices or see things that aren't there. Lithium was previously the most commonly used medication for bipolar disorder, but newer options also exist.

3. **Pain in the head or headache** (Neuralgia, Arthralgia, Cephalgia) is generally classified by type. **An intense, throbbing headache, usually one-sided** (Sciatica, Migraine, TIA), tension headache, and cluster headaches account for nearly 90% of all headaches. Other types of headaches include posttraumatic headaches, giant cell (temporal) arteritis, sinus headaches, brain tumor, and chronic daily headache. **Bleeding between the pia mater and arachnoid layers of the meninges caused by a ruptured blood vessel** (Cerebral thrombosis, Meningitis, Subarachnoid hemorrhage) may cause a headache that the patient describes as "the worst in my entire life."

4. In **process of recording the electrical activity of the brain** (electroencephalography, electrocardiography, myelography), electrodes are attached to areas of the patient's scalp. The electrical impulses are transmitted by an **instrument used for recording the electrical activity of the brain** (echocardiograph, electrocardiograph, electroencephalograph) that amplifies them and records them as brain waves on a moving strip of paper known as a(n) **record of electrical activity of the brain** (arteriogram, esophagram, electroencephalogram). The process of recording the electrical activity of the brain is used to diagnose intracranial lesions and to evaluate the brain's electrical activity in **sudden, abnormal surge of electrical activity in the brain** (multiple sclerosis, Parkinson disease, seizures), **injury to the brain caused by major or minor head trauma** (concussions, seizures, psychoses), **inflammation of the meninges** (meningioma, meningitis, meningocele), and **inflammation of the brain** (encephalitis, meningomyelitis, polyneuritis).

5. Common symptoms of a(n) **interruption of blood supply to a region of the brain**, (stroke, syncope, concussion) include **condition of without speech** (aphagia, dysphasia, aphasia), **condition of paralysis of half (of the body)** (quadriplegia, hemiplegia, myalgia), and facial drooping. Prompt diagnosis and treatment are critical. While the majority of strokes are ischemic, resulting from blockage in a **pertaining to the cerebrum** (cerebellar, celiac, cerebral) artery, some are hemorrhagic, caused by intracranial bleeding. A CT or MRI can usually help tell the difference. Early treatment with thrombolytic agents (which break up clots) can help save lives but can be very dangerous if given to a patient with a brain bleed. A **sudden deficient supply of blood to the brain lasting a short time** (SAH, CVA, TIA) usually does not require treatment.

6. The most common type of **cognitive impairment characterized by loss of intellectual brain function** (dementia, dysphasia, psychopathy) is caused by **degeneration of brain tissue and occurring more frequently after age 65** (Parkinson disease, multiple sclerosis, Alzheimer disease), accounting for 60% to 80% of all cases. Other types include vascular dementia, **chronic degenerative disease of the central nervous system** (Parkinson disease, encephalopathy, meningitis), normal pressure **water in the head (increased amount of cerebrospinal fluid in the brain)** (encephalitis, meningomyelitis, hydrocephalus), and Huntington disease.

EXERCISE R   Apply Medical Terms to the Case Study

Think back to Koji Kaneshiro, who was introduced in the case study at the beginning of the lesson. After working through Lesson 11 on the nervous system and behavioral health, consider the medical terms that might be used to describe his experience. List two terms relevant to the case study and their meanings. ◼

Medical Term   **Definition**

1. _____   _____

2. _____   _____

EXERCISE S   **Use Medical Terms in a Document**

The ambulance came and took Mr. Kaneshiro to the local emergency department. A neurology consultation was obtained. The neurologist's report is provided in the following medical record.

Use the definitions in numbers 1-11 to write medical terms within the document on the next page.

1. condition of without speech (or loss of the ability to speak)

2. condition of paralysis of half (of the body)

3. cognitive impairment characterized by loss of intellectual brain function

4. condition of difficulty with speech

5. bleeding between the pia mater and arachnoid layers of the meninges caused by a ruptured blood vessel

6. CVA

7. abnormal condition of a blood clot in the cerebrum

8. radiographic imaging of the blood vessels of the cerebrum

9. pertaining to the cerebrum

10. study of the nerves (nervous system)

11. physician who studies and treats diseases of the nervous system

Refer to the medical document to answer questions 12-13.

12. In the history section, Mrs. Kaneshiro describes an event that occurred about 1 year ago, in which her husband had a brief episode of partial paralysis. The medical term for this event is: _____

   _____ _____.

13. Identify two new medical terms in the medical record you would like to investigate. Use your medical dictionary or an online reference to look up the definition.

   Medical Term   **Definition**

   1. _____   _____

   2. _____   _____

0118003 KANESHIRO, Koji   _ □ ✕

File   Patient   Navigate   Custom Fields   Help

Chart Review | Encounters | Notes | Labs | Imaging | Procedures | Rx | Documents | Referrals | Scheduling | Billing

Name: **KANESHIRO, Koji**   MR#: 118003   Gender: M   **Allergies:** None known
                                 DOB: 12/08/19XX   Age: 78   **PCP:** Grace Yoshino MD

Neurology Consultation
Encounter Date: 05/22/20XX

History: This 78-year-old male presented to the emergency department after the sudden onset of (1.) _____, right (2.) _____, and facial droop. Symptoms began approximately 2 hours ago. He has a history of hypertension, for which he takes lisinopril, and high cholesterol, for which he takes atorvastatin. He does not take aspirin or any anticoagulants. His wife reports that he had a very brief episode of partial paralysis approximately 1 year ago; it resolved within a minute or two. His family history is significant for a father who had a heart attack and a mother who had (3.) _____.

Physical Examination: reveals an elderly Asian male who is alert and oriented × 3, but shows evidence of (4.) _____. Focused neurologic exam is significant for right-sided facial drooping with paralysis of the seventh cranial nerve. The rest of the cranial nerves appear normal. Deep tendon reflexes exhibit increased response on the right side as compared to the left. Motor strength is significantly diminished for the right arm and less so for the right leg. Sensation is also decreased on the right. Cerebellar exam is normal, though difficult to test on the right. Gait is not assessed due to the patient's weakness.

Diagnostic Studies: A CBC, chemistry panel, and prothrombin time are normal. ECG shows no acute changes. A CT of the head without contrast indicates no evidence of intercerebral or (5.) _____. No mass lesions or other abnormalities are noted.

Impression: (6.) _____, probably due to ischemia, likely caused by (7.) _____. Because this gentleman's stroke was diagnosed early, and he has no evidence of bleeding in the cerebrum, he is a good candidate for thrombolytic therapy.

Recommendation: Obtain blood for type and cross and coagulopathy panel. Administer rtPA at standard doses per protocol if patient meets all criteria. Consider (8.) _____ if symptoms do not improve. Monitor neurologic status continuously and also watch for any signs of bleeding. Monitor blood pressure and do not allow it to become too low, as this can decrease (9.) _____ perfusion. After discharge, he should follow up in our (10.) _____ clinic within 1 week.

Thank you for allowing me to participate in the care of Mr. Kaneshiro.
William Snyder, MD (11.) _____
Electronically signed by William Snyder, MD.

Start | Log On/Off | Print | Edit

| **EXERCISE T** | **Use Medical Language in Electronic Health Records Online** |

Select the correct medical terms to complete three medical records in one patient's electronic file.

🌐 Access online resources at evolve.elsevier.com > Evolve Resources > Practice Student Resources > Activities > Lesson 11 > Electronic Health Records

Topic: Multiple Sclerosis
Record 1: Ophthalmology Report
Record 2: Cytology Report
Record 3: Neurology Office Visit

❑ Check the box when complete.

 OBJECTIVE 6

Recall and assess knowledge of word parts, medical terms, and abbreviations.

| **EXERCISE U** | **Online Review of Lesson Content** |

🌐 *Recall and assess your learning from working through the lesson by completing online learning activities at evolve. elsevier.com > Evolve Resources > Student Resources.*

❑ Check the box when complete.

| **EXERCISE V** | **Lesson Content Quiz** |

Test your knowledge of the terms and abbreviations introduced in this lesson. Circle the letter for the medical term or abbreviation related to the words in italics.

1. The 71-year-old man with right leg pain was told he had *pain in the nerve(s)*.
   a. neuropathy
   b. neuralgia
   c. polyneuritis

2. An elderly gentleman was brought to the emergency department following an episode of *syncope*.
   a. confusion
   b. throbbing headache
   c. fainting

3. The linebacker on the high school football team sustained *an injury to the brain caused by head trauma* during yesterday's game.
   a. concussion
   b. seizure
   c. migraine

4. A 60-year-old man with type 2 diabetes was found to have peripheral *disease of the nerves* after undergoing a nerve conduction study.
   a. neuralgia
   b. neuropathy
   c. sciatica

5. A 55-year-old woman who complained of upper back and arm pain was diagnosed with *polymyalgia*.
   a. pain in one muscle
   b. disease of many muscles
   c. pain in many muscles

6. A diagnosis of *a chronic degenerative disease characterized by sclerotic patches along the brain and spinal cord* was made on a 32-year-old woman who presented with a history of leg weakness and muscle cramps.
   a. transient ischemic attack
   b. multiple sclerosis
   c. Parkinson disease

7. *Radiographic imaging of the blood vessels of the cerebrum* was performed on a 58-year-old man who presented with an acute onset of right arm and leg weakness.
   a. myelography
   b. cerebral thrombosis
   c. cerebral angiography

8. The 25-year-old man was diagnosed with a *major psychological disorder typified by a disturbance in mood.*
   a. depression
   b. bipolar disorder
   c. anxiety disorder

9. An 18-year-old female who presented with an acute onset of headache and fever of 102° F underwent a *diagnostic procedure performed by insertion of a needle into the subarachnoid space between vertebrae* to exclude acute meningitis.
   a. lumbar puncture
   b. epidural nerve block
   c. electroencephalography

10. An *ADL* scale is used to assess the ability to perform basic self-care tasks.
    a. activities of daily life
    b. acts of daily living
    c. activities of daily living

11. *Condition of difficult speech* was noted in a patient who had a CVA the previous week.
    a. dysphagia
    b. dysphasia
    c. dyspnea

12. Although recently associated with Zika virus, *small head* has also been linked to other diseases in pregnancy, including rubella, toxoplasmosis, and cytomegalovirus.
    a. microcephalus
    b. hydrocephalus
    c. encephalopathy

LESSON AT A GLANCE   **NERVOUS SYSTEM AND BEHAVIORAL HEALTH WORD PARTS**

COMBINING FORMS		PREFIXES	SUFFIX
cerebr/o	pleg/o	hemi-	-us
encephal/o	poli/o	micro-	
mening/o, meningi/o	psych/o		
myel/o	quadr/i		
phas/o			

SIGNS AND SYMPTOMS
aphasia
cephalgia
dysphasia
neuralgia
polyarthritis
polymyalgia
polyneuritis
seizure (Sz)
syncope

DISEASES AND DISORDERS
Alzheimer disease (AD)
anxiety disorder
bipolar disorder
cerebral thrombosis
concussion
dementia
depression
encephalitis
encephalopathy
hemiplegia
hydrocephalus
meningioma

meningitis
meningocele
meningomyelitis
microcephalus
migraine
multiple sclerosis (MS)
neuropathy
paraplegia
Parkinson disease (PD)
poliomyelitis
psychopathy
psychosis
quadriplegia
sciatica
stroke
subarachnoid hemorrhage (SAH)
transient ischemic attack (TIA)

**DIAGNOSTIC TESTS
AND EQUIPMENT**
cerebral angiography
electroencephalogram (EEG)
electroencephalograph
electroencephalography

lumbar puncture (LP)
myelogram
myelography

SURGICAL PROCEDURES
epidural nerve block

SPECIALTIES AND PROFESSIONS
neurologist
neurology
psychiatrist
psychologist
psychology

RELATED TERMS
cerebral
neural
psychogenic

ABBREVIATIONS

AD	CVA	PNS
ADHD	EEG	PTSD
ADL, ADLs	LP	SAH
CNS	MS	Sz
CP	OCD	TIA
CSF	PD	

CASE STUDY | Nascha Tohe

Nascha generally thinks of herself as being healthy. Lately, though, she's been really tired. She's also thirsty all the time and drinks 3-4 quarts of water every day. Now Nascha has to get up 2 or 3 times at night to go to the bathroom, and she goes more during the day, too. Her father has diabetes. He has to see a special doctor and have his sugar level tested all the time. She is worried that she might have the same problem. Her sister convinced her to come to the clinic to get checked out.

■ *Consider Nascha's situation as you work through the lesson on the endocrine system. We will return to this case study and identify medical terms used to describe and document her experiences.*

OBJECTIVES

1	■ Build, translate, pronounce, and spell medical terms built from word parts (p. 380).
2	■ Define, pronounce, and spell medical terms NOT built from word parts (p. 386).
3	■ Write abbreviations (p. 390).
4	■ Identify medical terms by clinical category (p. 391).
5	■ Use medical language in clinical statements, the case study, and a medical record (p. 393).
6	■ Recall and assess knowledge of word parts, medical terms, and abbreviations (p. 397).

INTRODUCTION TO THE ENDOCRINE SYSTEM

Anatomic Structures of the Endocrine System

adrenal glands (a-DRĒ-nal) (glans)	glands located above the kidneys that secrete various hormones, including cortisone and adrenaline
hormone (HŌR-mōn)	chemical substance secreted by an endocrine gland that is carried by the blood to a target tissue
islets of Langerhans (Ī-litz) (LAHNG-er-hahnz)	clusters of endocrine tissue found throughout the pancreas, made up of different cell types that secrete various hormones, including insulin (Figure 12.4)
metabolism (ma-TAB-a-liz-am)	sum total of all the chemical processes that take place in a living organism
pancreas (PAN-krē-as)	long organ that lies horizontally across the upper abdomen that has a role in digestion as well as hormone secretion; contains the islets of Langerhans, which perform endocrine functions
pituitary gland (pi-TOO-i-tār-ē) (gland)	pea-sized gland located at the base of the brain; produces hormones that stimulate the function of other endocrine glands

Continued

Anatomic Structures of the Endocrine System—cont'd	
thymus (THĬ-mas)	lymphatic organ located behind the sternum; plays an important role in the development of the body's immune system, particularly from infancy to puberty
thyroid gland (THĬ-roid) (gland)	butterfly-shaped gland located anteriorly in the neck and inferior to the larynx; secretes hormones that regulate the metabolism of carbohydrates, proteins, and fats needed for growth, development, and basal metabolic rate

Functions of the Endocrine System

- Regulates body activities
- Secretes hormones
- Influences growth, development, and metabolism

How the Endocrine System Works

The endocrine system is made up of glands that secrete hormones to assist in the regulation of body activities (see Figure 12.2). The nervous system also regulates body activities but does so through nerve impulses. Nervous system regulation takes place quickly, and the effects only last a short while. The endocrine system communicates through **hormones,** or chemical messengers, which take longer to produce results; however, the effects of endocrine system regulation usually last longer.

Hormones produced by endocrine glands are released directly into the bloodstream and are transported throughout the body. Target tissues are designed to respond to the specific hormone that influences their activities. Each endocrine gland secretes specialized hormones that affect various body systems. The **pituitary gland** is referred to as the master gland because it secretes several hormones that influence the activities of other endocrine glands. Testes and ovaries, presented in Lesson 6, are also considered endocrine glands because they secrete hormones.

CAREER FOCUS | Professionals Who Work with the Endocrine System

- **Medical assistants** are a critical part of the healthcare team. They work in physicians' offices, hospitals, nursing homes, or clinics. Responsibilities may include answering phones and scheduling appointments, greeting patients, taking vital signs, explaining procedures to patients, performing tests and labs, and maintaining electronic health records (EHRs).

- **Certified diabetes educators (CDEs)** are licensed healthcare professionals, such as nurses, dietitians, pharmacists, podiatrists, and exercise physiologists, who have received special training in teaching diabetes self-management skills.

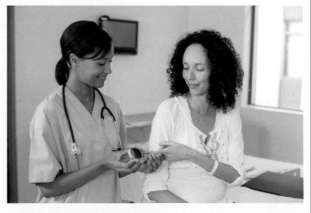

Figure 12.1 Medical assistant checking a patient's blood sugar with a glucometer.

OBJECTIVE 1

Build, translate, pronounce, and spell medical terms built from word parts.

WORD PARTS	Use the paper or online **flashcards** to familiarize yourself with the following word parts.

COMBINING FORM (WR + CV)	DEFINITION	COMBINING FORM (WR + CV)	DEFINITION
adrenal/o	adrenal gland	**glyc/o**	sugar
crin/o	to secrete	**thym/o**	thymus gland
dips/o	thirst	**thyroid/o**	thyroid gland
SUFFIX (S)	DEFINITION		
-ism	state of		

WORD PARTS PRESENTED IN PREVIOUS LESSONS	Used to Build Terms for the Endocrine System

COMBINING FORM (WR + CV)	DEFINITION	COMBINING FORM (WR + CV)	DEFINITION
acr/o	extremities	**path/o**	disease
aden/o	gland	**ur/o**	urine, urination, urinary tract
SUFFIX (S)	DEFINITION	SUFFIX (S)	DEFINITION
-e, -y	no meaning	**-itis**	inflammation
-ectomy	surgical removal, excision	**-logist**	one who studies and treats (specialist, physician)
-emia	in the blood	**-logy**	study of
-ia	diseased state, condition of	**-megaly**	enlargement
-ic	pertaining to	**-oma**	tumor
PREFIX (P)	DEFINITION	PREFIX (P)	DEFINITION
endo-	within	**hypo-**	below, deficient, under
hyper-	above, excessive	**poly-**	many, much

Refer to Appendix A, Word Parts Used in *Basic Medical Language*, for alphabetical lists of word parts and their meanings.

EXERCISE A	Build and Translate Terms Built from Word Parts

*Use the **Word Parts Tables** to complete the following questions. Check your responses with the Answer Key in Appendix C.*

1. LABEL: *Write the combining forms for anatomic structures of the endocrine system on Figure 12.2. These anatomic combining forms will be used to build and translate medical terms in Exercise A.*

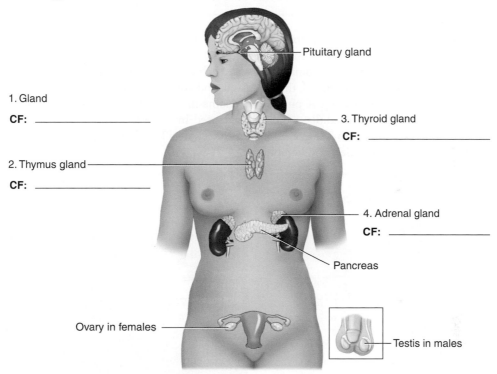

Pituitary gland

1. Gland

CF: _____

2. Thymus gland

CF: _____

3. Thyroid gland

CF: _____

4. Adrenal gland

CF: _____

Pancreas

Ovary in females

Testis in males

Figure 12.2 The endocrine system with combining forms.

2. MATCH: *Draw a line to match the word part with its definition.*

a.	acr/o	pertaining to
b.	-ic	tumor
c.	-itis	inflammation
d.	-ectomy	extremities
e.	-oma	enlargement
f.	-megaly	excision

3. BUILD: *Using the combining forms **acr/o**, **aden/o**, and **adrenal/o**, build the following terms. Remember, the definition usually starts with the meaning of the suffix.*

a. inflammation of the adrenal gland

_____ / _____

  wr   s

b. excision of the adrenal gland

_____ / _____

  wr   s

c. tumor composed of a gland (glandular tissue)

_____/_____
wr   s

d. enlargement of the extremities (and facial features)

_____/ o /_____
wr   cv   s

e. enlargement (of one or both) of the adrenal glands

_____/ o /_____
wr   cv   s

---

4. READ: **Adrenalitis** (a-drē-nal-Ī-tis) of autoimmune origin may lead to a primary adrenal insufficiency called Addison disease. An **adrenalectomy** (ad-rē-nal-EK-to-mē) may be performed to treat adrenal cancer or adrenal **adenoma** (ad-e-NŌ-ma). Adenomas are usually benign tumors and may occur in several locations in the body, including the pituitary gland, thyroid gland, and adrenal gland. They may also occur in organs such as the colon, breast, and kidney. A pituitary adenoma may excrete human growth hormone, causing **acromegaly** (ak-rō-MEG-a-lē) in adults, which is evidenced by enlarged hands, feet, and facial features. Causes of **adrenomegaly** (a-drē-nō-MEG-a-lē) include infections like tuberculosis, diseases like sarcoidosis, genetic abnormalities, malignancies, and hemorrhage.

---

5. LABEL: *Write word parts to complete Figure 12.3.*

Figure 12.3 _____/o/_____ is a hormonal disorder
                        wr   s
characterized by marked enlargement of the bones of the face, jaw, and extremities.

---

6. TRANSLATE: *Complete the definitions of the following terms describing the thymus gland and thyroid gland. Remember, the definition usually starts with the meaning of the suffix.*

a. thym/ic   _____ to the _____ gland

b. thym/oma   _____ of the thymus _____

c. thym/ectomy   _____ of the thymus gland

d. thyroid/ectomy   _____ of the thyroid _____

e. thyroid/itis   _____ of the _____ gland

7. READ: Thymectomy (thī-MEK-to-mē) is a surgical procedure that may be performed to treat **thymoma** (thī-MŌ-ma) and **thymic** (THĪ-mik) carcinoma. A **thyroidectomy** (thī-royd-EK-to-mē) may be performed to treat thyroid adenoma (nodules), thyroid cancer, goiter, and severe hyperthyroidism. **Thyroiditis** (thī-royd-Ī-tis) has many causes, including autoimmune diseases, viral and bacterial infections, drug reactions, and radiation therapy.

---

8. MATCH: *Draw a line to match the word part with its definition.*

a. hyper-   in the blood
b. hypo-   above, excessive
c. -emia   sugar
d. -ism   below, deficient, under
e. glyc/o   state of

---

9. BUILD: *Build the following terms using the combining form* **thyroid/o**.

a. state of excessive thyroid gland (activity)   _____/_____/_____
                                                                  p   wr   s

b. state of deficient thyroid gland (activity)   _____/_____/_____
                                                                  p   wr   s

---

10. READ: In **hyperthyroidism** (hī-per-THĪ-royd-izm), an excessive amount of thyroid hormone is released into the bloodstream, potentially leading to nervousness, sleep disruption, weight loss, goiter, and other symptoms. In **hypothyroidism** (hī-pō-THĪ-royd-izm), deficient amounts of thyroid hormone are produced, potentially leading to fatigue, depression, weight gain, increased sensitivity to cold, and other symptoms.

---

11. TRANSLATE: *Complete the definitions by using the meaning of word parts to fill in the blanks.*

a. glyc/emia   _____ in the blood
b. hyper/glyc/emia excessive _____ in the _____
c. hypo/glyc/emia   _____ sugar in the _____

---

12. READ: Glycemia (glī-SĒ-mē-a) refers to the sugar level in the blood and is measured by several lab tests, including glycosylated hemoglobin (HbA1c). **Hyperglycemia** (hī-per-glī-SĒ-mē-a) is most often associated with diabetes and occurs when insulin is not available to process sugar or when it is not used effectively. **Hypoglycemia** (hī-pō-glī-SĒ-mē-a) can be a result of an overproduction of insulin, alcohol consumption, systemic infection, or hormonal imbalances. It can also be an unwanted side effect of medications used to treat diabetes.

---

13. MATCH: *Draw a line to match the word part with its definition.*

a. poly-   thirst
b. ur/o   many, much
c. dips/o   diseased state, condition of
d. -ia   urination, urine, urinary tract

---

14. BUILD: *Write word parts to build the following terms.*

   a. condition of much thirst   _____ / _____ / _____

                                                     p   **wr**   **s**

   b. condition of much urine   _____ / _____ / _____

                                                       p   **wr**   **s**

15. READ: **Polydipsia** (pol-ē-DIP-sē-a), or excessive thirst, may be a symptom of hyperglycemia. **Polyuria** (pol-ē-Ū-rē-a) refers to increased amount of urine. Polydipsia and polyuria are common symptoms of diabetes mellitus.

16. MATCH: *Draw a line to match the word part with its definition.*

   a. endo-   to secrete

   b. crin/o   disease

   c. path/o   within

   d. -logist   one who studies and treats (specialist, physician)

   e. -logy   no meaning

   f. -e, -y   study of

17. TRANSLATE: *Complete the definitions by using the meaning of word parts to fill in the blanks.*

   a. endo/crin/e   to _____ within

   b. endo/crin/o/logy   _____ of the endocrine system

   c. endo/crin/o/logist   physician who _____ and treats diseases of the _____ system

   d. endo/crin/o/path/y (any) _____ of the endocrine _____

> **FYI** The combination of the prefix **endo-** and the combining form **crin/o** will be translated as **endocrine system** in terms with suffixes or combining forms that add meaning. Examples include: endocrinology, endocrinologist, and endocrinopathy.

18. READ: The **endocrine** (EN-dō-krin) system is made up of glands that "secrete within" the body by releasing hormones directly into the bloodstream. **Endocrinopathy** (en-dō-kri-NOP-a-thē) refers to disease processes of the endocrine system, which usually manifest as hormonal imbalances. **Endocrinology** (en-dō-kri-NOL-o-jē) is the subspecialty of internal medicine focused on diagnosing and treating endocrinopathies. An **endocrinologist** (en-dō-kri-NOL-o-jist) is a physician who cares for patients affected by disease and disorders of the endocrine system.

19. **REVIEW OF ENDOCRINE SYSTEM TERMS BUILT FROM WORD PARTS:** *The following is an alphabetical list of terms built and translated in the previous exercises.*

MEDICAL TERMS BUILT FROM WORD PARTS

TERM	DEFINITION	TERM	DEFINITION
1. **acromegaly** (ak-rō-MEG-a-lē)	enlargement of the extremities (and facial features) (Figure 12.3)	12. **hyperthyroidism** (hī-per-THĪ-royd-izm)	state of excessive thyroid activity
2. **adenoma** (ad-e-NŌ-ma)	tumor composed of a gland (glandular tissue)	13. **hypoglycemia** (hī-pō-glī-SĒ-mē-a)	deficient sugar in the blood
3. **adrenalectomy** (ad-rē-nal-EK-to-mē)	excision of the adrenal gland	14. **hypothyroidism** (hī-pō-THĪ-royd-izm)	state of deficient thyroid activity
4. **adrenalitis** (a-drē-nal-Ī-tis)	inflammation of the adrenal gland	15. **polydipsia** (pol-ē-DIP-sē-a)	condition of much thirst
5. **adrenomegaly** (a-drē-nō-MEG-a-lē)	enlargement (of one or both) of the adrenal glands	16. **polyuria** (pol-ē-Ū-rē-a)	condition of much urine
6. **endocrine** (EN-dō-krin)	to secrete within	17. **thymectomy** (thī-MEK-to-mē)	excision of the thymus gland
7. **endocrinologist** (en-dō-kri-NOL-o-jist)	physician who studies and treats diseases of the endocrine system	18. **thymic** (THĪ-mik)	pertaining to the thymus gland
8. **endocrinology** (en-dō-kri-NOL-o-jē)	study of the endocrine system	19. **thymoma** (thī-MŌ-ma)	tumor of the thymus gland
9. **endocrinopathy** (en-dō-kri-NOP-a-thē)	(any) disease of the endocrine system	20. **thyroidectomy** (thī-royd-EK-to-mē)	excision of the thyroid gland
10. **glycemia** (glī-SĒ-mē-a)	sugar in the blood	21. **thyroiditis** (thī-royd-Ī-tis)	inflammation of the thyroid gland
11. **hyperglycemia** (hī-per-glī-SĒ-mē-a)	excessive sugar in the blood		

EXERCISE B   Pronounce and Spell Terms Built from Word Parts

Practice pronunciation and spelling on paper and online.

1. **Practice on Paper**

    a. **Pronounce**: Read the phonetic spelling and say aloud the terms listed in the previous table, Review of Terms Built from Word Parts.

    b. **Spell**: Have a study partner read the terms aloud. Write the spelling of the terms on a separate sheet of paper.

2. **Practice Online**

    a. **Access** online learning resources. Go to evolve.elsevier.com > Evolve Resources > Practice Student Resources.

    b. **Pronounce**: Select Audio Glossary > Lesson 12 > Exercise B. Select a term to hear its pronunciation and repeat aloud.

    c. **Spell**: Select Activities > Lesson 12 > Spell Terms > Exercise B. Select the audio icon and type the correct spelling of the term.

❏   Check the box when complete.

OBJECTIVE 2

Define, pronounce, and spell medical terms NOT built from word parts.

The terms listed below may contain word parts, but are difficult to translate literally.

MEDICAL TERMS NOT BUILT FROM WORD PARTS

TERM	DEFINITION
1. **Addison disease** (AD-i-sun) (di-ZĒZ)	chronic syndrome resulting from a deficiency in the hormonal secretion of the adrenal gland, with symptoms of weight loss, hypotension, and skin darkening (also called **primary adrenal insufficiency**)
2. **diabetes mellitus (DM)** (dī-a-BĒ-tēz) (MEL-li-tus)	chronic disease involving a disorder of carbohydrate metabolism caused by underactivity of the insulin-producing islets of Langerhans (Figure 12.4) in the pancreas and characterized by elevated blood sugar; it can also be caused by resistance of the tissues to insulin.

FYI   Two major forms of diabetes mellitus are **type 1**, previously called insulin-dependent juvenile-onset diabetes, and **type 2**, previously called noninsulin-dependent diabetes mellitus (NIDDM) or adult-onset diabetes mellitus (AODM). Type 2 diabetes mellitus has reached epidemic proportions and is a major cause of cardiovascular disease.

TERM	DEFINITION
3. **fasting blood sugar (FBS)** (FAST-ing) (blud) (SHOO-ger)	blood test to determine the amount of glucose (sugar) in the blood after fasting for 8 to 10 hours. Elevation may indicate diabetes mellitus.
4. **fine needle aspiration (FNA)** (FĪN) (NĒ-del) (as-pi-RĀ-shen)	biopsy technique that uses a narrow hollow needle to obtain tiny amounts of tissue for pathologic examination. Thyroid nodules are frequently biopsied using FNA.
5. **glycosylated hemoglobin (HbA1c)** (glī-KŌ-sa-lāt-ad) (HĒ-mō-glō-bin)	blood test used to diagnose diabetes and monitor its treatment by measuring the amount of glucose (sugar) bound to hemoglobin in the blood; provides an indication of blood sugar level over the past three months, covering the 120-day lifespan of the red blood cell (also called **glycated hemoglobin**, **hemoglobin A1c**)
6. **goiter** (GOY-ter)	enlargement of the thyroid gland
7. **Graves disease** (grāvz) (di-ZĒZ)	disorder of the thyroid gland characterized by the presence of hyperthyroidism, goiter, and exophthalmos (protrusion of the eyes)
8. **metabolic syndrome** (met-a-BOL-ik) (SIN-drōm)	group of signs and symptoms including insulin resistance, obesity characterized by excessive fat around the area of the waist and abdomen, hypertension, hyperglycemia, elevated triglycerides, and low levels of the "good" cholesterol HDL (also called **syndrome X** and **insulin resistance syndrome**)

Islets of Langerhans

Figure 12.4 Pancreas, with islets of Langerhans.

TABLE 12.1	COMPARING TYPES OF DIABETES MELLITUS	
	TYPE 1	**TYPE 2**
Cause	beta cells of the pancreas that produce insulin are destroyed and eventually no insulin is produced	resistance of body cells to the action of insulin, which may eventually lead to a decrease in insulin secretion
Characteristics	abrupt onset, occurs primarily in childhood or adolescence; patients often are thin	slow onset, usually occurs in adults though it is becoming more common among teens; many patients are overweight or obese
Symptoms	polyuria, polydipsia, weight loss, hyperglycemia, acidosis, and ketosis	fatigue, blurred vision, polydipsia, and hyperglycemia; may have neural or vascular complications
Treatment	insulin injections and diet	diet, exercise, oral or injected medication, and perhaps insulin

TABLE 12.2	LONG-TERM COMPLICATIONS OF DIABETES MELLITUS	
MACROVASCULAR COMPLICATIONS		**MICROVASCULAR COMPLICATIONS**
coronary artery disease → myocardial infarction		diabetic retinopathy → loss of vision
cerebrovascular disease → stroke		diabetic nephropathy → chronic kidney disease, renal failure
peripheral artery disease → leg pain when walking (intermittent vascular claudication)		neuropathy → loss of feeling in extremities, amputation

EXERCISE C   Label

Write the medical terms pictured and defined using the previous table of Medical Terms NOT Built from Word Parts. Check your work with the Answer Key in Appendix C.

1. _____

disorder of the thyroid gland characterized by the presence of hyperthyroidism, goiter, and exophthalmos (protrusion of the eyes)

2. _____

group of signs and symptoms including insulin resistance, obesity characterized by excessive fat around the area of the waist and abdomen, hypertension, hyperglycemia, elevated triglycerides, and low levels of the "good" cholesterol HDL

3. _____

enlargement of the thyroid gland

4. _____

chronic syndrome resulting from a deficiency in the hormonal secretion of the adrenal gland, with symptoms of weight loss, hypotension, and skin darkening

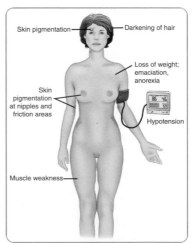

EXERCISE D Match

Match the terms in the first column with their correct descriptions in the second column.

_____ **1.** fine needle aspiration

_____ **2.** diabetes mellitus

_____ **3.** fasting blood sugar

_____ **4.** glycosylated hemoglobin

a. blood test that provides an indication of blood sugar level over the past three months, covering the 120-day lifespan of the red blood cell

b. biopsy technique that uses a narrow hollow needle to obtain tiny amounts of tissue for pathologic examination

c. chronic disease involving a disorder of carbohydrate metabolism caused by underactivity of the insulin-producing islets of Langerhans in the pancreas and characterized by elevated blood sugar

d. blood test to determine the amount of glucose (sugar) in the blood after fasting for 8 to 10 hours

EXERCISE E Learn Medical Terms NOT Built from Word Parts

Fill in the blanks with medical terms defined in bold using the Medical Terms NOT Built from Word Parts table. Answers are listed in Appendix C.

1. The **chronic disease involving a disorder of carbohydrate metabolism caused by underactivity of the insulin-producing islets of Langerhans in the pancreas and characterized by elevated blood sugar**, or _____, may be diagnosed based on the results of the glucose tolerance test, the **blood test to determine the amount of glucose (sugar) in the blood after fasting for 8 to 10 hours**, or _____, and the **blood test used to diagnose diabetes and monitor its treatment by measuring the amount of glucose (sugar) bound to hemoglobin in the blood**, or _____. After a diabetes diagnosis, the HbA1c will likely be ordered by a provider two to four times a year to monitor effectiveness of treatment over time.

2. **Enlargement of the thyroid gland**, or _____, may occur when the thyroid gland cannot produce enough hormones to meet the body's needs. If symptoms become significant, such as breathing difficulties, a thyroidectomy may be performed.

3. Goiter may be a symptom of a **disorder of the thyroid gland characterized by the presence of hyperthyroidism, goiter, and exophthalmos**, or _____. Goiter may also be caused by thyroiditis or a thyroid nodule, which is a mass on the thyroid gland that can sometimes be palpated.

4. A patient with a diagnosis of **chronic syndrome resulting from a deficiency in the hormonal secretion of the adrenal gland**, or _____, may have weakness, darkening of skin, loss of appetite, and/or depression.

5. **Biopsy technique that uses a narrow hollow needle to obtain tiny amounts of tissue for pathologic examination**, or _____, is frequently performed on thyroid nodules. Small biopsy needles are used to obtain multiple tissue samples, which are sent to the pathologist to evaluate for the possibility of malignant cells.

6. **Group of signs and symptoms including insulin resistance, obesity characterized by excessive fat around the area of the waist and abdomen, hypertension, hyperglycemia, elevated triglycerides, and low levels of the "good" cholesterol HDL**, or _____, increases the risks of developing type 2 diabetes mellitus, coronary artery disease, or stroke.

| EXERCISE F | Pronounce and Spell Terms NOT Built from Word Parts |

Practice pronunciation and spelling on paper and online.

1. **Practice on Paper**

   a. **Pronounce**: Read the phonetic spelling and say aloud the terms listed in the previous table, Medical Terms NOT Built from Word Parts.

   b. **Spell**: Have a study partner read the terms aloud. Write the spelling of the terms on a separate sheet of paper.

2. **Practice Online** 🌐

   a. **Access** online learning resources. Go to evolve.elsevier.com > Evolve Resources > Practice Student Resources.

   b. **Pronounce**: Select Audio Glossary > Lesson 12 > Exercise F. Select a term to hear its pronunciation and repeat aloud.

   c. **Spell**: Select Activities > Lesson 12 > Spell Terms > Exercise F. Select the audio icon and type the correct spelling of the term.

   ❏ Check the box when complete.

OBJECTIVE 3

Write abbreviations.

ABBREVIATIONS RELATED TO THE ENDOCRINE SYSTEM

Use the online **flashcards** to familiarize yourself with the following abbreviations.

ABBREVIATION	TERM	ABBREVIATION	TERM
DM	diabetes mellitus	HbA1c	glycosylated hemoglobin
FBS	fasting blood sugar	T1DM	type 1 diabetes mellitus
FNA	fine needle aspiration	T2DM	type 2 diabetes mellitus

| EXERCISE G | Abbreviate Medical Terms |

Write the correct abbreviation next to its medical term.

1. Diseases and Disorders:

   a. _____ diabetes mellitus

   b. _____ type 1 diabetes mellitus

   c. _____ type 2 diabetes mellitus

2. Diagnostic Tests:

   a. _____ fasting blood sugar

   b. _____ glycosylated hemoglobin

   c. _____ fine needle aspiration

OBJECTIVE 4

Identify medical terms by clinical category.

Now that you have worked through the lesson on the endocrine system, review and practice medical terms grouped by clinical category. Categories include signs and symptoms, diseases and disorders, diagnostic tests, surgical procedures, specialties and professions, and other terms related to the endocrine system. Check your responses with the Answer Key in Appendix C.

EXERCISE H   Signs and Symptoms

Write the medical terms for signs and symptoms next to their definitions.

1. _____   excessive sugar in the blood
2. _____   deficient sugar in the blood
3. _____   condition of much thirst
4. _____   condition of much urine
5. _____   enlargement (of one or both) of the adrenal glands

EXERCISE I   Diseases and Disorders

Write the medical terms for diseases and disorders next to their definitions.

1. _____   (any) disease of the endocrine system
2. _____   chronic syndrome resulting from a deficiency in the hormonal secretion of the adrenal gland
3. _____   inflammation of the adrenal gland
4. _____   disorder of the thyroid gland characterized by the presence of hyperthyroidism, goiter, and exophthalmos (protrusion of the eyes)
5. _____   enlargement of the thyroid gland
6. _____   state of excessive thyroid activity
7. _____   state of deficient thyroid activity
8. _____   tumor composed of a gland (glandular tissue)
9. _____   enlargement of the extremities (and facial features)
10. _____   tumor of the thymus gland
11. _____   inflammation of the thyroid gland

12. _____ chronic disease involving a disorder of carbohydrate
metabolism caused by underactivity of the insulin-producing
islets of Langerhans in the pancreas and characterized by
elevated blood sugar

13. _____ group of signs and symptoms including insulin resistance,
obesity characterized by excessive fat around the area of the
waist and abdomen, hypertension, hyperglycemia, elevated
triglycerides, and low levels of the "good" cholesterol HDL

EXERCISE J   Diagnostic Tests

Write the medical terms for diagnostic tests and equipment next to their definitions.

1. _____ blood test used to diagnose diabetes and monitor its treatment
by measuring the amount of glucose (sugar) bound to
hemoglobin in the blood

2. _____ blood test to determine the amount of glucose (sugar) in the
blood after fasting for 8 to 10 hours

3. _____ biopsy technique that uses a narrow hollow needle to obtain
tiny amounts of tissue for pathologic examination

EXERCISE K   Surgical Procedures

Write the medical terms for surgical procedures next to their definitions.

1. _____ excision of the adrenal gland

2. _____ excision of the thymus gland

3. _____ excision of the thyroid gland

EXERCISE L   Specialties and Professions

Write the medical terms for specialties and professions next to their definitions.

1. _____ physician who studies and treats diseases of the endocrine
system

2. _____ study of the endocrine system

EXERCISE M   Medical Terms Related to the Endocrine System

Write the medical terms related to the endocrine system next to their definitions.

1. _____ to secrete within

2. _____ sugar in the blood

3. _____ pertaining to the thymus gland

OBJECTIVE 5

Use medical language in clinical statements, the case study, and a medical record.

Check responses for the following exercises in Appendix C.

EXERCISE N Use Medical Terms in Clinical Statements

Circle the medical terms and abbreviations defined in the bolded phrases. For pronunciation practice, read the answers aloud.

1. A **biopsy technique that uses a narrow hollow needle to obtain tiny amounts of tissue for pathologic examination** (glycosylated hemoglobin, fine needle aspiration, fasting blood sugar) is frequently performed on thyroid nodules. Sonography is often used to localize the lesion. The procedure may be performed by a(n) **physician who studies and treats diseases of the endocrine system** (endocrinologist, pathologist, hematologist) or by a radiologist.

2. Unlike the results of **fasting blood sugar** (HbA1c, FNA, FBS), **glycosylated hemoglobin** (HbA1c, FNA, FBS) test results are not altered by what was eaten prior to the test.

3. **Condition of much thirst** (Polyuria, Polydipsia, Polyneuritis) and **condition of much urine** (polyuria, polydipsia, polyneuritis) may be caused by uncontrolled diabetes mellitus.

4. Graves disease is characterized by **state of excessive thyroid activity** (hypoglycemia, hyperthyroidism, hypothyroidism), **enlargement of the thyroid gland** (adenoma, goiter, acromegaly), and exophthalmos.

5. **Pertaining to the thymus gland** (Glycemia, Thymic, Endocrine) hypoplasia is a congenital condition caused by the absence or underdevelopment of the thymus gland.

6. A pituitary **tumor composed of a glandular tissue** (adrenalitis, thymoma, adenoma) can lead to an overproduction of growth hormone, which may cause **enlargement of the extremities** (thyroiditis, goiter, acromegaly) in adults, which primarily affects the bones of the hands, feet, and jaw.

7. Autoimmune **inflammation of the adrenal gland** (adenoma, thyroiditis, adrenalitis) is a common cause of **chronic syndrome resulting from a deficiency in the hormonal secretion of the adrenal gland** (diabetes mellitus, Addison disease, Graves disease).

EXERCISE O Apply Medical Terms to the Case Study

Think back to Nascha, introduced in the case study at the beginning of the lesson. After working through Lesson 12 on the endocrine system, consider the medical terms that might be used to describe her experiences. List two terms relevant to the case study and their meanings. ■

Medical Term	Definition
1. _____	_____
2. _____	_____

EXERCISE P   Use Medical Terms in a Document

Nascha was able to see a healthcare provider. The following medical record documents her experiences.

Use the definitions in numbers 1-9 to write medical terms within the history and physical report on the next page.

1. condition of much urine

2. condition of much thirst

3. disorder of the thyroid gland characterized by the presence of hyperthyroidism, goiter, and exophthalmos

4. chronic disease involving a disorder of carbohydrate metabolism and characterized by elevated blood sugar

5. blood test to determine the amount of glucose (sugar) in the blood after fasting for 8 to 10 hours

6. blood test used to diagnose diabetes and monitor its treatment by measuring the amount of glucose (sugar) bound to hemoglobin in the blood

7. excessive sugar in the blood

8. deficient sugar in the blood

9. study of the endocrine system

Refer to the History and Physical on the next page to answer questions 10 and 11.

10. Several terms used in the medical record were presented in previous lessons. Can you identify them and recall their meanings? Identify two.

    Medical Term   **Definition**

    1. _____   _____

    2. _____   _____

11. Identify two new medical terms in the medical record you would like to investigate. Use your medical dictionary or an online reference to look up the definitions.

    Medical Term   **Definition**

    1. _____   _____

    2. _____   _____

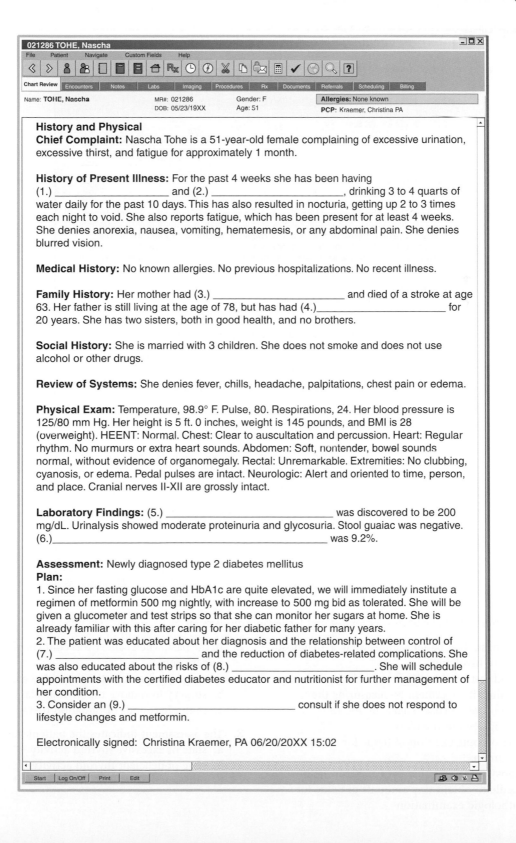

File   Patient   Navigate   Custom Fields   Help

Chart Review | Encounters | Notes | Labs | Imaging | Procedures | Rx | Documents | Referrals | Scheduling | Billing

Name: **TOHE, Nascha**   MR#: 021286   Gender: F   **Allergies:** None known
                                 DOB: 05/23/19XX   Age: 51   **PCP:** Kraemer, Christina PA

History and Physical

Chief Complaint: Nascha Tohe is a 51-year-old female complaining of excessive urination, excessive thirst, and fatigue for approximately 1 month.

History of Present Illness: For the past 4 weeks she has been having (1.) _____ and (2.) _____, drinking 3 to 4 quarts of water daily for the past 10 days. This has also resulted in nocturia, getting up 2 to 3 times each night to void. She also reports fatigue, which has been present for at least 4 weeks. She denies anorexia, nausea, vomiting, hematemesis, or any abdominal pain. She denies blurred vision.

Medical History: No known allergies. No previous hospitalizations. No recent illness.

Family History: Her mother had (3.) _____ and died of a stroke at age 63. Her father is still living at the age of 78, but has had (4.)_____ for 20 years. She has two sisters, both in good health, and no brothers.

Social History: She is married with 3 children. She does not smoke and does not use alcohol or other drugs.

Review of Systems: She denies fever, chills, headache, palpitations, chest pain or edema.

Physical Exam: Temperature, 98.9° F. Pulse, 80. Respirations, 24. Her blood pressure is 125/80 mm Hg. Her height is 5 ft. 0 inches, weight is 145 pounds, and BMI is 28 (overweight). HEENT: Normal. Chest: Clear to auscultation and percussion. Heart: Regular rhythm. No murmurs or extra heart sounds. Abdomen: Soft, nontender, bowel sounds normal, without evidence of organomegaly. Rectal: Unremarkable. Extremities: No clubbing, cyanosis, or edema. Pedal pulses are intact. Neurologic: Alert and oriented to time, person, and place. Cranial nerves II-XII are grossly intact.

Laboratory Findings: (5.) _____ was discovered to be 200 mg/dL. Urinalysis showed moderate proteinuria and glycosuria. Stool guaiac was negative. (6.)_____ was 9.2%.

Assessment: Newly diagnosed type 2 diabetes mellitus
Plan:
1. Since her fasting glucose and HbA1c are quite elevated, we will immediately institute a regimen of metformin 500 mg nightly, with increase to 500 mg bid as tolerated. She will be given a glucometer and test strips so that she can monitor her sugars at home. She is already familiar with this after caring for her diabetic father for many years.
2. The patient was educated about her diagnosis and the relationship between control of (7.) _____ and the reduction of diabetes-related complications. She was also educated about the risks of (8.) _____. She will schedule appointments with the certified diabetes educator and nutritionist for further management of her condition.
3. Consider an (9.) _____ consult if she does not respond to lifestyle changes and metformin.

Electronically signed: Christina Kraemer, PA 06/20/20XX 15:02

Start | Log On/Off | Print | Edit

EXERCISE Q   **Interpret Language Used in a Medical Record**

Read the medical record and answer the questions.

21152 WEBBER, Susan

File   Patient   Navigate   Custom Fields   Help

Chart Review | Encounters | Notes | Labs | Imaging | Procedures | Rx | Documents | Referrals | Scheduling | Billing

| Name: **WEBBER, Susan** | MR#: 21152 | Sex: F | **Allergies:** None |
| | DOB: 12/21/19xx | Age: 65 | PCP: Wong, Samuel MD |

Endocrinology Consultation
DATE: 06/04/20XX

SUBJECTIVE: This 65-year-old female was referred by her PCP due to a 3 month history of weight gain, fatigue, hair loss, dry skin, and cold intolerance. Approximately 3 years ago she had a painless thyroid nodule, and underwent thyroid sonography and fine needle aspiration at that time. A diagnosis of cancer was confirmed. She underwent a thyroidectomy and received thyroid replacement hormone thereafter. She remained in a normal thyroid state until she stopped taking the medication 4 months ago.

OBJECTIVE:

Vitals: T=96.4°F. P=56/min. R=16/min. BP=128/86 mm Hg. Wt=155 lbs. Ht=64 in.

Exam: Alert and oriented in no acute distress, though speech is slower than normal. Her face appears puffy, and hair and skin appear coarse and dry. Neck examination reveals no masses. Cardiac examination is significant for a decreased heart rate. Lungs are clear to auscultation. Extremities show bilateral edema.

Labs and Imaging: TSH was elevated at 30 uIU/mL, and T4 was low at 1.4 mIU/mL.

ASSESSMENT: Severe hypothyroidism and risk for myxedema coma due to lack of thyroid replacement therapy.

PLAN:
1. Restart levothyroxine therapy at 50 mcg po qd. We are starting with a lower dose due to her age and will increase it slowly for the same reason.
2. Repeat TSH in 4 weeks.
3. We will continue gradual adjustment of the levothyroxine dose until the TSH result is within normal limits.
4. Mrs. Webber was educated about the importance of continuing her thyroid medication and asked to contact us if she has any difficulty obtaining her prescriptions.

Electronically signed: Samuel Wong, MD, Endocrinologist on 04 June 20XX 14:15

Start | Log On/Off | Print | Edit

Circle the letter with the best answer for 1-4 and write your answers for 5.

1. In the past, the patient underwent a diagnostic procedure involving:
   a. blood test used to diagnose diabetes and monitor its treatment by measuring the amount of glucose (sugar) bound to hemoglobin in the blood
   b. laparoscopic excision of tissue for a biopsy specimen
   c. biopsy technique that uses a narrow hollow needle to obtain tiny amounts of tissue for pathologic examination

2. In the past, when cancer was confirmed, the patient underwent:
   a. surgery to remove the thyroid gland
   b. surgery to remove the thymus gland
   c. multiple rounds of radiation therapy

3. The assessment indicates the patient has severe:
   a. state of excessive thyroid activity
   b. state of deficient thyroid activity
   c. inflammation of the thyroid gland

4. Dr. Wong is a(n):
   a. physician who studies and treats diseases of the nervous system
   b. physician who studies and treats diseases of the endocrine system
   c. physician who studies and treats diseases of the skin

5. Identify one new medical term used in the report and research its meaning using a medical dictionary or reliable online source.

Term: _____

Definition: _____

Source: _____

EXERCISE R   **Use Medical Language in Electronic Health Records Online**

Select the correct medical terms to complete three medical records in one patient's electronic file

🌐 Access online resources at evolve.elsevier.com > Evolve Resources > Practice Student Resources > Activities > Lesson 12 > Electronic Health Records.

Topic: Thymoma
Record 1: Preoperative Note
Record 2: Radiology Report
Record 3: Pathology Report

❏ Check the box when complete.

 OBJECTIVE 6

Recall and assess knowledge of word parts, medical terms, and abbreviations.

EXERCISE S   **Online Review of Lesson Content**

🌐 *Recall and assess your learning from working through the lesson by completing learning activities at evolve.elsevier.com > Evolve Resources > Student Resources.*

❏ Check the box when complete.

EXERCISE T   **Lesson Content Quiz**

Test your knowledge of the terms and abbreviations introduced in this lesson. Circle the letter for the medical term or abbreviation related to the words in italics.

1. *Enlargement of the extremities (and facial features)* is usually a result of excess human growth hormone in adults, while gigantism is due to excess growth hormone before puberty.
   a. adrenomegaly
   b. acromegaly
   c. adrenalitis

2. Myasthenia gravis, an autoimmune disorder affecting the connection between nerves and muscles, is associated with thymus abnormalities. *Excision of the thymus gland* is frequently required in these patients.
   a. thymectomy
   b. thyroidectomy
   c. adrenalectomy

3. *Condition of much urine* and *condition of much thirst* are two common initial symptoms of diabetes mellitus.
   a. polydipsia; polyuria
   b. polyuria; polydipsia
   c. polysomnia; polydipsia

4. *A blood test to determine the amount of glucose (sugar) in the blood after fasting for 8-10 hours* is very important in helping patients manage their diabetes treatment.
   a. HbA1c
   b. FNA
   c. FBS

5. An increase in the risk of type 2 diabetes mellitus, coronary heart disease, and stroke is associated with *group of signs and symptoms including insulin resistance, obesity characterized by excessive fat around the area of the waist and abdomen, hypertension, hyperglycemia, elevated triglycerides, and low levels of the "good" cholesterol HDL.*
   a. metabolic syndrome
   b. Addison disease
   c. Graves disease

6. *Disorder of the thyroid gland characterized by the presence of hyperthyroidism, goiter, and exophthalmos* and Hashimoto thyroiditis are both autoimmune diseases affecting the thyroid.
   a. hyperglycemia
   b. Graves disease
   c. hypothyroidism

7. A(n) *physician who studies and treats diseases of the endocrine system* may treat thyroid disease, diabetes mellitus, or any other *disease of the endocrine system* such as Addison disease or Cushing syndrome.
   a. dermatologist; dermatopathy
   b. endocrinology; endocrinologist
   c. endocrinologist; endocrinopathy

8. A fine needle aspiration of the thyroid may be performed to help distinguish between a(n) *tumor composed of a gland* and thyroid carcinoma.
   a. adenoma
   b. thymoma
   c. hematoma

LESSON AT A GLANCE — ENDOCRINE SYSTEM WORD PARTS

COMBINING FORMS
adrenal/o   glyc/o
crin/o   thym/o
dips/o   thyroid/o

SUFFIX
-ism

LESSON AT A GLANCE — ENDOCRINE SYSTEM MEDICAL TERMS AND ABBREVIATIONS

SIGNS AND SYMPTOMS
adrenomegaly
hyperglycemia
hypoglycemia
polydipsia
polyuria

DISEASES AND DISORDERS
acromegaly
Addison disease
adenoma
adrenalitis
diabetes mellitus (DM)
endocrinopathy
goiter
Graves disease

hyperthyroidism
hypothyroidism
metabolic syndrome
thymoma
thyroiditis

DIAGNOSTIC TESTS AND EQUIPMENT
fasting blood sugar (FBS)
fine needle aspiration (FNA)
glycosylated hemoglobin (HbA1c)

SURGICAL PROCEDURES
adrenalectomy
thymectomy
thyroidectomy

SPECIALTIES AND PROFESSIONS
endocrinologist
endocrinology

RELATED TERMS
endocrine
glycemia
thymic

ABBREVIATIONS
DM   HbA1c
FBS   T1DM
FNA   T2DM

WORD PART	TYPE	DEFINITION	LESSON
a-	prefix	absence of, without	4
-a	suffix	no meaning	3
abdomin/o	combining form	abdomen, abdominal cavity	8
-ac	suffix	pertaining to	7
acr/o	combining form	extremities	3
-ad	suffix	toward	2
aden/o	combining form	gland(s); (node(s) when combined with lymph/o)	7
adrenal/o	combining form	adrenal gland	12
-al	suffix	pertaining to	1,2
-algia	suffix	pain	8
an-	prefix	absence of, without	4
an/o	combining form	anus	8
angi/o	combining form	blood vessel(s)	7
anter/o	combining form	front	2
append/o	combining form	appendix	8
appendic/o	combining form	appendix	8
arteri/o	combining form	artery (*s.*), arteries (*pl.*)	7
arthr/o	combining form	joint(s)	10
-ary	suffix	pertaining to	4
-asthenia	suffix	weakness	10
audi/o	combining form	hearing	9
blephar/o	combining form	eyelid	9
brady-	prefix	slow	7
bronch/o	combining form	bronchus (*s.*), bronchi (*pl.*)	4

WORD PART	TYPE	DEFINITION	LESSON
burs/o	combining form	bursa	10
capn/o	combining form	carbon dioxide	4
carcin/o	combining form	cancer	1
cardi/o	combining form	heart	7
carp/o	combining form	carpals, wrist (bone)	10
caud/o	combining form	tail (downward)	2
-cele	suffix	hernia, protrusion	6
-centesis	suffix	surgical puncture to remove fluid (with a sterile needle)	4
cephal/o	combining form	head (upward)	2
cerebr/o	combining form	cerebrum, brain	11
cervic/o	combining form	cervix (or neck)	6
chol/e	combining form	gall, bile	8
chondr/o	combining form	cartilage	10
col/o	combining form	colon (large intestine)	8
colon/o	combining form	colon (large intestine)	8
colp/o	combining form	vagina	6
cost/o	combining form	rib(s)	10
crani/o	combining form	skull (cranium)	10
crin/o	combining form	to secrete	12
cutane/o	combining form	skin	3

WORD PART	TYPE	DEFINITION	LESSON
cyan/o	combining form	blue	3
cyst/o	combining form	bladder, sac	5
cyt/o	combining form	cell(s)	1
derm/o	combining form	skin	3
dermat/o	combining form	skin	3
-desis	suffix	binding, fusion	10
dips/o	combining form	thirst	12
dist/o	combining form	away (from the point of attachment)	2
dors/o	combining form	back	2
duoden/o	combining form	duodenum (1st portion of the small intestine)	8
dys-	prefix	difficult, painful, abnormal	4
-e	suffix	no meaning	3
-eal	suffix	pertaining to	4
ech/o	combining form	sound	7
-ectomy	suffix	surgical removal, excision	4
electr/o	combining form	electrical activity	7
-emia	suffix	in the blood	5
encephal/o	combining form	brain	11
endo-	prefix	within	4
endometri/o	combining form	endometrium	6
enter/o	combining form	intestines (usually the small intestine)	8
epi-	prefix	on, upon, over	3
epitheli/o	combining form	epithelium, epithelial tissue	1
erythr/o	combining form	red	3
esophag/o	combining form	esophagus	8
femor/o	combining form	femur (upper leg bone)	10
gastr/o	combining form	stomach	8

WORD PART	TYPE	DEFINITION	LESSON
-genic	suffix	producing, originating, causing	1
gingiv/o	combining form	gums	8
gloss/o	combining form	tongue	8
glyc/o	combining form	sugar	12
-gram	suffix	record, radiographic image	4
-graph	suffix	instrument used to record	7
-graphy	suffix	process of recording, radiographic imaging	2
gynec/o	combining form	woman, female reproductive system	6
hem/o	combining form	blood	5
hemat/o	combining form	blood	5
hemi-	prefix	half	11
hepat/o	combining form	liver	8
hist/o	combining form	tissue(s)	1
hydr/o	combining form	water	5
hyper-	prefix	above, excessive	4
hypo-	prefix	below, deficient, under	3
hyster/o	combining form	uterus	6
-ia	suffix	diseased state, condition of	4
-iasis	suffix	condition	5
-ic	suffix	pertaining to	1, 2
ile/o	combining form	ileum (3rd portion of the small intestine)	8
ili/o	combining form	ilium (upper wing-shaped part on each side of the pelvis)	10
infer/o	combining form	below	2
inter-	prefix	between	10
intra-	prefix	within	3
-ior	suffix	pertaining to	2

WORD PART	TYPE	DEFINITION	LESSON
ir/o	combining form	iris	9
irid/o	combining form	iris	9
ischi/o	combining form	ischium (lower posterior portion of the pelvis on which one sits)	10
-ism	suffix	state of	12
-itis	suffix	inflammation	3
jejun/o	combining form	jejunum (2nd portion of the small intestine)	8
kerat/o	combining form	cornea (also means hard, horny tissue)	9
kinesi/o	combining form	movement, motion	10
kyph/o	combining form	hump (thoracic spine)	10
lapar/o	combining form	abdomen, abdominal cavity	8
laryng/o	combining form	larynx (voice box)	4
later/o	combining form	side	2
leuk/o	combining form	white	3
lingu/o	combining form	tongue	8
lip/o	combining form	fat, fat tissue	1
lith/o	combining form	stone(s), calculus (*pl.* calculi)	5
-logist	suffix	one who studies and treats (specialist, physician)	1
-logy	suffix	study of	1
lord/o	combining form	bent forward (lumbar spine)	10
lymph/o	combining form	lymph, lymphatic tissue	7
-lysis	suffix	dissolution, separating	3
-malacia	suffix	softening	10
mamm/o	combining form	breast	6
mast/o	combining form	breast	6

WORD PART	TYPE	DEFINITION	LESSON
meat/o	combining form	meatus (opening)	5
medi/o	combining form	middle	2
-megaly	suffix	enlargement	1
melan/o	combining form	black	3
men/o	combining form	menstruation, menstrual	6
mening/o	combining form	meninges	11
meningi/o	combining form	meninges	11
meta-	prefix	beyond	1
-meter	suffix	instrument used to measure	4
-metry	suffix	measurement	9
micro-	prefix	small	11
muc/o	combining form	mucus	4
my/o	combining form	muscle(s), muscle tissue	1
myc/o	combining form	fungus	3
myel/o	combining form	spinal cord	11
myring/o	combining form	eardrum (tympanic membrane)	9
nas/o	combining form	nose	4
necr/o	combining form	death	10
neo-	prefix	new	1
nephr/o	combining form	kidney	5
neur/o	combining form	nerve(s), nerve tissue	1
noct/i	combining form	night	5
-oid	suffix	resembling	1
olig/o	combining form	scanty, few	5
-oma	suffix	tumor	1
onc/o	combining form	tumor(s)	1
onych/o	combining form	nail	3

WORD PART	TYPE	DEFINITION	LESSON
oophor/o	combining form	ovary	6
ophthalm/o	combining form	eye	9
opt/o	combining form	vision	9
or/o	combining form	mouth	8
orchi/o	combining form	testis (testicle)	6
organ/o	combining form	organ	1
-osis	suffix	abnormal condition	3
oste/o	combining form	bone(s)	10
ot/o	combining form	ear	9
-ous	suffix	pertaining to	3
ox/i	combining form	oxygen	4
pancreat/o	combining form	pancreas	8
path/o	combining form	disease	1
-penia	suffix	abnormal reduction (in number)	7
peps/o	combining form	digestion	8
per-	prefix	through	3
-pexy	suffix	surgical fixation, suspension	6
phag/o	combining form	swallowing, eating	8
phalang/o	combining form	phalanx (pl. phalanges) (any bone of the fingers or toes)	10
pharyng/o	combining form	pharynx (throat)	4
phas/o	combining form	speech	11
phleb/o	combining form	vein(s)	7
-plasm	suffix	growth (substance or formation)	1
-plasty	suffix	surgical repair	5
pleg/o	combining form	paralysis	11

WORD PART	TYPE	DEFINITION	LESSON
-plegia	suffix	paralysis	9
-pnea	suffix	breathing	4
pneum/o	combining form	lung, air	4
pneumon/o	combining form	lung, air	4
poli/o	combining form	gray matter	11
poly-	prefix	many, much	4
poster/o	combining form	back, behind	2
proct/o	combining form	rectum	8
prostat/o	combining form	prostate gland	6
proxim/o	combining form	near (the point of attachment)	2
psych/o	combining form	mind	11
-ptosis	suffix	drooping, sagging, prolapse	9
pub/o	combining form	pubis (anterior portion of the pelvis)	10
pulmon/o	combining form	lung	4
py/o	combining form	pus	5
pyel/o	combining form	renal pelvis	5
quadr/i	combining form	four	11
rachi/o	combining form	vertebra, spine, vertebral column	10
radi/o	combining form	x-rays (ionizing radiation)	1, 2
rect/o	combining form	rectum	8
ren/o	combining form	kidney	5
retin/o	combining form	retina	9
rhin/o	combining form	nose	4
-rrhagia	suffix	excessive bleeding	4
-rrhaphy	suffix	suturing, repairing	6
-rrhea	suffix	flow, discharge	4
-rrhexis	suffix	rupture	6

WORD PART	TYPE	DEFINITION	LESSON
salping/o	combining form	fallopian tube (uterine tube)	6
sarc/o	combining form	flesh, connective tissue	1
-schisis	suffix	split, fissure	10
scler/o	combining form	sclera	9
-sclerosis	suffix	hardening	7
scoli/o	combining form	crooked, curved (spine)	10
-scope	suffix	instrument used for visual examination	4
-scopic	suffix	pertaining to visual examination	4
-scopy	suffix	visual examination	4
scrot/o	combining form	scrotum	6
sigmoid/o	combining form	sigmoid colon	8
sinus/o	combining form	sinus *(s.)*, sinuses *(pl.)*	4
somn/o	combining form	sleep	4
son/o	combining form	sound	2
spir/o	combining form	breathe, breathing	4
splen/o	combining form	spleen	7
spondyl/o	combining form	vertebra, spine, vertebral column	10
-stasis	suffix	control, stop	1
stern/o	combining form	sternum (breastbone)	10
-stomy	suffix	creation of an artifical opening	4
sub-	prefix	below, under	3
super/o	combining form	above	2
system/o	combining form	system	1
tachy-	prefix	rapid, fast	7
ten/o	combining form	tendon(s)	10
tendin/o	combining form	tendon(s)	10

WORD PART	TYPE	DEFINITION	LESSON
thorac/o	combining form	chest, chest cavity	4
-thorax	suffix	chest, chest cavity	4
thromb/o	combining form	blood clot	7
thym/o	combining form	thymus gland	12
thyroid/o	combining form	thyroid gland	12
tom/o	combining form	cut, section, or slice	2
-tomy	suffix	cut into, incision	4
trache/o	combining form	trachea (windpipe)	4
-trans	suffix	through, across, beyond	3
-tripsy	suffix	surgical crushing	5
troph/o	combining form	development	10
tympan/o	combining form	middle ear	9
ur/o	combining form	urination, urine, urinary tract	5
ureter/o	combining form	ureter	5
urethr/o	combining form	urethra	5
urin/o	combining form	urination, urine, urinary tract	5
-us	suffix	no meaning	11
vagin/o	combining form	vagina	6
vas/o	combining form	vessel, duct (in male reproductive system, refers to vas deferens)	6
ven/o	combining form	vein(s)	7
ventr/o	combining form	belly (front)	2
vertebr/o	combining form	vertebra, spine, vertebral column	10
viscer/o	combining form	internal organs	1
xanth/o	combining form	yellow	3
-y	suffix	no meaning	3

Topics include:

Common Medical Abbreviations, pp. e1-e6

Institute for Safe Medical Practices' (ISMP) List of Error-Prone Abbreviations, Symbols, and Dose Designations, includes The Joint Commission's "Do Not Use" list, pp. e7-e10

Abbreviations are written as they appear most commonly in the medical and healthcare environment. Some may also appear in both capital and lowercase letters and with or without periods. A plural is formed by adding a lower case s. Consult with the healthcare facility for an approved list of abbreviations.

COMMON MEDICAL ABBREVIATIONS	DEFINITION
A&P	auscultation and percussion; anatomy and physiology
A1c	glycosylated hemoglobin (see also HgbA1c)
a.c.	before meals
ABE	acute bacterial endocarditis
ABG	arterial blood gas
ACS	acute coronary syndrome
AD	Alzheimer disease
ADHD	attention deficit/hyperactivity disorder
ADL, ADLs	activities of daily living
AFib	atrial fibrillation
AICD	automatic implantable cardioverter-defibrillator
AIDS	acquired immune deficiency syndrome
AKA	above-knee amputation
AKI	acute kidney injury
ALL	acute lymphocytic leukemia
ALS	amyotrophic lateral sclerosis
AM	between midnight and noon
AMA	against medical advice; American Medical Association
AMB	ambulate, ambulatory
AMD	age-related macular degeneration
AMI	acute myocardial infarction
AML	acute myelocytic leukemia
amp	ampule
amt	amount
ant	anterior

COMMON MEDICAL ABBREVIATIONS	DEFINITION
AOM	acute otitis media
AP	anteroposterior
APR	abdominoperineal resection
ARDS	acute respiratory distress syndrome; adult respiratory distress syndrome
ARF	acute renal failure
AROM	artificial rupture of membranes
ASA	aspirin
as tol	as tolerated
AST	astigmatism
ASCVD	arteriosclerotic cardiovascular disease
ASD	atrial septal defect
ASHD	arteriosclerotic heart disease
AV	arteriovenous; atrioventricular
AVR	aortic valve replacement
ax	axillary
BA	bronchial asthma
BBB	bundle branch block
BCC	basal cell carcinoma
BE	barium enema
b.i.d.	twice a day
BKA	below-knee amputation
BM	bowel movement
BMI	body mass index
BOM	bilateral otitis media
BP	blood pressure
BPH	benign prostatic hyperplasia
BR	bed rest

COMMON MEDICAL ABBREVIATIONS	DEFINITION
BRP	bathroom privileges
BS	blood sugar; bowel sounds; breath sounds
BSO	bilateral salpingo-oophorectomy
BUN	blood urea nitrogen
Bx	biopsy
C	Celsius
C1-C7	cervical vertebrae
c̄	with
C&S	culture and sensitivity
c/o	complains of
Ca (or Ca⁺⁺)	calcium
CA	cancer, carcinoma
CA-MRSA	community-associated methicillin-resistant *Staphylococcus aureus*
CABG	coronary artery bypass graft
CAD	coronary artery disease
cal	calorie
cap	capsule
CAPD	continuous ambulatory peritoneal dialysis
cath	catheterization, catheter
CBC	complete blood count
CBC with diff	complete blood count and differential
CBR	complete bed rest
CC	chief complaint, cubic centimeter*
CCU	coronary care unit
CDE	certified diabetes educator
CDH	congenital dislocation of the hip
C. diff	*Clostridium difficile* (bacteria)
CEA	carcinoembryonic antigen
CF	cystic fibrosis
CHB	complete heart block
CHD	coronary heart disease
chemo	chemotherapy
CHF	congestive heart failure
CHO	carbohydrate
chol	cholesterol
circ	circumcision
CKD	chronic kidney disease
Cl (or Cl⁻)	chloride
cl liq	clear liquid
CLD	chronic liver disease

COMMON MEDICAL ABBREVIATIONS	DEFINITION
CLL	chronic lymphocytic leukemia
cm	centimeter
CMA	certified medical assistant
CML	chronic myelogenous leukemia
CMP	comprehensive metabolic panel
CMV	cytomegalovirus
CNA	certified nursing assistant
CNM	certified nurse midwife
CNS	central nervous system
CO	carbon monoxide
CO₂	carbon dioxide
comp	compound
COPD	chronic obstructive pulmonary disease
COVID-19	coronavirus disease
CP	cerebral palsy
CPAP	continuous positive airway pressure
CPK	creatine phosphokinase
CPR	cardiopulmonary resuscitation
creat	creatinine
CRF	chronic renal failure
CRP	C-reactive protein
CS, C-sect, C-section	cesarean section
CSF	cerebrospinal fluid
CT	computed tomography
CTC	computed tomography colonography
CTS	carpal tunnel syndrome
Cu	copper
CVA	cerebrovascular accident (stroke)
CVD	cardiovascular disease
CVP	central venous pressure
Cx	cervix
CXR	chest radiograph (chest x-ray)
D&C	dilation and curettage
D/S	dextrose in saline
D/W	dextrose in water
DAT	diet as tolerated
DC	doctor of chiropractic
DCIS	ductal carcinoma in situ
DERM	dermatology
DEXA	dual-energy x-ray absorptiometry (bone density test)

*CC, mistaken in pharmacology for "units," is used in laboratory, pathology, and prostate measurements.

COMMON MEDICAL ABBREVIATIONS	DEFINITION
DI	diabetes insipidus
diff	differential (part of complete blood count)
disch	discharge
DM	diabetes mellitus
DO	doctor of osteopathy
DOA	dead on arrival
DOB	date of birth
DRE	digital rectal examination
DSA	digital subtraction angiography
DVT	deep vein thrombosis
DW	distilled water
Dx	diagnosis
DXA	dual x-ray absorptiometry (bone density test)
EBL	estimated blood loss
ECG	electrocardiogram
ECHO	echocardiogram
ECT	electroconvulsive therapy
ED	erectile dysfunction; emergency department
EEG	electroencephalogram
EENT	eyes, ears, nose, and throat
EGD	esophagogastroduodenoscopy
EHR	electronic health record
EKG	electrocardiogram
elix	elixir
EMG	electromyogram
EMR	electronic medical record
ENG	electronystagmography
ENT	ears, nose, and throat; otolaryngologist
ERCP	endoscopic retrograde cholangiopancreatography
ESR	erythrocyte sedimentation rate
ESRD	end-stage renal disease
ESWL	extracorporeal shock wave lithotripsy
ET	endotracheal
exam	examination
F	Fahrenheit
FBS	fasting blood sugar
Fe	iron
FHT	fetal heart tones
flu	influenza
FNA	fine needle aspiration

COMMON MEDICAL ABBREVIATIONS	DEFINITION
Fr	French (catheter size)
FSH	follicle-stimulating hormone
FTT	failure to thrive
FUO	fever of undetermined origin
Fx	fracture
g	gram
GB	gallbladder
GERD	gastroesophageal reflux disease
GI	gastrointestinal
GSW	gunshot wound
gtt	drop
GTT	glucose tolerance test
GU	genitourinary
Gyn	gynecology
h	hour
H&H	hemoglobin and hematocrit
H&P	history and physical
H_2O	water
H_2O_2	hydrogen peroxide (hydrogen dioxide)
HA-MRSA	hospital-associated methicillin-resistant *Staphylococcus aureus*
HB	heart block
HbA1c	glycosylated hemoglobin
HBV	hepatitis B virus
HCl	hydrochloric acid
HCO_3	bicarbonate
Hct	hematocrit
HCVD	hypertensive cardiovascular disease
HD	hemodialysis
HgbA1c	glycosylated hemoglobin (see also HbA1c)
HF	heart failure
Hg	mercury
Hgb	hemoglobin
HHD	hypertensive heart disease
HIT	health information technology
HIV	human immunodeficiency virus
HMD	hyaline membrane disease
HNP	herniated nucleus pulposus
HOB	head of bed
HOH	hard of hearing
HPI	history of present illness
HPV	human papillomavirus
HRT	hormone replacement therapy
HSG	hysterosalpingogram

COMMON MEDICAL ABBREVIATIONS	DEFINITION
ht	height
HTN	hypertension
Hx	history
hypo	hypodermic
I&D	incision and drainage
I&O	intake and output
IBS	irritable bowel syndrome
ICU	intensive care unit
ID	intradermal
IDDM	insulin-dependent diabetes mellitus
IHD	ischemic heart disease
IM	intramuscular
inf	inferior
IOP	intraocular pressure
IPPB	intermittent positive pressure breathing
irrig	irrigation
isol	isolation
IUD	intrauterine device
IV	intravenous
IVC	inferior vena cava
IVP	intravenous pyelogram
K	potassium
KCl	potassium chloride
kg	kilogram
KUB	kidneys, ureters, bladder
KVO	keep vein open
L	liter
L1–L5	lumbar vertebrae
L&D	labor and delivery
lab	laboratory
lac	laceration
lat	lateral
LE	lupus erythematosus
LFT	liver function tests
lg	large
LLL	left lower lobe
LLQ	left lower quadrant
LMP	last menstrual period
LP	lumbar puncture
LPN	licensed practical nurse
LR	lactated Ringer (IV solution)
lt	left

COMMON MEDICAL ABBREVIATIONS	DEFINITION
LTB	laryngotracheobronchitis
LUL	left upper lobe
LUQ	left upper quadrant
MA	medical assistant
med	medial
MCH	mean corpuscular hemoglobin
MCV	mean corpuscular volume
MD	muscular dystrophy; medical doctor
mEq	milliequivalent
METS	metastasis, metastases
mg	milligram
MH	mental health
MI	myocardial infarction
mL	milliliter
mm	millimeter
MM	multiple myeloma
MOM	milk of magnesia
MR	magnetic resonance
MRI	magnetic resonance imaging
MRSA	methicillin-resistant *Staphylococcus aureus*
MS	multiple sclerosis
MVP	mitral valve prolapse
N&V	nausea and vomiting
NA	nursing assistant
Na	sodium
NaCl	sodium chloride (salt)
NAS	no added salt
NB	newborn
neg	negative
neuro	neurology
NG	nasogastric
NICU	neurologic intensive care unit; neonatal intensive care unit
NIDDM	noninsulin-dependent diabetes mellitus
NKDA	no known drug allergies
NM	nuclear medicine
noc, noct	night
NP	nurse practitioner
NPO	nothing by mouth
NS	normal saline
NSAID	nonsteroidal antiinflammatory drug

COMMON MEDICAL ABBREVIATIONS	DEFINITION
NSR	normal sinus rhythm
NVS	neurologic vital signs
O_2	oxygen
OA	osteoarthritis
OAB	overactive bladder
OB	obstetrics
OB/GYN	obstetrician-gynecologist
OBS	organic brain syndrome
OCD	obsessive-compulsive disorder
OD	overdose
oint	ointment
OM	otitis media
OOB	out of bed
OP	outpatient
Ophth	ophthalmology
OR	operating room
Ortho, ortho	orthopedics
OSA	obstructive sleep apnea
OT	occupational therapy
oz	ounce
P	pulse
$\bar{p}$	after
PA	posteroanterior; physician's assistant
PAC	premature atrial contraction
PAD	peripheral artery disease
PAT	paroxysmal atrial tachycardia
PATH	pathology
p.c.	after meals
PCI	percutaneous coronary intervention
PCP	primary care physician; *Pneumocystis carinii* pneumonia
PCT	patient care technician
PCU	progressive care unit
PCV	packed cell volume
PD	Parkinson disease
PDA	patent ductus arteriosus
PE	pulmonary edema; pulmonary embolism
Peds	pediatrics
PEEP	positive end-expiratory pressure
PEG	percutaneous endoscopic gastrostomy
per	by

COMMON MEDICAL ABBREVIATIONS	DEFINITION
PERRLA	pupils equal, round, reactive to light and accommodation
PET	positron emission tomography (scan)
PFTs	pulmonary function tests
PICU	pediatric intensive care unit
PID	pelvic inflammatory disease
PKD	polycystic kidney disease
PKU	phenylketonuria
PM	between noon and midnight
PMH	past medical history
PMR	polymyalgia rheumatica
PNS	peripheral nervous system
PO	orally; phone order
post	posterior
post-op	postoperatively
PP	postpartum; postprandial (after meals)
PPD	purified protein derivative
PRBC	packed red blood cells
PRN	as needed
PSA	prostate-specific antigen
PSG	polysomnography
pt	patient; pint
PT	physical therapy; prothrombin time
PTA	physical therapist assistant
PTCA	percutaneous transluminal coronary angioplasty
PT/INR	prothrombin time/international normalized ratio
PTSD	post-traumatic stress disorder
PTT	partial thromboplastin time (pro time)
PUL	percutaneous ultrasound lithotripsy, pulmonary
PVC	premature ventricular contraction
PVD	peripheral vascular disease
Px	prognosis
q	every
q_h	every number of hours (e.g., q2h)
qt	quart
R	respiration
RA	rheumatoid arthritis
RBC	erythrocyte; red blood cell count; red blood cell
RCP	respiratory care practitioner
RD	registered dietitian

COMMON MEDICAL ABBREVIATIONS	DEFINITION
reg	regular
REM	rapid eye movement
resp	respirations
RHD	rheumatic heart disease
RLL	right lower lobe
RLQ	right lower quadrant
RN	registered nurse
R/O	rule out
ROM	range of motion
ROS	review of systems
RP	radical prostatectomy
RR	recovery room
rt	right; routine
RT	respiratory therapist; radiologic technologist; respiratory therapy
RUL	right upper lobe
RUQ	right upper quadrant
Rx	prescription
s̄	without
SAH	subarachnoid hemorrhage
SBE	subacute bacterial endocarditis
SCC	squamous cell carcinoma
SH	social history
SIDS	sudden infant death syndrome
SLE	systemic lupus erythematosus
SMAC	sequential multiple analysis computer
SNF	skilled nursing facility
SO$_2$	oxygen saturation
SOAP	subjective, objective, assessment, plan (note format)
SOB	shortness of breath
SSE	soapsuds enema
staph	staphylococcus, staphylococci
stat	immediately
STD	sexually transmitted disease
STI	sexually transmitted infection
strep	streptococcus, streptococci
subcut	subcutaneous
sup	superior
SVN	small volume nebulizer
Sz	seizure
T	temperature
T1–T12	thoracic vertebrae

COMMON MEDICAL ABBREVIATIONS	DEFINITION
T1DM	type 1 diabetes mellitus
T2DM	type 2 diabetes mellitus
T&A	tonsillectomy and adenoidectomy
tab	tablet
TAH	total abdominal hysterectomy
TAH/BSO	total abdominal hysterectomy [and] bilateral salpingo-oophorectomy
TB	tuberculosis
TBI	traumatic brain injury
TCDB	turn, cough, deep breathe
TD	transdermal
temp	temperature
THA	total hip arthroplasty
TIA	transient ischemic attack
tid	three times a day
TKA	total knee arthroplasty
TPN	total parenteral nutrition
trach	tracheostomy
TRUS	transrectal ultrasound
TURP	transurethral resection of the prostate gland
TVH	total vaginal hysterectomy
TWE	tap water enema
Tx	treatment; traction
UA	urinalysis
UC	ulcerative colitis
UGI series	upper GI (gastrointestinal) series
UPPP	uvulopalatopharyngoplasty
URI	upper respiratory infection
US	ultrasonography
UTI	urinary tract infection
VA	visual acuity
vag	vaginal
VCUG	voiding cystourethrogram
VDRL	venereal disease research laboratory
v fib	ventricular fibrillation
V/Q scan	lung ventilation/perfusion scan
VRE	vancomycin-resistant *Enterococcus*
VS	vital signs
W/C	wheelchair
WA	while awake
WBC	leukocyte; white blood cell
wt	weight
XRT	radiation therapy

INSTITUTE FOR SAFE MEDICATION PRACTICES' LIST OF ERROR-PRONE ABBREVIATIONS, SYMBOLS, AND DOSE DESIGNATIONS

The abbreviations, symbols, and dose designations found in this table have been reported to ISMP through the ISMP National Medication Errors Reporting Program (ISMP MERP) as being frequently misinterpreted and involved in harmful medication errors. They should **NEVER** be used when communicating medical information. This includes internal communications, telephone/verbal prescriptions, computer-generated labels, labels for drug storage bins, medication administration records, as well as pharmacy and prescriber computer order entry screens.

The Joint Commission established a National Patient Safety Goal specifying certain abbreviations, acronyms, and symbols that must appear on an accredited organization's "do not use" list; these are called to your attention with a double asterisk (**). However, we hope that you consider others beyond the minimum Joint Commission requirements. By using and promoting safe practices, and by educating one another about hazards, we can better protect our patients.

ABBREVIATIONS	INTENDED MEANING	MISINTERPRETATION	CORRECTION
µg	Microgram	Mistaken as "mg"	Use "mcg"
AD, AS, AU	Right ear, left ear, each ear	Mistaken as OD, OS, OU (right eye, left eye, each eye)	Use "right ear," "left ear," or "each ear"
OD, OS, OU	Right eye, left eye, each eye	Mistaken as AD, AS, AU (right ear, left ear, each ear)	Use "right eye," "left eye," or "each eye"
BT	Bedtime	Mistaken as "BID" (twice daily)	Use "bedtime"
cc	Cubic centimeters	Mistaken as "u" (units)	Use "mL"
D/C	Discharge or discontinue	Premature discontinuation of medications if D/C (intended to mean "discharge") has been misinterpreted as "discontinued" when followed by a list of discharge medications	Use "discharge" and "discontinue"
IJ	Injection	Mistaken as "IV" or "intrajugular"	Use "injection"
IN	Intranasal	Mistaken as "IM" or "IV"	Use "intranasal" or "NAS"
HS	Half-strength	Mistaken as bedtime	Use "half-strength" or "bedtime"
hs	At bedtime, hours of sleep	Mistaken as half-strength	
IU**	International unit	Mistaken as IV (intravenous) or 10 (ten)	Use "units"
o.d. or OD	Once daily	Mistaken as "right eye" (OD-oculus dexter), leading to oral liquid medications administered in the eye	Use "daily"
OJ	Orange juice	Mistaken as OD or OS (right or left eye); drugs meant to be diluted in orange juice may be given in the eye	Use "orange juice"
Per os	By mouth, orally	The "os" can be mistaken as "left eye" (OS-oculus sinister)	Use "PO," "by mouth," or "orally"
q.d. or QD**	Every day	Mistaken as q.i.d., especially if the period after the "q" or the tail of the "q" is misunderstood as an "i"	Use "daily"
qhs	Nightly at bedtime	Mistaken as "qhr" or every hour	Use "nightly"
qn	Nightly or at bedtime	Mistaken as "qh" (every hour)	Use "nightly" or "at bedtime"
q.o.d. or QOD**	Every other day	Mistaken as "q.d." (daily) or "q.i.d." (four times daily) if the "o" is poorly written	Use "every other day"

ABBREVIATIONS	INTENDED MEANING	MISINTERPRETATION	CORRECTION
q1d	Daily	Mistaken as q.i.d. (four times daily)	Use "daily"
q6PM, etc.	Every evening at 6 PM	Mistaken as every 6 hours	Use "daily at 6 PM" or "6 PM daily"
SC, SQ, sub q	Subcutaneous	SC mistaken as SL (sublingual); SQ mistaken as "5 every;" the "q" in "sub q" has been mistaken as "every" (e.g., a heparin dose ordered "sub q 2 hours before surgery" misunderstood as every 2 hours before surgery)	Use "subcut" or "subcutaneously"
ss	Sliding scale (insulin) or ½ (apothecary)	Mistaken as "55"	Spell out "sliding scale;" use "one-half" or "½"
SSRI	Sliding scale regular insulin	Mistaken as selective-serotonin reuptake inhibitor	Spell out "sliding scale (insulin)"
SSI	Sliding scale insulin	Mistaken as Strong Solution of Iodine (Lugol's)	
i/d	One daily	Mistaken as "tid"	Use "1 daily"
TIW or tiw	3 times a week	Mistaken as "3 times a day" or "twice in a week"	Use "3 times weekly"
U or u**	Unit	Mistaken as the number 0 or 4, causing a 10-fold overdose or greater (e.g., 4U seen as "40" or 4u seen as "44"); mistaken as "cc" so dose given in volume instead of units (e.g., 4u seen as 4cc)	Use "unit"
UD	As directed ("ut dictum")	Mistaken as unit dose (e.g., diltiazem 125 mg IV infusion "UD" misinterpreted as meaning to give the entire infusion as a unit [bolus] dose)	Use "as directed"

DOSE DESIGNATIONS AND OTHER INFORMATION	INTENDED MEANING	MISINTERPRETATION	CORRECTION
Trailing zero after decimal point (e.g., 1.0 mg)**	1 mg	Mistaken as 10 mg if the decimal point is not seen	Do not use trailing zeros for doses expressed in whole numbers
"Naked" decimal point (e.g., .5 mg)**	0.5 mg	Mistaken as 5 mg if the decimal point is not seen	Use zero before a decimal point when the dose is less than a whole unit
Abbreviations such as mg. or mL. with a period following the abbreviation	mg mL	The period is unnecessary and could be mistaken as the number 1 if written poorly	Use mg, mL, etc. without a terminal period
Dose Designations and Other Information	**Intended Meaning**	**Misinterpretation**	**Correction**
Drug name and dose run together (especially problematic for drug names that end in "l" such as Inderal 40 mg; Tegretol 300 mg)	Inderal 40 mg Tegretol 300 mg	Mistaken as Inderal 140 mg Mistaken as Tegretol 1300 mg	Place adequate space between the drug name, dose, and unit of measure

DOSE DESIGNATIONS AND OTHER INFORMATION	INTENDED MEANING	MISINTERPRETATION	CORRECTION
Numerical dose and unit of measure run together (e.g., 10mg, 100mL)	10 mg 100 mL	The "m" is sometimes mistaken as a zero or two zeros, risking a 10- to 100-fold overdose	Place adequate space between the dose and unit of measure
Large doses without properly placed commas (e.g., 100000 units; 1000000 units)	100,000 units 1,000,000 units	100000 has been mistaken as 10,000 or 1,000,000; 1000000 has been mistaken as 100,000	Use commas for dosing units at or above 1,000, or use words such as 100 "thousand" or 1 "million" to improve readability

DRUG NAME ABBREVIATIONS	INTENDED MEANING	MISINTERPRETATION	CORRECTION
To avoid confusion, do not abbreviate drug names when communicating medical information. Examples of drug name abbreviations involved in medication errors include:			
APAP	acetaminophen	Not recognized as acetaminophen	Use complete drug name
ARA A	vidarabine	Mistaken as cytarabine (ARA C)	Use complete drug name
AZT	zidovudine (Retrovir)	Mistaken as azathioprine or aztreonam	Use complete drug name
CPZ	Compazine (prochlorperazine)	Mistaken as chlorpromazine	Use complete drug name
DPT	Demerol-Phenergan-Thorazine	Mistaken as diphtheria-pertussis-tetanus (vaccine)	Use complete drug name
DTO	Diluted tincture of opium, or deodorized tincture of opium (Paregoric)	Mistaken as tincture of opium	Use complete drug name
HCl	hydrochloric acid or hydrochloride	Mistaken as potassium chloride (The "H" is misinterpreted as "K")	Use complete drug name unless expressed as a salt of a drug
HCT	hydrocortisone	Mistaken as hydrochlorothiazide	Use complete drug name
HCTZ	hydrochlorothiazide	Mistaken as hydrocortisone (seen as HCT250 mg)	Use complete drug name
MgSO4**	magnesium sulfate	Mistaken as morphine sulfate	Use complete drug name
MS, MSO4**	morphine sulfate	Mistaken as magnesium sulfate	Use complete drug name
MTX	methotrexate	Mistaken as mitoxantrone	Use complete drug name
PCA	procainamide	Mistaken as patient-controlled analgesia	Use complete drug name
PTU	propylthiouracil	Mistaken as mercaptopurine	Use complete drug name
T3	Tylenol with codeine No. 3	Mistaken as liothyronine	Use complete drug name
TAC	triamcinolone	Mistaken as tetracaine, Adrenalin, cocaine	Use complete drug name
TNK	TNKase	Mistaken as "TPA"	Use complete drug name
ZnSO4	zinc sulfate	Mistaken as morphine sulfate	Use complete drug name

STEMMED DRUG NAMES	INTENDED MEANING	MISINTERPRETATION	CORRECTION
"Nitro" drip	nitroglycerin infusion	Mistaken as sodium nitroprusside infusion	Use complete drug name
"Norflox"	norfloxacin	Mistaken as Norflex	Use complete drug name
"IV Vanc"	intravenous vancomycin	Mistaken as Invanz	Use complete drug name

SYMBOLS	INTENDED MEANING	MISINTERPRETATION	CORRECTION
ℨ	Dram	Symbol for dram mistaken as "3"	Use the metric system
ℳ	Minim	Symbol for minim mistaken as "mL"	
x3d	For three days	Mistaken as "3 doses"	Use "for three days"
> and **<**	Greater than and less than	Mistaken as opposite of intended; mistakenly use incorrect symbol; "< 10" mistaken as "40"	Use "greater than" or "less than"
/ (slash mark)	Separates two doses or indicates "per"	Mistaken as the number 1 (e.g., "25 units/ 10 units" misread as "25 units and 110" units)	Use "per" rather than a slash mark to separate doses
@	At	Mistaken as "2"	Use "at"
&	And	Mistaken as "2"	Use "and"
+	Plus or and	Mistaken as "4"	Use "and"
°	Hour	Mistaken as a zero (e.g., q2° seen as q 20)	Use "hr," "h," or "hour"
Φ or ⊘	zero, null sign	Mistaken as numerals 4, 6, 8, and 9	Use 0 or zero, or describe intent using whole words

Visit www.jointcommission.org for more information about this Joint Commission requirement.

APPENDIX C

Answer Key

LESSON 1

Exercise A

Identify Origins of Medical Language

1. a; 2. c; 3. d; 4. b
5. a. acronym; MRSA
   b. eponym; Parkinson disease
   c. modern language; posttraumatic stress disorder
   d. Greek and Latin; arthritis

Exercise B

Define Word Parts, Combining Forms, and Categories of Medical Terms

A.
1. c; 2. e; 3. a; 4. g; 5. f; 6. b; 7. d
B.
1. word root; 2. end; beginning;
3. suffix; prefix; pertaining to within a vein; 4. combining vowel; inflammation of the bone and joint

Exercise C

Build and Translate Terms Built from Word Parts

1. **Match:** a. -al; pertaining to;
   b. -logy; study of; c. -oma; tumor
2. **Label:** Figure 1.3, (1) hist/o; (2) cyt/o; (3) organ/o; (4) system/o
3. **Translate:** hist/o/logy; study of tissue(s)
4. **Reading Exercise**
5. **Label:** Figure 1.4, (1) neur/o, (2) epitheli/o; (3) sarc/o; (4) my/o
6. **Build:** a. my/oma; b. epitheli/oma; c. sarc/oma
7. **Reading Exercise**
8. **Match:** a. lip/o; fat, fat tissue;
   b. carcin/o; cancer; c. -oma; tumor; d. -oid; resembling
9. **Translate:** a. lip/oma; tumor (composed of) fat tissue; b. lip/oid; resembling fat; c. carcin/oid; resembling cancer
10. **Reading Exercise**
11. **Label:** Figure 1.5, lip/oma
12. **Label:** Figure 1.6, 1. viscer/o
13. **Match:** a. -al; pertaining to; b. -megaly; enlargement; c. -ic; pertaining to;

d. organ/o; organ; e. epitheli/o; epithelium; f. system/o; system
14. **Build:** a. viscer/al; b. epitheli/al; c. system/ic; d. organ/o/megaly
15. **Reading Exercise**
16. **Match:** a. path/o; disease; b. -genic; producing, originating, causing; c. -logy; study of; d. -logist; one who studies and treats (specialist, physician)
17. **Translate:** a. path/o/logist; physician who studies disease; b. path/o/genic; producing disease; c. path/o/logy; study of disease
18. **Reading Exercise**
19. a. radi/o/logy; b. radi/o/logist
20. **Reading Exercise**
21. **Match:** a. carcin/o; cancer; b. -oma; tumor; c. -genic; producing, originating, causing; d. meta-; beyond; e. neo-; new; f. -plasm; growth (substance or formation); g. -stasis; control, stop
22. **Build:** a. neo/plasm; b. meta/stasis; c. carcin/o/genic; d. carcin/oma
23. **Reading Exercise**
24. **Label:** Figure 1.7, carcin/oma
25. **Reading Exercise**
26. **Label:** Figure 1.8, meta/stasis
27. **Match:** a. onc/o; tumor(s); b. -logy; study of; c. -logist; one who studies and treats (specialist, physician)
28. **Translate:** a. onc/o/logy; study of tumors; b. onc/o/logist; physician who studies and treats tumors
29. **Reading Exercise**
30. **Term Table: Review of Body Structure and Oncology Terms Built from Word Parts**

Exercise D

Pronounce and Spell Terms Built from Word Parts

1. Check responses with the Table for Terms Built from Word Parts
2. Check answers with online resources

Exercise E

Label

1. staphylococcus (s.); staphylococci (pl.);
2. streptococcus (s.); streptococci (pl.);
3. infection; 4. biopsy;
5. chemotherapy; 6. radiation therapy;
7. malignant; 8. chemistry panel;
9. genetic testing; 10. specimen

Exercise F

Match

1. c; 2. d; 3. a; 4. f; 5. g; 6. e; 7. b

Exercise G

Learn Medical Terms NOT Built from Word Parts

1. benign; malignant; biopsy;
2. diagnosis; prognosis;
3. chemotherapy; radiation therapy; biological therapy; remission;
4. inflammation; 5. infection; staphylococcus; streptococcus;
6. chemistry panel; complete blood count with differential; CBC with diff;
7. genetic testing; specimen

Exercise H

Pronounce and Spell Terms NOT Built from Word Parts

1. Check responses with the Table for Terms NOT Built from Word Parts
2. Check answers with online resources

Exercise I

Abbreviate Medical Terms

1. Diseases and disorders: CA
2. Descriptive of the disease process: a. METS; b. Dx; c. Px
3. Surgical procedures: Bx
4. Laboratory terms: CBC with diff
5. Treatments: a. XRT; b. chemo
6. Specialties: PATH
7. Related terms: a. lab; b. staph; c. strep

Exercise J

Body Structure Terms

1. lipoid; 2. epithelial;
3. visceral; 4. systemic

Copyright © 2024 by Elsevier, Inc. All rights reserved.

Exercise K

Oncology Terms
Signs and Symptoms
 1. inflammation; 2. organomegaly
Diseases and Disorders
 3. neoplasm; 4. epithelioma;
 5. neuroma; 6. sarcoma; 7. lipoma;
 8. myoma; 9. carcinoma; 10. infection
Descriptive of Disease and Disease
    Processes
 11. diagnosis; 12. prognosis;
 13. malignant; 14. benign; 15. remission;
 16. metastasis
Treatments
 17. radiation therapy; 18. chemotherapy;
 19. biological therapy
Specialties and Professions
 20. pathologist; 21. oncologist;
 22. oncology; 23. histology;
 24. pathology; 25. cytology;
 26. radiology; 27. radiologist
Related Terms
 28. carcinogenic; 29. pathogenic;
 30. streptococcus; 31. staphylococcus;
 32. carcinoid

Exercise L

Laboratory Terms
 1. biopsy; 2. chemistry panel;
 3. complete blood count with differential;
 4. genetic testing; 5. specimen

Exercise M

Use Medical Terms in Clinical Statements
 1. Pathogenic; carcinogenic; 2. diagnosis;
 CA; oncologist; 3. neoplasm; cytology;
 benign; malignant; 4. pathologist; lipoid;
 5. pathology; sarcoma; metastasis;
 oncology; Px; 6. infection; systemic

Exercise N

Apply Medical Terms to Case Study
Answers will vary and may include:
diagnosis, prognosis, and remission along
with their respective definitions.

Exercise O

Use Medical Terms in a Document
 1. biopsy; 2. cytology; 3. pathologist;
 4. diagnosis; 5. carcinoma;
 6. inflammation; 7. metastasis;
 8. malignant; 9. oncologist;
 10. chemotherapy; 11. prognosis;
 12. radiation therapy; 13. F; "no evidence
 of metastasis" (beyond control)
 means the cancer has not spread to
 surrounding organs.
 14. F; prognosis means "prediction of
 a possible outcome of a disease";

diagnosis means "identification of a
disease."
 15. F; an oncologist treats patients with
 cancer; a pathologist studies body
 changes caused by disease, usually
 from a specimen.
 16. Answers will vary and may include:
 Bx, biopsy; Dx, diagnosis; METS,
 metastasis; chemo, chemotherapy;
 Px, prognosis; XRT, radiation therapy;
 CA, cancer
 17. Research exercise; answers
 will vary

Exercise P

*Interpret Language Used in a Medical
Record*
 1. c; 2. b; 3. a; 4. Research exercise;
 answers will vary

Exercise Q

Online Review of Lesson Content
Completed with online resources

Exercise R

Lesson Content Quiz
 1. b; 2. a; 3. c; 4. a; 5. c; 6. b; 7. b;
 8. a; 9. c; 10. b; 11. a; 12. b

LESSON 2

Exercise A

Build and Translate Directional Terms
 1. **Match:** a. -al, -ic, -ior; pertaining to;
 b. -ad; toward
 2. **Label:** Figure 2.3, (1) dors/o;
 (2) poster/o; (3) anter/o; (4) ventr/o
 3. **Translate:** a. ventr/al; pertaining to
 the belly; b. dors/al; pertaining to the
 back; c. anter/ior; pertaining to the
 front; d. poster/ior; pertaining to
 the back (behind)
 4. **Reading Exercise**
 5. **Label:** Figure 2.4, (1) dors/al,
 poster/ior; (2) anter/ior; (3) ventr/al
 6. **Translate:** a. poster/o/anter/ior (PA);
 pertaining to the back and to the
 front; b. anter/o/poster/ior (AP);
 pertaining to the front and to the
 back
 7. **Reading Exercise**
 8. **Label:** Figure 2.5, a. poster/o/anter/
 ior; b. anter/o/poster/ior
 9. **Label:** Figure 2.6, (1) super/o;
 (2) cephal/o; (3) caud/o; (4) infer/o
 10. **Translate:** a. super/ior; pertaining to
 above; b. infer/ior; pertaining to

below; c. anter/o/super/ior; pertaining
to the front and above
 11. **Reading Exercise**
 12. **Translate:** a. cephal/ic; pertaining to
 the head; b. caud/al; pertaining to the
 tail; c. cephal/ad; toward the head;
 d. caud/ad; toward the tail
 13. **Reading Exercise**
 14. **Label:** Figure 2.7, (1) super/ior;
 (2) cephal/ic; (3) cephal/ad;
 (4) caud/ad; (5) infer/ior; (6) caud/al
 15. **Label:** Figure 2.8, (1) later/o;
 (2) medi/o; (3) proxim/o; (4) dist/o
 16. **Build:** a. proxim/al; b. dist/al
 17. **Reading Exercise**
 18. **Build:** a. medi/al; b. later/al
 19. **Reading Exercise**
 20. **Label:** Figure 2.11, later/al
 21. **Build:** a. medi/o/later/al;
 b. anter/o/medi/al; c. poster/o/later/al;
 d. super/o/later/al; e. infer/o/later/al;
 f. anter/o/later/al
 22. **Term Table: Review of Directional
 Terms**

Exercise B

Pronounce and Spell Directional Terms
 1. Check responses with the Term Table
 in Exercise A, #22
 2. Check answers with online resources

Exercise C

*Learn Anatomic Planes, Abdominopelvic
Regions, and Patient Positions*
 1. **Label:** Figure 2.14, (1) axial;
 (2) coronal; (3) sagittal
 2. **Label:** Figure 2.16, (1) Right
 hypochondriac region; (2) Right
 lumbar region; (3) Right iliac region;
 (4) Hypogastric region; (5) Epigastric
 region; (6) Left hypochondriac region;
 (7) Umbilical region; (8) Left lumbar
 region; (9) Left iliac region
 3. **Label:** Figure 2.17, (1) supine position;
 (2) prone position; (3) sitting position;
 (4) orthopnea position; (5) lateral
 position; (6) semiprone position;
 (7) Trendelenburg position

Exercise D

*Pronounce and Spell Anatomic Planes,
Abdominopelvic Regions, and Patient
Positions*
 1. Check responses with the Term Tables
 for Anatomic Planes, Abdominopelvic
 Regions, and Patient Positions
 2. Check answers with online
 resources

Copyright © 2024 by Elsevier, Inc. All rights reserved.

Exercise E

Learn Diagnostic Imaging Terms

1. **Match:** a. radi/o; x-rays (ionizing radiation); b. tom/o; slice(s); c. son/o; sound; d. -graphy; process of recording
2. **Translate:** a. son/o/graphy; process of recording sound; b. radi/o/graphy; process of recording x-rays; c. tom/o/graphy; process of recording slices
3. **Label:** A. radi/o/graphy; B. son/o/graphy; C. tom/o/graphy
4. **Reading Exercise**
5. **Identify:** a. nuclear medicine, NM; b. magnetic resonance imaging, MRI
6. **Label:** A. magnetic resonance imaging; B. nuclear medicine
7. **Reading Exercise**

Exercise F

Pronounce and Spell Diagnostic Imaging Terms

1. Check responses with the Term Table for Diagnostic Imaging Terms
2. Check answers with online resources

Exercise G

Abbreviate Medical Terms

1. Directional Terms
   a. sup; b. inf; c. med; d. lat; e. PA; f. AP; g. post; h. ant
2. Abdominopelvic Quadrants
   a. RUQ; b. RLQ; c. LUQ; d. LLQ
3. Diagnostic Imaging
   a. US; b. NM; c. MRI

Exercise H

Directional Terms

1. cephalic; 2. superior; 3. superolateral; 4. posterolateral; 5. posteroanterior; 6. posterior; 7. dorsal; 8. mediolateral; 9. anteromedial; 10. medial; 11. lateral; 12. inferolateral; 13. inferior; 14. proximal; 15. distal; 16. caudad; 17. cephalad; 18. caudal; 19. ventral; 20. anterior; 21. anterosuperior; 22. anteroposterior; 23. anterolateral

Exercise I

Anatomic Planes

1. axial; 2. coronal; 3. sagittal

Exercise J

Abdominopelvic Regions

1. umbilical; 2. epigastric; 3. hypogastric; 4. hypochondriac; 5. lumbar; 6. iliac

Exercise K

Patient Positions

1. supine; 2. prone; 3. orthopnea; 4. Trendelenburg; 5. semiprone; 6. sitting; 7. lateral

Exercise L

Diagnostic Imaging

1. radiology; 2. tomography; 3. sonography; 4. magnetic resonance imaging; 5. nuclear medicine

Exercise M

Use Medical Terms in Clinical Statements

1. Underlined Terms: distal, lateral, anterior, medial, inferior, anterolateral, proximal, inferior, medial, anterosuperior, posterior, inferior, medial, dorsal, lateral 2. b; 3. a; 4. a; 5. AP; 6. lateral; sagittal; 7. nuclear medicine; 8. lumbar; 9. anterior; 10. coronal; axial; 11. orthopnea; 12. Trendelenburg; 13. Dorsal; 14. cephalic

Exercise N

Apply Medical Terms to the Case Study
Answers will vary and may include: distal, proximal, ventral, anterior, dorsal, posterior, umbilical region, iliac region(s), and lumbar region(s) along with their respective definitions.

Exercise O

Use Medical Terms in a Document

1. iliac; 2. lumbar; 3. distal; 4. medial; 5. lateral; 6. proximal; 7. tomography; 8. superolaterally; pertaining to above and to the side; 9. anteroposterior; pertaining to the front and to the back

Exercise P

Online Review of Lesson Content
Completed with online resources

Exercise Q

Lesson Content Quiz
1. c; 2. a; 3. b; 4. c; 5. b; 6. c; 7. a; 8. b; 9. b; 10. c; 11. a; 12. c

LESSON 3

Exercise A

Build and Translate Terms Built from Word Parts

1. **Label:** Figure 3.2, cutane/o; dermat/o; derm/o
2. **Match:** a. -logist, one who studies and treats (specialist, physician);

b. -logy, study of; c. path/o, disease; d. -itis, inflammation; e. -y, no meaning
3. **Translate:** a. dermat/o/logy, study of the skin; b. dermat/o/logist, physician who studies and treats diseases of the skin; c. dermat/o/path/y, (any) disease of the skin; d. dermat/itis, inflammation of the skin; e. dermat/o/path/o/logist, physician who (microscopically) studies diseases of the skin
4. **Reading Exercise**
5. **Label:** Figure 3.3, dermat/itis
6. **Match:** a. epi-, on, upon, over; b. hypo-, below, deficient, under; c. intra-, within; d. trans-, through, across, beyond; e. -al, -ic, pertaining to
7. **Build:** a. derm/al; b. epi/derm/al; c. intra/derm/al; d. trans/derm/al; e. hypo/derm/ic;
8. **Reading Exercise**
9. **Label:** Figure 3.4, trans/derm/al
10. **Match:** a. per-, through; b. -ous, pertaining to; c. -sub, below, under
11. **Translate:** a. cutane/ous, pertaining to the skin; b. sub/cutane/ous, pertaining to under the skin; c. per/cutane/ous, pertaining to through the skin
12. **Reading Exercise**
13. **Label:** Figure 3.5, hypo/derm/ic; sub/cutane/ous
14. **Label:** Figure 3.6, onych/o
15. **Match:** a. -osis; abnormal condition; b. -lysis; separation; c. myc/o; fungus
16. **Build:** a. onych/osis; b. onych/o/myc/osis; c. onych/o/lysis
17. **Reading Exercise**
18. **Label:** Figure 3.7, onych/o/myc/osis
19. **Term Table: Review of Integumentary System Terms Built from Word Parts**

Exercise B

Pronounce and Spell Terms Built from Word Parts

1. Check responses with the Term Table in Exercise A, #19
2. Check answers with online resources

Exercise C

Build and Translate MORE Terms Built from Word Parts

1. **Label:** Figure 3.8, A. erythr/o; B. xanth/o; C. melan/o; D. leuk/o; E. cyan/o
2. **Match:** a. derm/o, skin; b. -a, no meaning

Copyright © 2024 by Elsevier, Inc. All rights reserved.

3. **Translate:** a. leuk/o/derm/a, white skin; b. melan/o/derm/a, black skin; c. erythr/o/derm/a, red skin; d. xanth/o/derm/a, yellow skin
4. **Reading Exercise**
5. **Label:** Figure 3.9, A. leuk/o/derm/a; B. erythr/o/derm/a; C. xanth/o/derm/a
6. **Match:** a. -osis, abnormal condition; b. -oma, tumor; c. acr/o, extremities
7. **Build:** a. xanth/osis; b. cyan/osis; c. acr/o/cyan/osis; d. xanth/oma; e. melan/oma
8. **Reading Exercise**
9. **Label:** Figure 3.10, a. melan/oma; b. cyan/osis
10. **Match:** a. cyt/o, cell(s); b. -e, no meaning
11. **Translate:** a. leuk/o/cyt/e, white (blood) cell; b. erythr/o/cyt/e, red (blood) cell
12. **Reading Exercise**
13. **Label:** Figure 3.11, a. erythr/o/cyt/e(s); b. leuk/o/cyt/e(s)
14. **Term Table: Review of MORE Integumentary System Terms Built from Word Parts**

Exercise D

Pronounce and Spell MORE Terms Built from Word Parts
1. Check responses with the Term Table in Exercise C, #14
2. Check answers with online resources

Exercise E

Label
1. basal cell carcinoma; 2. squamous cell carcinoma; 3. pressure injury; 4. cellulitis; 5. herpes; 6. nevus; 7. impetigo; 8. laceration; 9. edema; 10. eczema

Exercise F

Match
1. b; 2. f; 3. d; 4. a; 5. e; 6. c

Exercise G

Learn Medical Terms NOT Built from Word Parts
1. Lesion; 2. Pressure injuries; 3. abscess; 4. Laceration; 5. Edema; 6. nevus; 7. basal cell carcinoma; squamous cell carcinoma; 8. herpes; 9. Impetigo; 10. cellulitis, erythema; 11. Pallor; 12. Jaundice; 13. Methicillin-resistant *Staphylococcus aureus*.; 14. Eczema

Exercise H

Pronounce and Spell Terms NOT Built from Word Parts
1. Check responses with the Table for Terms NOT Built from Word Parts
2. Check answers with online resources

Exercise I

Abbreviate Medical Terms
1. a. lac; b. SCC; c. BCC;
2. a. DERM; b. hypo; c. MRSA; d. WBC; e. RBC; f. TD; g. ID; h. subcut

Exercise J

Learn Plural Endings
1. thoraces; -aces; 2. appendices; -ices; 3. cervices; -ices; 4. diagnoses; -ses; 5. prognoses; -ses; 6. metastases; -ses; 7. pelves; -es; 8. testes; -es; 9. bronchi; -i; 10. nevi; -i; 11. streptococci; -i; 12. fungi; -i; 13. bacteria; -a; 14. ova; -a; 15. sarcomata; -mata; 16. fibromata; -mata; 17. pharynges; -nges; 18. larynges; -nges; 19. apices; -ices; 20. cortices; -ices; 21. ganglia; -a; 22. spermatozoa; -a; 23. pleurae; -ae; 24. sclerae; -ae; 25. bursae; -ae

Exercise K

Signs and Symptoms
1. edema; 2. lesion; 3. pallor; 4. jaundice; 5. erythema; 6. acrocyanosis; 7. cyanosis; 8. melanoderma; 9. leukoderma; 10. xanthoderma; 11. erythroderma; 12. xanthosis

Exercise L

Diseases and Disorders
1. abscess; 2. cellulitis; 3. pressure injury; 4. laceration; 5. onychosis; 6. dermatopathy; 7. dermatitis; 8. eczema; 9. onychomycosis; 10. impetigo; 11. herpes; 12. xanthoma; 13. melanoma; 14. squamous cell carcinoma; 15. basal cell carcinoma; 16. methicillin-resistant *Staphylococcus aureus*; 17. onycholysis; 18. nevus

Exercise M

Specialties and Professions
1. dermatology; 2. dermatologist; 3. dermatopathologist

Exercise N

Medical Terms Related to the Integumentary System and Colors
1. erythrocyte; 2. leukocyte; 3. a. cutaneous; b. dermal; 4. epidermal; 5. intradermal; 6. a. hypodermic;

b. subcutaneous; 7. a. percutaneous; b. transdermal

Exercise O

Use Medical Terms in Clinical Statements
1. pressure injury, erythema; 2. lesions, impetigo; 3. erythroderma, dermatologist, dermatitis; 4. onychomycosis; 5. intradermal; 6. melanoma, metastasis, hypodermic, subcutaneous; 7. basal cell carcinoma, squamous cell carcinoma; 8. MRSA, cellulitis, abscess; 9. a. metastases; b. emboli; c. ovum; d. testes; e. lipomata

Exercise P

Apply Medical Terms to Case Study
Answers will vary and may include lesion, nevus, melanoma, biopsy, basal cell carcinoma, squamous cell carcinoma, and dermatologist along with their respective definitions.

Exercise Q

Use Medical Terms in a Document
1. pathology; 2. melanoma; 3. basal cell carcinoma; 4. nevus; 5. biopsy; 6. proximal; 7. epidermal; 8. anterior; 9. benign; 10. dermatopathologist; 11. b; 12. a. melanoma, S; b. melanomata, P; c. nevi, P; d. nevus, S; e. metastasis, S; f. metastases, P; g. biopsy, S; h. biopsies, P; 13. Research exercise; answers vary.

Exercise R

Online Review of Lesson Content
Completed with online resources

Exercise S

Lesson Content Quiz
1. b; 2. c; 3. a; 4. c; 5. a; 6. b; 7. c; 8. a; 9. b; 10. b; 11. a; 12. b; 13. b; 14. a

LESSON 4

Exercise A

Build and Translate Terms Built from Word Parts
1. **Match:** a. -rrhea, flow, discharge; b. -rrhagia, excessive bleeding; c. -itis, inflammation
2. **Label:** Figure 4.3, (1) sinus/o; (2) nas/o, rhin/o; (3) laryng/o; (4) pharyng/o

Copyright © 2024 by Elsevier, Inc. All rights reserved.

3. **Build:** a. rhin/itis; b. rhin/o/rrhea; c. rhin/o/rrhagia
4. **Reading Exercise**
5. **Match:** a. -tomy, cut into, incision; b. -al, -ous, pertaining to; c. muc/o, mucus; d. -itis, inflammation;
6. **Translate:** a. nas/al, pertaining to the nose; b. muc/ous, pertaining to mucus; c. sinus/itis, inflammation of the sinus (membranes); d. sinus/o/tomy, incision of a sinus
7. **Reading Exercise**
8. **Label:** Figure 4.4, sinus/itis
9. **Match:** a. -itis, inflammation; b. -eal, pertaining to; c. -ectomy, surgical removal, excision; d. -scope, instrument used for visual examination; e. -scopy, visual examination
10. **Build:** a. pharyng/itis; b. nas/o/pharyng/itis; c. laryng/itis
11. **Reading Exercise**
12. **Build:** a. pharyng/eal; b. laryng/eal
13. **Translate:** a. laryng/o/scope, instrument used for visual examination of the larynx; b. laryng/o/scopy, visual examination of the larynx; c. laryng/ectomy, excision of the larynx
14. **Reading Exercise**
15. **Match:** a. a-, an-, absence of, without; b. dys-, difficult, painful, abnormal; c. hyper-, above, excessive; d. hypo-, below, deficient, under; e. -pnea, breathing
16. **Translate:** a. a/pnea, absence of breathing; b. dys/pnea, difficult breathing; c. hypo/pnea, deficient breathing; d. hyper/pnea, excessive breathing
17. **Reading Exercise**
18. **Match:** a. -ia, condition of; b. -meter, instrument used to measure; c. hyper-, above, excessive; d. hypo-, below, deficient, under; e. capn/o, carbon dioxide; f. ox/i, oxygen; g. spir/o, breathing
19. **Build:** a. hyper/ox/ia; b. hyper/capn/ia; c. hypo/capn/ia; d. hyp/ox/ia [the **o** from the prefix **hypo-** has been dropped]
20. **Reading Exercise**
21. **Translate:** a. capn/o/meter, instrument used to measure carbon dioxide; b. ox/i/meter, instrument used to measure oxygen; c. spir/o/meter, instrument used to measure breathing

22. **Reading Exercise**
23. **Label:** Figure 4.5, A. pulse ox/i/meter; B. capn/o/meter; C. spir/o/meter
24. **Term Table: Review of Respiratory System Terms Built from Word Parts**

Exercise B
Pronounce and Spell Terms Built from Word Parts
1. Check responses with the Term Table in Exercise A, #24
2. Check answers with online resources

Exercise C
Build and Translate MORE Medical Terms Built from Word Parts
1. **Label:** Figure 4.6, (1) trache/o; (2) bronch/o; (3) pneum/o, pneumon/o, pulmon/o; (4) thorac/o, -thorax
2. **Match:** a. -stomy, creation of an artificial opening; b. -tomy, cut into, incision; c. endo-, within; d. -al, pertaining to; e. -scope, instrument used for visual examination
3. **Translate:** a. trache/o/tomy, incision of the trachea; b. trache/o/stomy, creation of an artificial opening into the trachea; c. endo/trache/al, pertaining to within the trachea
4. **Reading Exercise**
5. **Label:** Figure 4.7, endo/trache/al, laryng/o/scope
6. **Reading Exercise**
7. **Label** Figure 4.8, trache/o/stomy
8. **Match:** a. -scope, instrument used for visual examination; b. -scopy, visual examination; c. -itis, inflammation
9. **Build:** a. bronch/itis; b. bronch/o/scope; c. bronch/o/scopy
10. **Reading Exercise**
11. **Label:** Figure 4.9, bronch/o/scopy
12. **Match:** a. -ia, diseased state, condition of; b. -ectomy, surgical removal, excision; c. -ary, pertaining to; d. -logy, study of; e. -logist, one who studies and treats (specialist, physician)
13. **Translate:** a. pulmon/ary, pertaining to the lung; b. pulmon/o/logy, study of the lung; c. pulmon/o/logist, physician who studies and treats diseases of the lung
14. **Reading Exercise**
15. **Build:** a. pneumon/ia; b. bronch/o/pneumon/ia; c. pneumon/ectomy
16. **Reading Exercise**

17. **Match:** a. -tomy, cut into, incision; b. -centesis, surgical puncture to remove fluid (with a sterile needle); c. -thorax, thorac/o; chest, chest cavity; d. pneum/o, lung, air
18. **Build:** a. pneum/o/thorax; b. thorac/o/tomy; c. thora/centesis
19. **Label:** Figure 4.10, pneum/o/thorax
20. **Reading Exercise**
21. **Label:** Figure 4.11, thora/centesis
22. **Match:** a. thorac/o, chest, chest cavity; b. endo-, within; c. -scope, instrument used for visual examination; d. -scopy, visual examination; e. -scopic, pertaining to visual examination; f. -ic, pertaining to
23. **Translate:** a. endo/scope, instrument used for visual examination within (a hollow organ or body cavity); b. endo/scopic, pertaining to visual examination within (a hollow organ or body cavity); c. endo/scopy, visual examination within (a hollow organ or body cavity)
24. **Reading Exercise**
25. **Build:** a. thorac/ic; b. thorac/o/scopy; c. thorac/o/scope; d. thorac/o/scopic
26. **Reading Exercise**
27. **Label:** Figure 4.12, thorac/o/scopic
28. **Match:** a. -graphy, process of recording; b. -gram, record; c. poly-, many; d. somn/o, sleep
29. **Translate:** a. poly/somn/o/graphy, process of recording many sleep (tests); b. poly/somn/o/gram, record of many sleep (tests)
30. **Reading Exercise**
31. **Label:** Figure 4.13, A. poly/somn/o/graphy; B. poly/somn/o/gram
32. **Term Table: Review of MORE Terms Built from Word Parts**

Exercise D
Pronounce and Spell MORE Terms Built from Word Parts
1. Check responses with the Term Table in Exercise C, #32
2. Check answers with the online resources

Exercise E
Match
1. e; 2. d; 3. f; 4. a; 5. b; 6. c

Exercise F
Label
1. computed tomography; 2. radiograph; 3. obstructive sleep apnea;

Copyright © 2024 by Elsevier, Inc. All rights reserved.

4. emphysema; 5. upper respiratory infection; 6. culture and sensitivity

Exercise G

Learn Medical Terms NOT Built from Word Parts

1. chronic obstructive pulmonary disease; radiograph; 2. asthma; 3. upper respiratory infection; influenza; 4. tuberculosis; sputum; culture and sensitivity; 5. emphysema; 6. computed tomography; 7. obstructive sleep apnea; OSA; 8. coronavirus disease

Exercise H

Pronounce and Spell Medical NOT Terms Built from Word Parts

1. Check responses with the Table for Terms NOT Built from Word Parts
2. Check answers with online resources

Exercise I

Abbreviate Medical Terms

1. Signs and Symptoms
   SOB
2. Diseases and Disorders
   a. TB; b. COPD; c. flu; d. URI; e. OSA; f. COVID-19
3. Diagnostic Tests and Equipment
   a. C&S; b. CT; c. CXR; d. V/Q scan; e. PSG; f. PFTs; g. ABG
4. Professions
   RT
5. Medical Record Abbreviations
   a. VS; b. T; c. P; d. R; e. BP; f. SOAP
6. Related Terms
   a. CPAP; b. CO_2; c. ET; d. O_2

Exercise J

Signs and Symptoms

1. apnea; 2. dyspnea; 3. hyperpnea; 4. hypopnea; 5. hyperoxia; 6. hypoxia; 7. hypocapnia; 8. hypercapnia; 9. rhinorrhea; 10. rhinorrhagia

Exercise K

Diseases and Disorders

1. sinusitis; 2. laryngitis; 3. pharyngitis; 4. nasopharyngitis; 5. upper respiratory infection; 6. rhinitis; 7. influenza; 8. tuberculosis; 9. pneumothorax; 10. pneumonia; 11. bronchopneumonia; 12. bronchitis; 13. emphysema; 14. chronic obstructive pulmonary

disease; 15. obstructive sleep apnea; 16. asthma; 17. coronavirus disease

Exercise L

Diagnostic Tests and Equipment

1. capnometer; 2. oximeter; 3. spirometer; 4. endoscopic; 5. thoracoscopy; 6. laryngoscopy; 7. bronchoscopy; 8. endoscope; 9. laryngoscope; 10. bronchoscope; 11. thoracoscope; 12. endoscopy; 13. thoracoscopic; 14. radiograph; 15. computed tomography; 16. culture and sensitivity; 17. polysomnography; 18. polysomnogram

Exercise M

Surgical Procedures

1. thoracentesis; 2. thoracotomy; 3. sinusotomy; 4. tracheotomy; 5. tracheostomy; 6. laryngectomy; 7. pneumonectomy

Exercise N

Specialties and Professions

1. pulmonology; 2. pulmonologist

Exercise O

Medical Terms Related to the Respiratory System

1. thoracic; 2. pulmonary; 3. nasal; 4. laryngeal; 5. pharyngeal; 6. endotracheal; 7. mucous; 8. sputum

Exercise P

Use Medical Terms in Clinical Statements

1. hypopnea; apnea; acrocyanosis
2. bronchoscopy; carcinoma; metastasis; thoracentesis; pneumonectomy
3. dyspnea; pneumothorax; thoracotomy
4. Sinusitis; rhinitis; rhinorrhea; Endoscopic; 5. radiograph; tuberculosis; pneumonia; COPD; pulmonary;
6. oximeter; radiograph; computed tomography; emphysema; Hypercapnia
7. ABG; O_2; CO_2; SOB; 8. V/Q scan; pulmonary; 9. polysomnography; polysomnogram, pulmonologist;
10. OSA; CPAP

Exercise Q

Apply Medical Terms to Case Study

Answers will vary and may include dyspnea, pharyngitis, rhinorrhea, upper

respiratory infection, and/or sputum along with their respective definitions.

Exercise R

Use Medical Language in Documents

1. dyspnea; 2. sputum; 3. rhinorrhea; 4. nasal; 5. edema; 6. cyanosis; 7. radiographs; 8. pneumonia; 9. upper respiratory infection; 10. T: 101.2° F; P: 80/min; R: 14/min; BP:130/74 mm Hg; 11. mucous; resembling; 12. oximeter; radiographs; 13. posteroanterior; back to the front; 14. Research exercise; answers vary.

Exercise S

Use Medical Language in Online Electronic Health Records

Completed with online resources.

Exercise T

Online Review of Lesson Content

Completed with online resources.

Exercise U

Lesson Content Quiz

1. b; 2. a; 3. a; 4. a; 5. b; 6. c; 7. b; 8. a; 9. c; 10. a; 11. b; 12. c; 13. c; 14. a

LESSON 5

Exercise A

Build and Translate Medical Terms Built from Word Parts

1. **Label:** Figure 5.3, (1) cyst/o; (2) urethr/o
2. **Match:** a. -gram; record, radiographic image; b. -graphy; process of recording, radiographic imaging; c. -itis; inflammation; d. -iasis; condition; e. lith/o; stone(s), calculus (*pl.* calculi)
3. **Build:** a. cyst/itis; b. cyst/o/graphy; c. cyst/o/gram; d. cyst/o/lith/iasis
4. **Reading exercise**
5. **Label:** Figure 5.4, A. cyst/o/gram; B. cyst/o/lith/iasis
6. **Match:** a. -stomy; creation of an artificial opening; b. -scope; instrument used for visual examination; c. -scopy; visual examination; d. -tomy; cut into, incision; e. -plasty; surgical repair; f. lith/o; stone(s), calculus (*pl.* calculi)
7. **Translate:** a. cyst/o/stomy; creation of an artificial opening into the bladder; b. cyst/o/scope; instrument

Copyright © 2024 by Elsevier, Inc. All rights reserved.

used for visual examination of the bladder; c. cyst/o/scopy; visual examination of the bladder; d. cyst/o/lith/o/tomy; incision into the bladder to remove stone(s)

8. **Reading Exercise**
9. **Build:** a. urethr/o/scope; b. urethr/o/cyst/itis; c. cyst/o/urethr/o/graphy; d. urethr/o/plasty
10. **Reading Exercise**
11. **Label:** Figure 5.5, cyst/o/urethr/o/graphy
12. **Match:** a. ur/o; urine, urination, urinary tract; b. hem/o, hemat/o; blood; c. py/o; pus; d. dys-; difficult, painful, abnormal; e. -ia; diseased state, condition of
13. **Translate:** a. hemat/ur/ia; condition of blood in the urine; b. py/ur/ia; condition of pus in the urine; c. dys/ur/ia; condition of difficult or painful urination
14. **Reading Exercise**
15. **Match:** a. a-, an-; absence of, without; b. noct/i; night; c. olig/o; few, scanty; d. -emia; in the blood; e. ur/o; urine, urination, urinary tract
16. **Build:** a. an/ur/ia; b. noct/ur/ia; c. olig/ur/ia; d. ur/emia
17. **Reading Exercise**
18. **Label:** Figure 5.6, (1) nephr/o, ren/o; (2) pyel/o
19. **Match:** a. lith/o; stone(s), calculus (*pl.* calculi); b. -tripsy; surgical crushing; c. -iasis; condition
20. **Translate:** a. lith/o/tripsy; surgical crushing of stone(s); b. nephr/o/lith/iasis; condition of stone(s) in the kidney; c. pyel/o/lith/o/tomy; incision into the renal pelvis to remove stone(s)
21. **Reading Exercise**
22. **Label:** Figure 5.7, pyel/o/lith/o/tomy
23. **Term Table: Review of Urinary System Terms Built from Word Parts**

Exercise B

Pronounce and Spell Terms Built from Word Parts

1. Check responses with the Term Table in Exercise A, #23
2. Check answers with online resources

Exercise C

Build and Translate MORE Medical Terms Built from Word Parts

1. **Label:** Figure 5.8, 1. ureter/o; 2. meat/o
2. **Match:** a. -itis; inflammation; b. -osis; abnormal condition; c. -al; pertaining to; d. hydr/o; water

3. **Translate:** a. nephr/itis; inflammation of the kidney; b. ren/al; pertaining to kidney; c. hydr/o/nephr/osis; abnormal condition of water (urine) in the kidney; d. pyel/o/nephr/itis; inflammation of the renal pelvis and kidney
4. **Reading Exercise**
5. **Label:** Figure 5.9, pyel/o/nephr/itis
6. **Reading Exercise**
7. **Label:** Figure 5.10, hydr/o/nephr/osis
8. **Match:** a. pyel/o; renal pelvis; b. -ectomy; surgical removal, excision; c. -stomy; creation of an artificial opening; d. -tomy; cut into, incision
9. **Build:** a. nephr/ectomy; b. nephr/o/stomy; c. nephr/o/tomy
10. **Reading Exercise**
11. **Label:** Figure 5.11, nephr/o/stomy
12. **Match:** a. -itis; inflammation; b. -tomy; cut into, incision; c. -iasis; condition; d. -plasty; surgical repair; e. lith/o; stone(s), calculus (*pl.* calculi)
13. **Translate:** a. ureter/o/lith/iasis; condition of stone(s) in the ureter; b. ureter/o/pyel/o/nephr/itis; inflammation of the ureter, renal pelvis, and kidney; c. ureter/o/lith/o/tomy; incision into the ureter to remove stone(s)
14. **Reading Exercise**
15. **Build:** a. ureter/ectomy; b. ureter/o/plasty
16. **Reading Exercise**
17. **Label:** Figure 5.12, ureter/o/plasty
18. **Match:** a. -al; pertaining to; b. -scopy; visual examination; c. -tomy; cut into, incision
19. **Translate:** a. meat/al; pertaining to the meatus; b. meat/o/scopy; visual examination of the meatus; c. meat/o/tomy; incision into the meatus (to enlarge it)
20. **Reading Exercise**
21. **Match:** a. -gram; record, radiographic image; b. -logist; one who studies and treats (specialist, physician); c. -logy; study of; d. -stomy; creation of an artificial opening
22. **Build:** a. ur/o/gram; b. ur/o/logist; c. ur/o/logy; d. ur/o/stomy
23. **Reading Exercise**
24. **Label:** Figure 5.13, ur/o/gram
25. **Translate:** a. nephr/o/logist; physician who studies and treats diseases of the kidney; b. nephr/o/logy; study of the kidney
26. **Reading Exercise**

27. **Term Table: Review of MORE Urinary System Terms Built from Word Parts**

Exercise D

Pronounce and Spell Terms MORE Built from Word Parts

1. Check responses with the Term Table in Exercise C, #27
2. Check answers with the online resources

Exercise E

Label

1. urinary catheterization;
2. extracorporeal shock wave lithotripsy;
3. dialysis; 4. renal calculi; 5. urinalysis;
6. renal transplant

Exercise F

Match

1. d; 2. b; 3. a; 4. e; 5. c

Exercise G

Learn Medical Terms NOT Built from Word Parts

1. incontinence; void; urinary tract infection; urinalysis; urinary catheterization
2. chronic kidney disease; renal failure
3. dialysis; renal transplant
4. renal calculi; extracorporeal shock wave lithotripsy

Exercise H

Pronounce and Spell Medical Terms NOT Built from Word Parts

1. Check responses with the Table for Terms NOT Built from Word Parts
2. Check answers with the online resources

Exercise I

Write abbreviations

1. Diseases and Disorders: a. CKD; b. UTI; c. PKD; d. OAB
2. Diagnostic Tests: a. UA; b. VCUG
3. Surgical Procdures: a. ESWL; b. HD
4. Specialties and Professions: PCT
5. Related Term: cath

Exercise J

Signs and Symptoms

1. anuria; 2. dysuria; 3. hematuria;
4. nocturia; 5. oliguria; 6. pyuria;
7. incontinence

Copyright © 2024 by Elsevier, Inc. All rights reserved.

Exercise K

Diseases and Disorders

1. cystitis; 2. cystolithiasis;
3. hydronephrosis; 4. nephrolithiasis
(or renal calculi); 5. nephritis;
6. pyelonephritis; 7. urethrocystitis;
8. renal calculi (or nephrolithiasis);
9. renal failure; 10. urinary tract infection;
11. uremia; 12. ureterolithiasis;
13. ureteropyelonephritis;
14. chronic kidney disease

Exercise L

Diagnostic Tests and Equipment

1. cystogram; 2. cystography;
3. cystoscope; 4. cystoscopy;
5. cystourethrography; 6. meatoscopy;
7. urethroscope; 8. urinalysis;
9. urogram

Exercise M

Surgical Procedures

1. cystolithotomy; 2. cystostomy;
3. extracorporeal shock wave lithotripsy;
4. lithotripsy; 5. meatotomy;
6. nephrectomy; 7. ureteroplasty;
8. nephrostomy; 9. nephrotomy;
10. pyelolithotomy; 11. renal transplant;
12. ureterectomy; 13. urostomy;
14. ureterolithotomy;
15. urethroplasty

Exercise N

Specialties and Professions

1. nephrology; 2. nephrologist;
3. urology; 4. urologist

Exercise O

Medical Terms Related to the Urinary System

1. meatal; 2. renal; 3. dialysis;
4. urinary catheterization; 5. void

Exercise P

Use Medical Terms in Clinical Statements

1. nephrectomy; renal; nephritis
2. dysuria; hematuria; urinalysis; pyuria; cystitis
3. urethrocystitis; urogram; cystourethrography
4. Lithotripsy; ureterolithiasis
5. incontinence; urologist; urethroplasty
6. cystourethrography; urinary tract infection
7. nephrologist; CKD (chronic kidney disease); dialysis; ureterolithotomy

Exercise Q

Apply Medical Terms to the Case Study

Answers will vary and may include hematuria, urinary tract infection, dysuria, nephrolithiasis and/or renal calculi along with their respective definitions.

Exercise R

Use Medical Terms in a Document

1. hematuria; 2. nephrolithiasis or renal calculi; 3. urinary tract infection; 4. renal;
5. dialysis; 6. urinalysis; 7. pyuria
8. ureterolithiasis; 9. hydronephrosis
10. urine, urination, urinary tract; diseased state, condition of; blood; condition of blood in the urine
11. may include pyuria, nocturia, oliguria, anuria, dysuria
12. chronic kidney disease
13. pertaining to away; ureter (Away means far from the kidney in this case)
14. Dictionary and use of online resources exercise; answers vary

Exercise S

Interpret Language Used in a Medical Record

1. a; 2. b; 3. a; 4. b; 5. answers vary

Exercise T

Use Medical Language in Electronic Health Records Online

Completed with online resources.

Exercise U

Online Review of Lesson Content

Completed with online resources.

Exercise V

Lesson Content Quiz

1. b; 2. a; 3. c; 4. a; 5. c; 6. b; 7. a;
8. b; 9. c; 10. b; 11. a; 12. c

LESSON 6

Exercise A

Build and Translate Terms Built from Word Parts

1. **Label:** Figure 6.2, A. (1) oophor/o, (2) salping/o, (3) endometri/o, (4) cervic/o
   B. (1) colp/o, vagin/o; (2) hyster/o
2. **Match:** a. -al, pertaining to; b. -itis, inflammation; c. -osis, abnormal condition

3. **Build:** a. vagin/itis; b. salping/itis; c. oophor/itis; d. cervic/itis
4. **Translate:** a. vagin/al, pertaining to the vagina; b. cervic/al, pertaining to the cervix; c. endometri/al, pertaining to the endometrium; d. endometr/itis, inflammation of the endometrium; e. endometri/osis, abnormal condition of the endometrium (growth of endometrial tissue outside of the uterus)
5. **Reading exercise**
6. **Label:** Figure 6.3, (1) endometr/itis, (2) cervic/itis, (3) vagin/itis, (4) salping/itis
7. **Reading exercise**
8. **Label:** Figure 6.4, endometri/osis
9. **Match:** a. -logy, study of; b. -logist, one who studies and treats (physician, specialist); c. -scope, instrument used for visual examination; d. -scopy, visual examination; e. gynec/o, woman (women)
10. **Build:** a. colp/o/scope; b. colp/o/scopy; c. gynec/o/logy; d. gynec/o/logist
11. **Reading exercise**
12. **Match:** a. -cele, hernia, protrusion; b. -pexy, surgical fixation
13. **Translate:** a. cyst/o/cele, protrusion of the (urinary) bladder (through anterior vaginal wall); b. hyster/o/pexy, surgical fixation of the uterus
14. **Reading exercise**
15. **Label:** Figure 6.5, cyst/o/cele
16. **Match:** a. -gram, record, radiographic image; b. -pexy, surgical fixation; c. -ectomy, surgical removal, excision; d. -rrhexis, rupture; e. -rrhaphy, suturing, repairing
17. **Build:** a. hyster/ectomy; b. oophor/o/pexy; c. hyster/o/rrhexis; d. hyster/o/rrhaphy
18. **Reading exercise**
19. **Translate:** a. cervic/ectomy, excision of the cervix; b. oophor/ectomy, excision of the ovary; c. hyster/o/salping/o/-oophor/ectomy, excision of the uterus, fallopian tube(s), and ovaries; d. hyster/o/salping/o/gram, radiographic image of the uterus and fallopian tubes
20. **Reading exercise**
21. **Label:** Figure 6.6, hyster/o/salping/o/gram
22. **Reading exercise**
23. **Label:** Figure 6.7, A. hyster/ectomy; B. oophor/ectomy; C. hyster/o/salping/o/-oophor/ectomy

Copyright © 2024 by Elsevier, Inc. All rights reserved.

24. **Match:** a. a-, without, absence of; b. dys-, difficult, painful, abnormal; c. men/o, menstruation, menstrual; d. -rrhea, flow, discharge; e. -rrhagia, excessive bleeding
25. **Translate:** a. a/men/o/rrhea, without menstrual flow; b. dys/men/o/rrhea, painful menstrual flow; c. men/o/rrhea, flow at menstruation; d. men/o/rrhagia, excessive bleeding at menstruation
26. **Reading exercise**
27. **Match:** a. -gram, record, radiographic image; b. -graphy, process of recording, radiographic imaging; c. -plasty, surgical repair; d. -ectomy, surgical removal, excision; e. mamm/o, mast/o, breast; f. -pexy, surgical fixation
28. **Build:** a. mast/ectomy; b. mast/o/pexy; c. mamm/o/gram; d. mamm/o/graphy; e. mamm/o/plasty
29. **Reading exercise**
30. **Label:** Figure 6.8, A. mamm/o/graphy; B. mamm/o/gram
31. **Review of Female Reproductive System Terms Built from Word Parts**

Exercise B

Pronounce and Spell Terms Built from Word Parts

1. Check responses with the Term Table in Exercise A, #31
2. Check answers with the online resources

Exercise C

Build and Translate MORE Medical Terms Built from Word Parts

1. **Label:** Figure 6.9, 1. prostat/o, 2. scrot/o, 3. orchi/o
2. **Match:** a. cyst/o, bladder, sac; b. lith/o, stone(s), calculus (*pl.* calculi); c. -itis, inflammation; d. -ectomy, surgical removal, excision; e. -ic, pertaining to
3. **Translate:** a. prostat/itis, inflammation of the prostate gland; b. prostat/o/cyst/itis, inflammation of the prostate gland and the (urinary) bladder; c. prostat/ic, pertaining to the prostate gland; d. prostat/o/lith, stone(s) in the prostate gland; e. prostat/ectomy, excision of the prostate gland
4. **Reading exercise**
5. **Label:** Figure 6.10, prostat/ic

6. **Match:** a. -itis, inflammation; b. -ectomy, surgical removal, excision; c. -pexy, surgical fixation; d. -al, pertaining to; e. -plasty, surgical repair
7. **Build:** a. orch/itis [the i from the combining form orchi/o has been dropped], b. orchi/o/pexy, c. orchi/ectomy; d. scrot/al; e. scrot/o/plasty
8. **Reading Exercise**
9. **Match:** a. vas/o, vessel, duct; b. -ectomy, surgical removal, excision; c. -stomy, creation of an artificial opening
10. **Translate:** a. vas/ectomy, excision of the duct (vas deferens); b. creation of an artificial opening between ducts
11. **Reading Exercise**
12. **Label:** 6.11, vas/ectomy
13. **Review of Male Reproductive System Terms Built from Word Parts**

Exercise D

Pronounce and Spell MORE Terms Built from Word Parts

1. Check responses with the Term Table in Exercise C, #13
2. Check answers with the online resources

Exercise E

Label

1. Pap test; 2. dilation and curettage; 3. uterine fibroid; 4. uterovaginal prolapse; 5. pelvic inflammatory disease; 6. obstetrics; 7. transurethral resection of the prostate gland; 8. circumcision; 9. benign prostatic hyperplasia

Exercise F

Match

1. d; 2. c; 3. e; 4. a; 5. b

Exercise G

Learn Medical Terms NOT Built from Word Parts

1. Pap test; 2. sexually transmitted infection; 3. uterine fibroids; 4. pelvic inflammatory disease; 5. dilation and curettage; 6. prostate-specific antigen assay; digital rectal examination; 7. benign prostatic hyperplasia; transurethral resection of the prostate gland; 8. erectile dysfunction;

9. circumcision; 10. semen analysis; 11. obstetrics; 12. uterovaginal prolapse

Exercise H

Pronounce and Spell Terms NOT Built from Word Parts

1. Check responses with the Table for Terms NOT Built from Word Parts
2. Check answers with the online resources.

Exercise I

Abbreviate Medical Terms

1. Diseases and Disorders: a. STI; b. STD; c. PID; d. BPH; e. HPV; f. ED
2. Diagnostic Tests: a. DRE; b. PSA; c. HSG; d. TRUS
3. Surgical Procedures: a. D&C; b. TURP; c. TAH/BSO; d. RP
4. Specialties and Professions: a. OB/GYN
5. Related Terms: Cx

Exercise J

Signs and Symptoms

1. menorrhagia; 2. amenorrhea; 3. dysmenorrhea

Exercise K

Diseases and Disorders

1. benign prostatic hyperplasia; 2. erectile dysfunction; 3. sexually transmitted infection; 4. cervicitis; 5. cystocele; 6. endometritis; 7. endometriosis; 8. uterovaginal prolapse; 9. mastitis; 10. oophoritis; 11. salpingitis; 12. vaginitis; 13. orchitis; 14. prostatitis; 15. prostatocystitis; 16. prostatolith; 17. pelvic inflammatory disease; 18. uterine fibroid

Exercise L

Surgical Procedures

1. orchiectomy; 2. orchiopexy; 3. prostatectomy; 4. scrotoplasty; 5. vasectomy; 6. vasovasostomy; 7. cervicectomy; 8. hysterectomy; 9. hysteropexy; 10. hysterorrhaphy; 11. hysterorrhexis; 12. hysterosalpingo-oophorectomy; 13. mammoplasty; 14. mastectomy; 15. oophorectomy; 16. oophoropexy; 17. transurethral resection of the prostate gland; 18. dilation and curettage; 19. mastopexy

Copyright © 2024 by Elsevier, Inc. All rights reserved.

Exercise M

Diagnostic Tests and Equipment
1. colposcope; 2. colposcopy;
3. hysterosalpingogram; 4. mammogram;
5. mammography; 6. Pap test;
7. digital rectal examination; 8. prostate-specific antigen assay; 9. semen analysis

Exercise N

Specialties and Professions
1. gynecology; 2. gynecologist;
3. obstetrics

Exercise O

Medical Terms Related to the Reproductive Systems
1. menorrhea; 2. vaginal; 3. cervical;
4. endometrial; 5. scrotal; 6. prostatic

Exercise P

Use Medical Terms in Clinical Statements
1. colposcopy; Pap test
2. vaginal; vaginitis
3. mammography; mammogram; mastectomy; mammoplasty
4. BPH; prostatitis; prostatic; prostatectomy
5. scrotal; orchiectomy, orchiopexy

Exercise Q

Apply Medical Terms to Case Study
Answers will vary, and may include menorrhea, dysmenorrhea, menorrhagia, sexually transmitted infection, orchiopexy, and corresponding definitions.

Exercise R

Use Medical Terms in a Document
1. orchiopexy; 2. menorrhea;
3. dysmenorrhea; 4. menorrhagia;
5. Pap test; 6. prostatitis; 7. sexually transmitted infections; 8. cervicitis;
9. pelvic inflammatory disease
10. semen analysis
11. hysterosalpingogram
12. scrot/o, scrotum; -cele, hernia, protrusion; scrotocele, hernia of the scrotum
13. DRE, digital rectal examination; BPH, benign prostatic hyperplasia
14. Dictionary exercise; answers will vary

Exercise S

Use Medical Language in Electronic Health Records Online
Completed with online resources.

Exercise T

Online Review of Lesson Content
Completed with online resources.

Exercise U

Lesson Content Quiz
1. b; 2. a; 3. c; 4. a; 5. a; 6. c; 7. b;
8. a; 9. b; 10. c; 11. b; 12. a

LESSON 7

Exercise A

Build and Translate Medical Terms Built from Word Parts
1. **Label:** Figure 7.5, (1) arteri/o;
(2) cardi/o; (3) angi/o
2. **Match:** a. -logist; one who studies and treats (specialist, physician);
b. -logy; study of; c. -ac; pertaining to; d. -megaly; enlargement
3. **Build:** a. cardi/ac; b. cardi/o/logy;
c. cardi/o/logist; d. cardi/o/megaly
4. **Reading Exercise**
5. **Match:** a. -gram; record, radiographic image; b. -graph; instrument used to record; c. -graphy; process of recording, radiographic imaging
6. **Translate:** a. electr/o/cardi/o/gram, record of the electrical activity of the heart; b. electr/o/cardi/o/graph, instrument used to record the electrical activity of the heart;
c. electr/o/cardi/o/graphy, process of recording the electrical activity of the heart
7. **Reading Exercise**
8. **Label:** Figure 7.6, electr/o/cardi/o/gram
9. **Match:** a. my/o; muscle; b. ech/o; sound; c. tachy-; rapid, fast;
d. brady-; slow; e. -pnea; breathing;
f. path/o; disease; g. -a, -y; no meaning
10. **Build:** a. ech/o/cardi/o/gram;
b. brady/cardi/a;
c. cardi/o/my/o/path/y
11. **Reading Exercise**
12. **Label:** Figure 7.7, ech/o/cardi/o/gram
13. **Translate:** a. my/o/cardi/al, pertaining to the muscle of the heart;
b. tachy/cardi/a, rapid heart rate;
c. tachy/pnea, rapid breathing
14. **Reading Exercise**

15. **Match:** a. -ectomy; surgical removal, excision; b. -al; pertaining to; c. -gram; record, radiographic image;
d. -sclerosis; hardening; e. endo-; within
16. **Build:** a. end/arter/ectomy [the o from the prefix endo- has been dropped];
b. arteri/al; c. arteri/o/sclerosis;
d. arteri/o/gram
17. **Reading Exercise**
18. **Label:** Figure 7.8, arteri/o/gram;
Figure 7.9, end/arter/ectomy [the o from the prefix endo- has been dropped]
19. **Match:** a. -graphy; process of recording, radiographic imaging;
b. -plasty; surgical repair
20. **Translate:** a. angi/o/graphy, radiographic imaging of the blood vessels; b. angi/o/plasty, surgical repair of the blood vessels
21. **Reading Exercise**
22. **Label:** Figure 7.10, angi/o/plasty
23. **Term Table: Review of Cardiovascular and Lymphatic System Terms Built from Word Parts**

Exercise B

Pronounce and Spell Terms Built from Word Parts
1. Check responses with the Term Table in Exercise A, #23
2. Check answers with online resources

Exercise C

Build and Translate MORE Medical Terms Built from Word Parts
1. **Label:** Figure 7.11, phleb/o, ven/o
2. **Match:** a. -ous; pertaining to;
b. -gram; record, radiographic image;
c. -intra; within
3. **Build:** a. intra/ven/ous; b. ven/o/gram
4. **Reading Exercise**
5. **Label:** Figure 7.12 A. ven/o/gram;
B. intra/ven/ous
6. **Match:** a. -itis; inflammation;
b. -tomy; cut into, incision;
c. thromb/o; blood clot;
d. -osis; abnormal condition
7. **Translate:** a. phleb/itis, inflammation of the veins; b. phleb/o/tomy, incision into the vein (with a needle to remove or instill fluid); c. thromb/osis, abnormal condition of a blood clot;
d. thromb/o/phlebitis, inflammation of the veins associated with blood clots
8. **Reading Exercise**

Copyright © 2024 by Elsevier, Inc. All rights reserved.

9. **Label:** Figure 7.13, thromb/osis
10. **Match:** a. cyt/o; cell; b. -e; no meaning; c. -penia; abnormal reduction (in number); d. leuk/o; white; e. thromb/o; blood clot
11. **Translate:** a. thromb/o/cyt/e, blood clotting cell; b. thromb/o/cyt/o/penia, abnormal reduction of blood clotting cells; c. leuk/o/cyt/o/penia, abnormal reduction of white blood cells
12. **Reading Exercise**
13. **Label:** Figure 7.14, (1) lymph/o; (2) splen/o
14. **Match:** a. -ectomy; surgical removal, excision; b. -megaly; enlargement
15. **Build:** a. splen/o/megaly; b. splen/ectomy
16. **Reading Exercise**
17. **Match:** a. -itis; inflammation; b. path/o; disease; c. -oma; tumor; d. aden/o; gland(s); node(s); e. -y; no meaning
18. **Translate:** a. lymph/aden/o/path/y, disease of the lymph nodes; b. lymph/aden/itis, inflammation of the lymph nodes; c. lymph/oma, tumor of lymphatic tissue
19. **Reading Exercise**
20. **Match:** a. -logist; one who studies and treats (specialist, physician); b. -logy; study of; c. -oma; tumor; d. -stasis; control, stop; e. -lysis; dissolution, separating
21. **Build:** a. hemat/o/logy; b. hemat/o/logist; c. hemat/oma; d. hem/o/stasis; e. hem/o/lysis
22. **Reading Exercise**
23. **Label:** Figure 7.15, hemat/oma
24. **Term Table: Review of MORE Cardiovascular and Lymphatic System Terms Built from Word Parts**

Exercise D

Pronounce and Spell MORE Terms Built from Word Parts

1. Check responses with the Term Table in Exercise C, #24
2. Check answers with the online resources

Exercise E

Label

1. cardiac catheterization; 2. coronary artery bypass graft; 3. varicose veins; 4. complete blood count; 5. aneurysm; 6. cardiopulmonary resuscitation; 7. stethoscope; 8. blood pressure

Exercise F

Match

1. e; 2. c; 3. b; 4. a; 5. d

Exercise G

Match

1. f; 2. c; 3. d; 4. e; 5. a; 6. b

Exercise H

Learn Medical Terms NOT Built from Word Parts

1. complete blood count; CBC; 2. blood pressure; BP; pulse; P; 3. stethoscope; sphygmomanometer; hypertension; HTN; hypotension; 4. coronary artery disease; CAD; myocardial infarction; MI; cardiac catheterization; 5. aneurysm; 6. anemia; hemorrhage; leukemia; 7. heart failure; HF; cardiopulmonary resuscitation; CPR; 8. embolus; coronary artery bypass graft; CABG; 9. varicose veins

Exercise I

Pronounce and Spell Terms NOT Built from Word Parts

1. Check responses with the Table for Medical Terms NOT Built from Word Parts
2. Check answers with the online resources

Exercise J

Abbreviate Medical Terms

1. Diseases and Disorders:
   a. CAD; b. HF; c. MI; d. HTN; e. PAD; f. HHD; g. DVT
2. Diagnostic Tests and Equipment:
   a. BP; b. CBC; c. ECHO; d. ECG, EKG; e. VS; f. P; g. DSA
3. Surgical Procedures: a. CABG; b. PTCA
4. Related Terms: a. CPR; b. IV

Exercise K

Signs and Symptoms

1. bradycardia; 2. cardiomegaly; 3. hemorrhage; 4. hypertension; 5. hypotension; 6. splenomegaly; 7. tachycardia; 8. tachypnea

Exercise L

Diseases and Disorders

1. anemia; 2. aneurysm; 3. arteriosclerosis; 4. cardiomyopathy; 5. coronary artery disease; 6. embolus; 7. heart failure; 8. hematoma; 9. hemolysis; 10. leukemia;

11. leukocytopenia; 12. lymphadenitis; 13. lymphadenopathy; 14. lymphoma; 15. myocardial infarction; 16. phlebitis; 17. thrombocytopenia; 18. thrombophlebitis; 19. thrombosis; 20. varicose veins

Exercise M

Diagnostic Tests and Equipment

1. angiography; 2. arteriogram; 3. blood pressure; 4. cardiac catheterization; 5. complete blood count; 6. echocardiogram; 7. electrocardiogram; 8. electrocardiograph; 9. electrocardiography; 10. pulse; 11. sphygmomanometer; 12. stethoscope; 13. venogram

Exercise N

Surgical Procedures

1. angioplasty; 2. coronary artery bypass graft; 3. endarterectomy; 4. phlebotomy; 5. splenectomy

Exercise O

Specialties and Professions

1. cardiologist; 2. cardiology; 3. hematologist; 4. hematology

Exercise P

Medical Terms Related to Cardiovascular and Lymphatic Systems

1. arterial; 2. cardiac; 3. cardiopulmonary resuscitation; 4. hemostasis; 5. intravenous; 6. myocardial; 7. thrombocyte

Exercise Q

Use Medical Terms in Clinical Statements

1. heart failure; electrocardiography; cardiac
2. thrombophlebitis; embolus
3. Thrombocytopenia; hemorrhage; hemostasis; anemia
4. Tachycardia; pulse; hypotension
5. Arteriosclerosis; arterial
6. complete blood count; leukemia; hematologist
7. Coronary artery disease; angioplasty; coronary artery bypass graft

Exercise R

Apply Medical Terms to the Case Study

Answers will vary and may include blood pressure, hypertension, tachycardia, and tachypnea, along with their corresponding definitions.

Copyright © 2024 by Elsevier, Inc. All rights reserved.

Exercise S

Use Medical Terms in a Document

1. hypertension; 2. varicose veins;
3. cardiologist; 4. coronary artery bypass graft (CABG); 5. aneurysm;
6. Phlebotomy;
7. Electrocardiogram (ECG, EKG);
8. myocardial infarction (MI);
9. Cardiac catheterization;
10. fatty plaque; vessel wall; producing, originating, causing; causing a fatty plaque deposit on a vessel wall;
11. HF; 12. coronary; 13. Dictionary and use of online references

Exercise T

Use Medical Language in Electronic Health Records Online

Complete with online resources

Exercise U

Online Review of Lesson Content

Complete with online resources

Exercise V

Lesson Content Quiz

1. a; 2. c; 3. b; 4. c; 5. c; 6. b; 7. a;
8. c; 9. a; 10. c; 11. b; 12. a

LESSON 8

Exercise A

Build and Translate Medical Terms Built from Word Parts

1. **Label:** Figure 8.3, (1) gloss/o; lingu/o; (2) gingiv/o; (3) or/o; (4) esophag/o; (5) gastr/o
2. **Match:** a. -algia; pain; b. -itis; inflammation
3. **Build:** a. gingiv/algia; b. gingiv/itis
4. **Reading Exercise**
5. **Label:** Figure 8.4, gingiv/itis
6. **Match:** a. -itis; inflammation; b. -al; pertaining to; c. sub-; below, under
7. **Translate:** a. gloss/itis; inflammation of the tongue; b. sub/lingu/al; pertaining to under the tongue
8. **Build:** or/al
9. **Reading Exercise**
10. **Label:** Figure 8.5, sub/lingu/al
11. **Match:** a. peps/o; digestion; b. phag/o; swallowing, eating; c. enter/o; intestines (usually the small intestine); d. -ia; diseased state, condition of; e. -y; no meaning; f. a-; without

12. **Build:** a. dys/enter/y; b. dys/peps/ia; c. dys/phag/ia
13. **Translate:** a/phag/ia; condition of without swallowing
14. **Reading Exercise**
15. **Match:** a. -eal; pertaining to; b. -itis; inflammation
16. **Build:** a. esophag/eal; b. esophag/itis
17. **Reading Exercise**
18. **Label:** Figure 8.6, esophag/itis
19. **Match:** a. enter/o; intestines (usually the small intestine); b. -itis; inflammation; c. -logist; one who studies and treats (specialist, physician); d. -logy; study of
20. **Build:** a. gastr/o/enter/o/logist; b. gastr/o/enter/o/logy; c. gastr/o/enter/itis
21. **Match:** a. -ectomy; excision; b. -itis; inflammation; c. -eal, -ic; pertaining to
22. **Translate:** a. gastr/itis; inflammation of the stomach; b. gastr/ic; pertaining to the stomach; c. gastr/ectomy; excision of the stomach; d. gastr/o/esophag/eal; pertaining to the stomach and esophagus
23. **Reading Exercise**
24. **Label:** Figure 8.7, gastr/ectomy
25. **Match:** a. -scope; instrument used for visual examination; b. -stomy; creation of an artificial opening; c. -scopy; visual examination
26. **Build:** a. gastr/o/scope; b. gastr/o/scopy; c. gastr/o/stomy
27. **Reading Exercise**
28. **Label:** Figure 8.8, A. gastr/o/scopy; B. gastr/o/scope
29. **Match:** a. -scope; instrument used for visual examination; b. -scopic; pertaining to visual examination; c. -scopy; visual examination; d. abdomin/o, lapar/o; abdomen, abdominal cavity
30. **Translate:** a. lapar/o/scope; instrument used for visual examination of the abdominal cavity; b. lapar/o/scopic; pertaining to visual examination of the abdominal cavity; c. lapar/o/scopy; visual examination of the abdominal cavity
31. **Reading Exercise**
32. **Label:** Figure 8.9, Lapar/o/scopic
33. **Match:** a. -centesis; surgical puncture to remove fluid; b. -tomy; incision
34. **Translate:** a. abdomin/o/centesis; surgical puncture to remove fluid from the abdominal cavity; b. lapar/o/tomy; incision into the abdominal cavity

35. **Reading Exercise**
36. **Term Table: Review of Digestive System Terms Built from Word Parts**

Exercise B

Pronounce and Spell Terms Built from Word Parts

1. Check responses with the Term Table in Exercise A, #36
2. Check answers with the online resources

Exercise C

Build and Translate MORE Medical Terms Built from Word Parts

1. **Label:** Figure 8.10, (1) chol/e, cyst/o; (2) duoden/o; (3) ile/o; (4) append/o, appendic/o; (5) proct/o, rect/o; (6) hepat/o; (7) pancreat/o; (8) col/o, colon/o; (9) jejun/o; (10) sigmoid/o; (11) an/o
2. **Match:** a. -stomy; creation of an artificial opening; b. -al; pertaining to; c. -scopy; visual examination
3. **Translate:** a. esophag/o/gastr/o/duoden/o/scopy; visual examination of the esophagus, stomach, and duodenum; b. duoden/al; pertaining to the duodenum
4. **Reading Exercise**
5. **Build:** a. ile/o/stomy; b. jejun/o/stomy
6. **Reading Exercise**
7. **Match:** a. -oma; tumor; b. -itis; inflammation; c. -megaly; enlargement
8. **Translate:** a. hepat/itis; inflammation of the liver; b. hepat/oma; tumor of the liver; c. hepat/o/megaly; enlargement of the liver
9. **Reading Exercise**
10. **Label:** Figure 8.11, hepat/oma
11. **Match:** a. -itis; inflammation; b. -ectomy; excision; c. cyst/o; bladder, sac; d. lith/o; stone(s), calculus (*pl.* calculi)
12. **Translate:** a. chol/e/cyst/itis; inflammation of the gallbladder; b. chol/e/cyst/ectomy; excision of the gallbladder; c. chol/e/lith/iasis; condition of gallstone(s)
13. **Reading Exercise**
14. **Label:** Figure 8.12, chol/e/lith/iasis
15. **Match:** a. -ic; pertaining to; b. -itis; inflammation
16. **Build:** a. pancreat/ic; b. pancreat/itis
17. **Reading Exercise**
18. **Match:** a. -itis; inflammation; b. -ectomy; excision

Copyright © 2024 by Elsevier, Inc. All rights reserved.

19. **Translate:** a. append/ectomy; excision of the appendix; b. appendic/itis; inflammation of the appendix
20. **Reading Exercise**
21. **Label:** Figure 8.13, appendic/itis
22. **Match:** a. -itis; inflammation; b. -stomy; creation of an artificial opening; c. -ectomy; excision; d. -graphy; process of recording, radiographic imaging; e. -scopy; visual examination
23. **Build:** a. colon/o/scopy; b. CT colon/o/graphy
24. **Reading Exercise**
25. **Label:** Figure 8.14, colon/o/graphy
26. **Build:** a. col/itis; b. col/o/stomy; c. col/ectomy
27. **Reading Exercise**
28. **Label:** Figure 8.15, Col/o/stomy
29. **Match:** a. -scopy; visual examination; b. -cele; hernia, protrusion; c. -al; pertaining to; d. -scope; instrument used for visual examination
30. **Translate:** a. sigmoid/o/scopy; visual examination of the sigmoid colon; b. proct/o/scope; instrument used for visual examination of the rectum; c. proct/o/scopy; visual examination of the rectum
31. **Reading Exercise**
32. **Label:** Figure 8.16, Sigmoid/o/scopy
33. **Build:** a. rect/o/cele; b. rect/al
34. **Translate:** an/al; pertaining to the anus
35. **Reading Exercise**
36. **Term Table: Review of MORE Digestive System Terms Built from Word Parts**

Exercise D

Pronounce and Spell MORE Terms Built from Word Parts

1. Check responses with the Term Table in Exercise C, #36
2. Check answers with online resources.

Exercise E

Label

1. endoscopic retrograde cholangiopancreatography; 2. peptic ulcer; 3. gastroesophageal reflux disease; 4. barium enema; 5. polyp; 6. stoma; 7. bariatric surgery; 8. hemorrhoids; 9. cirrhosis; 10. irritable bowel syndrome

Exercise F

Match

1. c; 2. a; 3. g; 4. e; 5. d; 6. b; 7. f

Exercise G

Learn Medical Terms NOT Built from Word Parts

1. gastroesophageal reflux disease; GERD; 2. irritable bowel syndrome; IBS; constipation; diarrhea; 3. polyp; barium enema; 4. endoscopic retrograde cholangiopancreatography; 5. ulcerative colitis; stoma; Crohn disease; 6. cirrhosis; 7. peptic ulcer; upper GI series; 8. celiac disease; parenteral; 9. bariatric surgery; 10. hemorrhoids

Exercise H

Pronounce and Spell Terms NOT Built from Word Parts

1. Check responses with the Table for Medical Terms NOT Built from Word Parts
2. Check answers with online resources.

Exercise I

Abbreviate Medical Terms

1. Diseases and Disorders: a. GERD; b. IBS; c. UC
2. Diagnostic Tests and Equipment: a. BE; b. EGD; c. ERCP; d. UGI series; e. CTC
3. Surgical Procedures: PEG
4. Related Terms: a. BM; b. GI; c. TPN

Exercise J

Signs and Symptoms

1. aphagia; 2. constipation; 3. diarrhea; 4. dyspepsia; 5. dysphagia; 6. gingivalgia; 7. hepatomegaly

Exercise K

Diseases and Disorders

1. appendicitis; 2. cholecystitis; 3. cholelithiasis; 4. colitis; 5. Crohn disease; 6. dysentery; 7. esophagitis; 8. gastritis; 9. gastroenteritis; 10. gastroesophageal reflux disease; 11. gingivitis; 12. glossitis; 13. hemorrhoids; 14. hepatitis; 15. hepatoma; 16. celiac disease; 17. irritable bowel syndrome; 18. pancreatitis; 19. peptic ulcer; 20. polyp; 21. rectocele; 22. ulcerative colitis; 23. cirrhosis

Exercise L

Diagnostic Tests and Equipment

1. barium enema; 2. colonoscopy; 3. CT colonography; 4. endoscopic retrograde cholangiopancreatography; 5. esophagogastroduodenoscopy; 6. gastroscope; 7. gastroscopy; 8. laparoscope; 9. laparoscopic; 10. laparoscopy; 11. proctoscope; 12. proctoscopy; 13. sigmoidoscopy; 14. upper GI series

Exercise M

Surgical Procedures

1. abdominocentesis; 2. appendectomy; 3. bariatric surgery; 4. cholecystectomy; 5. colectomy; 6. colostomy; 7. gastrectomy; 8. gastrostomy; 9. ileostomy; 10. jejunostomy; 11. laparotomy

Exercise N

Specialties and Professions

1. gastroenterologist; 2. gastroenterology

Exercise O

Medical Terms Related to the Digestive System

1. anal; 2. duodenal; 3. esophageal; 4. gastric; 5. gastroesophageal; 6. oral; 7. pancreatic; 8. rectal; 9. sublingual; 10. parenteral; 11. stoma

Exercise P

Use Medical Terms in Clinical Statements

1. cholecystitis; laparoscopy; cholecystectomy; 2. gastrostomy; esophageal; 3. esophagogastroduodenoscopy; gastroenterologist; peptic ulcer; 4. Hepatomegaly; hepatitis; hepatoma; cirrhosis; 5. GERD, gastroesophageal; dysphagia; esophagitis; 6. oral; gingivitis; glossitis; sublingual; 7. Ulcerative colitis; colectomy; ileostomy

Exercise Q

Apply Medical Terms to the Case Study

Answers will vary and may include gastric, dyspepsia, gastroesophageal reflux disease, dysphagia, and gastroenterologist, along with their respective definitions.

Copyright © 2024 by Elsevier, Inc. All rights reserved.

Exercise R

Use Medical Terms in a Document

1. dyspepsia;
2. esophagogastroduodenoscopy;
3. intravenous; 4. lateral;
5. gastroscope; 6. gastric; 7. distal;
8. gastritis; 9. duodenal; 10. blood;
vomiting; vomiting blood; 11. causing
(producing, originating) ulcers;
12. dictionary/online exercise

Exercise S

*Use Medical Language in Electronic
Health Records Online*

Completed with online resources.

Exercise T

Online Review of Lesson Content

Completed with online resources.

Exercise U

Lesson Content Quiz

1. a; 2. a; 3. b; 4. a; 5. c; 6. b; 7. b;
8. c; 9. a; 10. c; 11. a; 12. b

LESSON 9

Exercise A

*Build and Translate Terms Built from
Word Parts*

1. **Label:** Figure 9.5, A. (1) ophthalm/o,
   (2) blephar/o, (3) scler/o, (4) ir/o,
   irid/o; B. (1) kerat/o, (2) retin/o
2. **Match:** a. -logy, study of; b. -scope,
   instrument used for visual
   examination; c. -logist, one who
   studies and treats (specialist,
   physician); d. -meter, instrument used
   to measure; e. -itis, inflammation
3. **Build:** a. ophthalm/o/logy;
   b. ophthalm/o/logist
4. **Translate:** A. ophthalm/o/scope,
   instrument used for visual
   examination of the eye; B. kerat/o/
   meter, instrument used to measure
   (the curvature of) the cornea
5. **Label:** Figure 9.6, ophthalm/o/scope
6. **Reading exercise**
7. **Translate:** a. blephar/itis,
   inflammation of the eyelid;
   b. ir/itis, inflammation of the iris;
   c. retin/itis, inflammation of the
   retina; d. scler/itis, inflammation of
   the sclera
8. **Label:** Figure 9.7, A. scler/itis,
   B. blephar/itis
9. **Reading exercise**

10. **Match:** a. -ptosis, drooping, sagging,
    prolapse; b. -plegia, paralysis;
    c. -ectomy, excision; d. -plasty,
    surgical repair
11. **Build:** a. irid/ectomy; b. blephar/o/
    plasty; c. kerat/o/plasty
12. **Translate:** a. irid/o/plegia, paralysis of
    the iris; b. blephar/o/ptosis, drooping
    of the eyelid
13. **Label:** Figure 9.8, blephar/o/ptosis
14. **Reading exercise**
15. **Match:** a. -al, -ic, pertaining to;
    b. -metry, measurement; c. opt/o,
    vision
16. **Build:** a. opt/o/metry; b. opt/ic;
    c. ophthalm/ic
17. **Translate:** a. scler/al, pertaining to
    the sclera; b. retin/al, pertaining to
    the retina
18. **Reading exercise**
19. **Review of Eye Terms Built from
    Word Parts**

Exercise B

*Pronounce and Spell Terms Built from
Word Parts*

1. Check responses with the Term Table
   in Exercise A, #19
2. Check answers with the online
   resources

Exercise C

*Build and Translate MORE Medical
Terms Built from Word Parts*

1. **Label:** Figure 9.9. 1. ot/o;
   2. myring/o; 3. tympan/o
2. **Match:** a. -rrhea, flow, discharge;
   b. -plasty, surgical repair; c. -scope,
   instrument used for visual
   examination; d. -itis, inflammation
3. **Translate:** a. ot/o/rrhea, discharge
   from the ear; b. ot/o/scope,
   instrument used for visual
   examination of the ear; c. ot/o/plasty,
   surgical repair of the (outer) ear
4. **Label:** Figure 9.10, ot/o/scope
5. **Build:** a. ot/itis, b. myring/itis
6. **Reading exercise**
7. **Label:** Figure 9.11, ot/itis
8. **Match:** a. -ic, pertaining to, b. -tomy,
   incision; c. -plasty, surgical repair;
   d. -logy, study of; e. -logist, one
   who studies and treats (specialist,
   physician); f. laryng/o, larynx
   (voice box)
9. **Build:** a. tympan/ic; b. tympan/o/
   plasty

10. **Translate:** a. myring/o/tomy, incision
    of the eardrum; b. myring/o/plasty,
    surgical repair of the eardrum
11. **Reading exercise**
12. **Label:** Figure 9.12, myring/o/tomy
13. **Build:** a. ot/o/laryng/o/logy,
    b. ot/o/laryng/o/logist
14. **Reading exercise**
15. **Match:** a. audi/o, hearing; b. -logy,
    study of; c. -logist, one who studies
    and treats (specialist, physician);
    d. -meter, instrument used to
    measure; e. -metry, measurement
16. **Translate:** a. audi/o/logy, study of
    hearing; b. audi/o/logist, specialist
    who studies and treats (impaired)
    hearing; c. audi/o/meter, instrument
    used to measure hearing; d. audi/o/
    metry, measurement of hearing
17. **Reading exercise**
18. **Label:** Figure 9.13, audi/o/meter
19. **Review of Ear Terms Built from
    Word Parts**

Exercise D

*Pronounce and Spell MORE Terms Built
from Word Parts*

1. Check responses with the Term Table
   in Exercise C, #19
2. Check answers with the online
   resources

Exercise E

Label

1. cataract; 2. retinal detachment;
3. macular degeneration; 4. LASIK;
5. optometrist; 6. tinnitus;
7. A. presbyopia; B. presbycusis

Exercise F

Match

1. e; 2. d; 3. a; 4. b; 5. c

Exercise G

*Learn Medical Terms NOT Built from
Word Parts*

1. LASIK; astigmatism; hyperopia; myopia;
2. glaucoma; 3. cataract; optometrist;
4. macular degeneration; age-related;
5. retinal detachment; 6. otitis media;
7. tinnitus; 8. presbyopia; presbycusis

Exercise H

*Pronounce and Spell Terms NOT Built
from Word Parts*

1. Check responses with the Table for
   Terms NOT Built from Word Parts
2. Check answers with the online
   resources

Copyright © 2024 by Elsevier, Inc. All rights reserved.

Exercise I

Abbreviate medical terms.

1. Signs and Symptoms: a. IOP; b. HOH
2. Diseases and Disorders: a. OM; b. AST; c. AMD
3. Diagnostic Test: VA
4. Specialties and Professions: a. Ophth, b. ENT
5. Related: ENT

Exercise J

Signs and Symptoms

1. otorrhea; 2. tinnitus

Exercise K

Diseases and Disorders

1. astigmatism; 2. otitis media; 3. myopia; 4. hyperopia; 5. cataract; 6. macular degeneration; 7. retinal detachment; 8. glaucoma; 9. presbycusis; 10. presbyopia; 11. blepharitis; 12. blepharoptosis; 13. iridoplegia; 14. iritis; 15. scleritis; 16. retinitis; 17. myringitis; 18. otitis

Exercise L

Diagnostic Tests and Equipment

1. ophthalmoscope; 2. keratometer; 3. audiometer; 4. otoscope; 5. audiometry

Exercise M

Surgical Procedures

1. blepharoplasty; 2. iridectomy; 3. keratoplasty; 4. LASIK; 5. myringoplasty; 6. myringotomy; 7. otoplasty; 8. tympanoplasty

Exercise N

Specialties and Professions

1. ophthalmologist; 2. ophthalmology; 3. optometry; 4. optometrist; 5. audiologist; 6. audiology; 7. otolaryngologist; 8. otolaryngology

Exercise O

Medical Terms Related to the Eye and Ear

1. ophthalmic; 2. optic; 3. retinal; 4. scleral; 5. tympanic

Exercise P

Use Medical Terms in Clinical Statements

1. ophthalmologist
2. LASIK; hyperopia
3. iridectomy; glaucoma

4. blepharoplasty; blepharoptosis
5. keratometer
6. Presbyopia; optometrist
7. iritis
8. otoscope; audiometer
9. otolaryngologist; myringotomy
10. Myringoplasty; tympanoplasty
11. Presbycusis; audiologist

Exercise Q

Apply Medical Terms to Case Study

Answers will vary and may include presbyopia, presbycusis, glaucoma, ophthalmologist, otolaryngologist, and otitis media along with corresponding definitions.

Exercise R

Use Medical Terms in a Document

1. ENT; 2. tinnitus; 3. otitis media;
4. tympanoplasty; 5. glaucoma;
6. ophthalmologist; 7. optometrist;
8. otoscope; 9. tympanic; 10. otorrhea;
11. audiologist; 12. otitis; 13. audiology;
14. otolaryngologist;
15. ocul/o, eye; -ar, pertaining to; ocul/ar, pertaining to the eye;
16. any visible change in tissue resulting from injury or disease;
17. Research activity. Answers will vary.

Exercise S

Use Medical Language in Electronic Health Records Online

Completed with online resources.

Exercise T

Online Review of Lesson Content

Completed with online resources.

Exercise U

Lesson Content Quiz

1. a; 2. c; 3. b; 4. c; 5. b; 6. c; 7. b; 8. a; 9. a; 10. c; 11. b; 12. b

LESSON 10

Exercise A

Build and Translate Medical Terms Built from Word Parts

1. **Label:** Figure 10.2, (1) rachi/o, spondyl/o, vertebr/o; (2) carp/o; (3) phalang/o
2. **Match:** a. -al; pertaining to; b. -ectomy; excision; c. -plasty; surgical repair; d. inter-; between

3. **Build:** a. vertebr/al; b. inter/vertebr/al; c. vertebr/ectomy; d. vertebr/o/plasty
4. **Label:** Figure 10.3: inter/vertebr/al
5. **Reading Exercise**
6. **Match:** a. -schisis; split, fissure; b. -tomy; incision; c. -itis; inflammation; d. arthr/o; joint(s)
7. **Translate:** a. rachi/schisis; fissure of the vertebral column; b. rachi/o/tomy; incision into the vertebral column
8. **Build:** a. spondyl/arthr/itis
9. **Reading Exercise**
10. **Match:** a. -osis; abnormal condition; b. kyph/o; hump (thoracic spine); c. lord/o; bent forward (lumbar spine); d. scoli/o; crooked, curved (spine)
11. **Translate:** a. scoli/osis; abnormal condition of crooked, curved (spine); b. kyph/osis; abnormal condition of a hump (thoracic spine); c. lord/osis; abnormal condition of bent forward (lumbar spine)
12. **Label:** Figure 10.5, A. lord/osis; B. kyph/osis; C. scoli/osis
13. **Match:** a. -al, -eal; pertaining to; b. -ectomy; excision
14. **Build:** a. carp/al; b. carp/ectomy
15. **Reading Exercise**
16. **Translate:** a. phalang/eal; pertaining to a phalanx; b. phalang/ectomy; excision of a phalanx
17. **Reading Exercise**
18. **Match:** a. a-; absence of, without; b. dys-; difficult, painful, abnormal; c. hyper-; above, excessive; d. -y; no meaning; e. -ic; pertaining to
19. **Build:** a. dys/troph/y; b. a/troph/y; c. hyper/troph/y; d. hyper/troph/ic
20. **Reading Exercise**
21. **Label:** Figure 10.7, hyper/troph/ic
22. **Label:** Figure 10.8, burs/o
23. **Match:** a. -itis; inflammation; b. -ectomy; excision; c. -tomy; incision
24. **Translate:** a. burs/ectomy; excision of a bursa; b. burs/itis; inflammation of the bursa; c. burs/o/tomy; incision into a bursa
25. **Reading Exercise**
26. **Label:** Figure 10.9, burs/itis
27. **Label:** Figure 10.10, (1) ili/o; (2) pub/o; (3) ischi/o
28. **Match:** a. -al, -ac, -ic; pertaining to; b. femor/o; femur
29. **Translate:** a. ili/ac; pertaining to the ilium; b. femor/al; pertaining to the femur; c. ili/o/femor/al; pertaining to

Copyright © 2024 by Elsevier, Inc. All rights reserved.

the ilium and the femur; d. ischi/al; pertaining to the ischium; e. ischi/o/pub/ic; pertaining to the ischium and the pubis

30. **Reading Exercise**
31. **Match:** a. -algia; pain; b. -asthenia; weakness; c. -gram; record, radiographic image; d. electr/o; electrical activity; e. my/o; muscle(s), muscle tissue
32. **Build:** a. my/algia; b. my/asthenia; c. electr/o/my/o/gram
33. **Reading Exercise**
34. **Label:** Figure 10.11, electr/o/my/o/gram
35. **Match:** a. brady-; slow; b. dys-; difficult, painful, abnormal; c. -a; no meaning
36. **Build:** a. brady/kinesi/a; b. dys/kinesi/a
37. **Reading Exercise**
38. **Term Table: Review of Musculoskeletal System Terms Built from Word Parts**

Exercise B

Pronounce and Spell Medical Terms Built from Word Parts

1. Check responses with the Term Table in Exercise A, #38
2. Check answers with the online resources

Exercise C

Build and Translate MORE Medical Terms Built from Word Parts

1. **Label:** Figure 10.12, (1) crani/o; (2) stern/o; (3) cost/o
2. **Match:** a. -tomy; incision; b. intra-; within; c. -schisis; split, fissure; d. -malacia; softening; e. -al; pertaining to; f. -ia; diseased state, condition of
3. **Build:** a. intra/crani/al; b. crani/o/schisis; c. crani/o/tomy; d. crani/o/malacia
4. **Reading Exercise**
5. **Label:** Figure 10.13, intra/crani/al
6. **Match:** a. -al; pertaining to; b. inter-; between; c. sub-; below, under
7. **Translate:** a. stern/al; pertaining to the sternum; b. stern/o/cost/al; pertaining to the sternum and the ribs
8. **Reading Exercise**
9. **Label:** Figure 10.14, stern/al
10. **Build:** a. inter/cost/al; b. sub/cost/al
11. **Reading Exercise**

12. **Label:** Figure 10.15, (1) ten/o, tendin/o; (2) chondr/o; (3) oste/o; (4) arthr/o
13. **Match:** a. -itis; inflammation; b. -ectomy; excision; c. -malacia; softening; d. -al; pertaining to
14. **Translate:** a. cost/o/chondr/al; pertaining to the ribs and cartilage; b. chondr/itis; inflammation of cartilage; c. chondr/ectomy; excision of cartilage; d. chondr/o/malacia; softening of cartilage
15. **Reading Exercise**
16. **Label:** Figure 10.16, cost/o/chondr/al
17. **Match:** a. -osis; abnormal condition; b. -itis; inflammation; c. necr/o; death
18. **Build:** a. necr/osis; b. oste/o/necr/osis; c. oste/o/chondr/itis
19. **Reading Exercise**
20. **Match:** a. path/o; disease; b. -malacia; softening; c. -penia; abnormal reduction; d. -y; no meaning
21. **Translate:** a. oste/o/path/y; disease of the bone; b. oste/o/penia; abnormal reduction of bone mass; c. oste/o/malacia; softening of the bone
22. **Reading Exercise**
23. **Match:** a. sarc/o; flesh, connective tissue; b. -oma; tumor; c. -itis; inflammation
24. **Build:** a. oste/o/arthr/itis; b. oste/o/sarc/oma
25. **Reading Exercise**
26. **Label:** Figure 10.17, oste/o/sarc/oma
27. **Match:** a. -algia; pain; b. -desis; binding, fusion; c. -plasty; surgical repair; d. -itis; inflammation
28. **Translate:** a. arthr/algia; pain in the joint; b. arthr/itis; inflammation of the joint(s); c. arthr/o/desis; fusion of a joint; d. arthr/o/plasty; surgical repair of a joint
29. **Reading Exercise**
30. **Match:** a. -centesis; surgical puncture to remove fluid; b. -gram; record, radiographic image; c. -scopy; visual examination; d. -scopic; pertaining to visual examination
31. **Build:** a. arthr/o/centesis; b. arthr/o/gram; c. arthr/o/scopy; d. arthr/o/scopic
32. **Label:** Figure 10.18, arthr/o/scopy, arthr/o/scopic
33. **Match:** a. -desis; binding, fusion; b. -itis; inflammation; c. -plasty; surgical repair

34. **Translate:** a. tendin/itis; inflammation of the tendon(s); b. ten/o/plasty; surgical repair of a tendon; c. ten/o/desis; binding of a tendon (to a bone or ligament)
35. **Reading Exercise**
36. **Term Table: Review of MORE Musculoskeletal Terms Built from Word Parts**

Exercise D

Pronounce and Spell More Medical Terms Built from Word Parts

1. Check responses with the Term Table in Exercise C, #36
2. Check answers with the online resources

Exercise E

Label

1. Lyme disease; 2. carpal tunnel syndrome; 3. fracture; 4. gout; 5. osteoporosis; 6. herniated disk; 7. spinal stenosis; 8. plantar fasciitis; 9. dual x-ray absorptiometry; 10. orthopedist; 11. rheumatoid arthritis

Exercise F

Match

1. b; 2. d; 3. c; 4. a

Exercise G

Learn Medical Terms NOT Built from Word Parts

1. Orthopedics; orthopedist; fracture; herniated disk; spinal stenosis; 2. rheumatoid arthritis; 3. Gout; 4. muscular dystrophy; 5. carpal tunnel syndrome; plantar fasciitis 6. osteoporosis; dual x-ray absorptiometry; 7. hernia; 8. chiropractic; 9. Lyme disease

Exercise H

Pronounce and Spell Medical Terms NOT Built from Word Parts

1. Check responses with the Table for Terms NOT Built from Word Parts
2. Check answers with the online resources

Exercise I

Abbreviate Medical Terms

1. Diseases and Disorders: a. CTS; b. Fx; c. MD; d. OA; e. RA
2. Diagnostic Tests and Equipment: a. EMG; b. DXA; c. DEXA

Copyright © 2024 by Elsevier, Inc. All rights reserved.

3. Surgical Procedures:
   a. TKA; b. THA
4. Specialties and Professions:
   a. ortho; b. PT; c. DO; d. OT;
   e. DC
5. Related Terms:
   a. C1-C7; b. L1-L5; c. T1-T12;
   d. ROM

Exercise J

Signs and Symptoms

1. arthralgia; 2. atrophy; 3. bradykinesia;
4. dyskinesia; 5. dystrophy;
6. hypertrophy; 7. myalgia;
8. myasthenia

Exercise K

Diseases and Disorders

1. arthritis; 2. plantar fasciitis;
3. bursitis; 4. carpal tunnel syndrome;
5. chondritis; 6. chondromalacia;
7. craniomalacia; 8. cranioschisis;
9. fracture; 10. gout; 11. herniated
disk; 12. kyphosis; 13. lordosis;
14. muscular dystrophy;
15. necrosis; 16. osteoarthritis;
17. osteochondritis; 18. osteomalacia;
19. osteonecrosis; 20. osteopathy;
21. osteopenia; 22. osteoporosis;
23. osteosarcoma; 24. rachischisis;
25. rheumatoid arthritis; 26. scoliosis;
27. spondylarthritis; 28. tendinitis;
29. spinal stenosis; 30. Lyme disease;
31. hernia

Exercise L

Diagnostic Tests and Equipment

1. arthrogram; 2. arthroscopic;
3. arthroscopy; 4. electromyogram;
5. dual x-ray absorptiometry

Exercise M

Surgical Procedures

1. arthrocentesis; 2. arthrodesis;
3. arthroplasty; 4. bursectomy;
5. bursotomy; 6. carpectomy;
7. chondrectomy; 8. craniotomy;
9. phalangectomy; 10. rachiotomy;
11. tenodesis; 12. tenoplasty;
13. vertebrectomy; 14. vertebroplasty

Exercise N

Specialties and Professions

1. orthopedics; 2. orthopedist;
3. chiropractic

Exercise O

Medical Terms Related to the Musculoskeletal System

1. carpal; 2. costochondral; 3. femoral;
4. hypertrophic; 5. iliac; 6. iliofemoral;
7. intercostal; 8. intervertebral;
9. intracranial; 10. ischial;
11. ischiopubic; 12. phalangeal;
13. sternal; 14. sternocostal;
15. subcostal; 16. vertebral

Exercise P

Use Medical Terms in Clinical Statements

1. arthritis; fracture; arthrodesis
2. arthrogram; arthroscopy; arthroscopic
3. arthroplasty; osteoarthritis
4. scoliosis; lordosis; kyphosis;
   osteoporosis
5. muscular dystrophy; electromyogram
6. orthopedist; tendinitis; tenoplasty
7. Bursitis; arthritis; bursotomy
8. Chondromalacia; Osteomalacia
9. Hypertrophy; atrophy
10. chiropractic; spinal stenosis
11. intracranial; intercostal; subcostal;
    ischiopubic; iliac; sternocostal;
    vertebral; femoral; sternal

Exercise Q

Apply Medical Terms to A Case Study

Answers will vary and may include
phalangeal, carpal, iliac, myalgia, and
contusion, along with their respective
definitions.

Exercise R

Use Medical Terms in a Document

1. orthopedics; 2. fracture;
3. myalgia; 4. kyphosis;
5. vertebral; 6. iliac;
7. carpal; 8. phalangeal;
9. osteoporosis
10. a. radi/al;
    b. uln/ar
11. student exercise; 12. bruise
13. dictionary/online exercise

Exercise S

Use Medical Language in Electronic Health Records Online

Complete with online resources

Exercise T

Online Review of Lesson Content

Complete with online resources

Exercise U

Lesson Content Quiz

1. b; 2. a; 3. b; 4. c; 5. a; 6. b; 7. c;
8. b; 9. a; 10. c; 11. b; 12. c

LESSON 11

Exercise A

Build and Translate Medical Terms Built from Word Parts

1. **Label:** Figure 11.3, 1. cerebr/o;
   2. encephal/o
2. **Match:** a. -al; pertaining to; b. angi/o;
   blood vessel(s); c. -graphy; process
   of recording, radiographic imaging;
   d. thromb/o; blood clot; e. -osis;
   abnormal condition
3. **Build:** a. cerebr/al; b. cerebral angi/o/
   graphy; c. cerebral thromb/osis
4. **Reading Exercise**
5. **Label:** Figure 11.4, cerebr/al angi/o/
   graphy
6. **Match:** a. -itis; inflammation;
   b. -y; no meaning; c. path/o; disease
7. **Build:** a. encephal/o/path/y;
   b. encephal/itis
8. **Reading Exercise**
9. **Match:** a. electr/o; electrical activity;
   b. -graphy; process of recording,
   radiographic imaging; c. -graph;
   instrument used to record; d. -gram;
   record, radiographic image
10. **Translate:** a. electr/o/encephal/o/
    gram; record of electrical activity of
    the brain; b. electr/o/encephal/o/
    graph; instrument used to record
    electrical activity of the brain;
    c. electr/o/encephal/o/graphy; process
    of recording the electrical activity of
    the brain
11. **Reading Exercise**
12. **Label:** Figure 11.5, electr/o/encephal/o/
    graphy
13. **Match:** a. -al; pertaining to;
    b. -algia; pain
14. **Build:** a. neur/al; b. neur/algia
15. **Reading Exercise**
16. **Label:** Figure 11.6, neur/algia
17. **Match:** a. -logist; one who studies
    and treats (specialist, physician);
    b. -logy; study of; c. path/o; disease;
    d. -y; no meaning
18. **Translate:** a. neur/o/logist;
    physician who studies and treats
    diseases of the nervous system;
    b. neur/o/logy: study of the nerves
    (nervous system); c. neur/o/path/y;

Copyright © 2024 by Elsevier, Inc. All rights reserved.

disease of the nerves (nervous system)
19. **Reading Exercise**
20. **Match:** a. -itis; inflammation; b. -algia; pain; c. arthr/o; joint(s); d. my/o; muscle(s); e. neur/o; nerve(s)
21. **Build:** a. poly/my/algia; b. poly/arthr/itis; c. poly/neur/itis
22. **Reading Exercise**
23. **Term Table: Review of Nervous System and Behavioral Health Terms Built from Word Parts**

Exercise B

Pronounce and Spell Medical Terms Built from Word Parts
1. Check responses with the Term Table in Exercise A, #23
2. Check answers with online resources

Exercise C

Build and Translate MORE Medical Terms Built from Word Parts
1. **Label:** Figure 11.7, 1. myel/o; 2. mening/o, meningi/o
2. **Match:** a. -oma; tumor; b. -itis; inflammation; c. -cele; hernia, protrusion
3. **Build:** a. mening/o/cele; b. mening/itis; c. meningi/oma
4. **Reading Exercise**
5. **Label:** Figure 11.8, meningi/oma
6. **Match:** a. -itis; inflammation; b. poli/o; gray matter
7. **Translate:** a. mening/o/myel/itis; inflammation of the meninges and spinal cord; b. poli/o/myel/itis; inflammation of the gray matter of the spinal cord
8. **Reading Exercise**
9. **Match:** a. -graphy; process of recording, radiographic imaging; b. -gram; record, radiographic image
10. **Build:** a. myel/o/gram; b. myel/o/graphy
11. **Reading Exercise**
12. **Label:** Figure 11.9, myel/o/graphy
13. **Match:** a. -algia; pain; b. -us; no meaning; c. hydr/o; water; d. micro-; small
14. **Translate:** a. micro/cephal/us; small head; b. hydr/o/cephal/us; water (cerebrospinal fluid) in the head (brain); c. ceph/algia; pain in the head (headache). *Note: In ceph/algia, the* **al** *is dropped from the combining form cephal/o.*
15. **Reading Exercise**

16. **Match:** a. a-; absence of, without; b. dys-; difficult, painful, abnormal; c. hemi-; half; d. quadr/i; four; e. -ia; diseased state, condition of
17. **Build:** a. a/phas/ia; b. dys/phas/ia
18. **Reading Exercise**
19. **Translate:** a. hemi/pleg/ia; condition of paralysis of half (right or left side of the body); b. quadr/i/pleg/ia; condition of paralysis of four (limbs)
20. **Reading Exercise**
21. **Label:** Figure 11.10, A. hemi/pleg/ia; C. quadr/i/pleg/ia
22. **Match:** a. -genic; producing, originating, causing; b. path/o; disease; c. -y; no meaning; d. -osis; abnormal condition
23. **Build:** a. psych/o/genic; b. psych/o/path/y; c. psych/osis
24. **Reading Exercise**
25. **Match:** a. -logist; one who studies and treats (specialist, physician); b. -logy; study of
26. **Translate:** a. psych/o/logist; specialist who studies and treats the mind; b. psych/o/logy; study of the mind
27. **Reading Exercise**
28. **Term Table: Review of MORE Nervous System and Behavioral Health Terms Built from Word Parts**

Exercise D

Pronounce and Spell MORE Terms Built from Word Parts
1. Check responses with the Term Table in Exercise C, #28
2. Check answers with online resources

Exercise E

Label
1. transient ischemic attack; 2. stroke; 3. subarachnoid hemorrhage; 4. dementia; 5. Alzheimer disease; 6. lumbar puncture; 7. paraplegia; 8. sciatica; 9. migraine; 10. psychiatrist

Exercise F

Match
1. c; 2. b; 3. e; 4. a; 5. d

Exercise G

Match
1. d; 2. c; 3. a; 4. b

Exercise H

Learn Medical Terms NOT Built from Word Parts
1. multiple sclerosis; MS; 2. Parkinson disease; PD; 3. dementia; Alzheimer disease; 4. concussion; seizure; 5. sciatica; epidural nerve block; 6. migraine; 7. lumbar puncture; LP; 8. stroke; CVA; 9. subarachnoid hemorrhage; 10. transient ischemic attack; TIA; syncope; 11. paraplegia; 12. anxiety disorder; 13. depression; 14. bipolar disorder; 15. psychiatrist; 16. syncope

Exercise I

Pronounce and Spell Terms NOT Built from Word Parts
1. Check responses with the Table for Terms NOT Built from Word Parts
2. Check answers with online resources

Exercise J

Abbreviate Medical Terms
1. Signs and Symptoms:
   a. Sz
2. Diseases and Disorders:
   a. AD; b. CVA; c. MS; d. PD; e. SAH; f. TIA; g. OCD; h. CP; i. PTSD
3. Diagnostic Tests and Equipment:
   a. EEG; b. LP
4. Related Terms:
   a. CNS; b. CSF; c. PNS; d. ADL, ADLs

Exercise K

Signs and Symptoms
1. aphasia; 2. cephalgia; 3. dysphasia; 4. neuralgia; 5. polyarthritis; 6. polymyalgia; 7. polyneuritis; 8. seizure; 9. syncope

Exercise L

Diseases and Disorders
1. Alzheimer disease; 2. anxiety disorder; 3. bipolar disorder; 4. cerebral thrombosis; 5. concussion; 6. dementia; 7. depression; 8. encephalitis; 9. encephalopathy; 10. hemiplegia; 11. hydrocephalus; 12. meningioma; 13. meningitis; 14. meningocele; 15. meningomyelitis; 16. migraine; 17. multiple sclerosis; 18. neuropathy; 19. paraplegia; 20. Parkinson disease;

Copyright © 2024 by Elsevier, Inc. All rights reserved.

21. poliomyelitis; 22. psychopathy;
23. psychosis; 24. quadriplegia;
25. sciatica; 26. stroke (cerebrovascular accident); 27. subarachnoid hemorrhage;
28. transient ischemic attack;
29. microcephalus

Exercise M

Diagnostic Tests and Equipment
1. cerebral angiography
2. electroencephalogram
3. electroencephalograph
4. electroencephalography
5. lumbar puncture
6. myelogram
7. myelography

Exercise N

Surgical Procedure
epidural nerve block

Exercise O

Specialties and Professions
1. neurologist; 2. neurology;
3. psychologist; 4. psychology;
5. psychiatrist

Exercise P

Medical Terms Related to the Nervous System and Behavioral Health
1. cerebral; 2. neural; 3. psychogenic

Exercise Q

Use Medical Terms in Clinical Statements
1. Depression; psychology; anxiety disorder; psychiatrist, psychologist
2. bipolar disorder; psychosis
3. Cephalgia; Migraine; Subarachnoid hemorrhage
4. electroencephalography; electroencephalograph; electroencephalogram; seizures; concussions; meningitis; encephalitis
5. stroke; aphasia; hemiplegia; cerebral; TIA
6. dementia; Alzheimer disease; Parkinson disease; hydrocephalus

Exercise R

Apply Medical Terms to A Case Study
Answers will vary and may include aphasia, dysphasia, hemiplegia, stroke, or cerebrovascular accident, along with their respective definitions.

Exercise S

Use Medical Terms in a Document
1. aphasia; 2. hemiplegia; 3. dementia;
4. dysphasia; 5. subarachnoid hemorrhage; 6. cerebrovascular accident (or stroke); 7. cerebral thrombosis;
8. cerebral angiography; 9. cerebral;
10. neurology; 11. neurologist;
12. transient ischemic attack;
13. dictionary/online exercise

Exercise T

Use Medical Language in Electronic Health Records on Evolve
Complete with online resources

Exercise U

Online Review of Lesson Content
Complete with online resources

Exercise V

Lesson Content Quiz
1. b; 2. c; 3. a; 4. b; 5. c; 6. b; 7. c;
8. b; 9. a; 10. c; 11. b; 12. a

LESSON 12

Exercise A

Build and Translate Terms Built from Word Parts
1. **Label:** Figure 12.2, (1) aden/o; (2) thym/o; (3) thyroid/o; (4) adrenal/o
2. **Match:** a. acr/o, extremities; b. -ic, pertaining to; c. -itis, inflammation; d. -ectomy, excision; e. -oma, tumor; f. -megaly, enlargement
3. **Build:** a. adrenal/itis; b. adrenal/ectomy; c. aden/oma; d. acr/o/megaly; e. adren/o/megaly
4. **Reading exercise**
5. **Label:** Figure 12.3, acr/o/megaly
6. **Translate:** a. thym/ic, pertaining to the thymus gland; b. thym/oma, tumor of the thymus gland; c. thym/ectomy, excision of the thymus gland; d. thyroid/ectomy, excision of the thyroid gland; e. thyroid/itis, inflammation of the thyroid gland
7. **Reading exercise**
8. **Match:** a. hyper-, above, excessive; b. hypo-, below, deficient, under; c. -emia, in the blood; d. -ism, state of; e. glyc/o, sugar
9. **Build:** a. hyper/thyroid/ism; b. hypo/thyroid/ism

10. **Reading exercise**
11. **Translate:** glyc/emia, sugar in the blood; b. hyper/glyc/emia, excessive sugar in the blood; c. hypo/glyc/emia, deficient sugar in the blood
12. **Reading exercise**
13. **Match:** a. poly-, many, much; b. ur/o, urination, urine, urinary tract; c. dips/o, thirst; d. -ia, diseased state, condition of
14. **Build:** a. poly/dips/ia; b. poly/ur/ia
15. **Reading exercise**
16. **Match:** a. endo-, within; b. crin/o, to secrete; c. path/o, disease; d. -logist, one who studies and treats (specialist, physician), e. -logy, study of; f. -e, -y, no meaning
17. **Translate:** a. endo/crin/e, to secrete within; b. endo/crin/o/logy, study of the endocrine system; c. endo/crin/o/logist, physician who studies and treats diseases of the endocrine system; d. endo/crin/o/path/y, (any) disease of the endocrine system
18. **Reading Exercise**
19. **Term Table: Review of Endocrine System Terms Built from Word Parts**

Exercise B

Pronounce and Spell Terms Built from Word Parts
1. Check responses with the Term Table in Exercise A, #19
2. Check answers with the online resources

Exercise C

Label
1. Graves disease
2. metabolic syndrome
3. goiter
4. Addison disease

Exercise D

Match
1. b; 2. c; 3. d; 4. a

Exercise E

Learn Medical Terms NOT Built from Word Parts
1. diabetes mellitus; fasting blood sugar; glycosylated hemoglobin; 2. goiter;
3. Graves disease; 4. Addison disease;
5. fine needle aspiration; 6. metabolic syndrome

Copyright © 2024 by Elsevier, Inc. All rights reserved.

Exercise F
Pronounce and Spell Terms NOT Built from Word Parts
1. Check responses with the Table for Terms NOT Built from Word Parts
2. Check answers with the online resources

Exercise G
Abbreviate Medical Terms
1. Diseases and Disorders: a. DM; b. T1DM; c. T2DM;
2. Diagnostic Tests: a. FBS; b. HbA1c; c. FNA

Exercise H
Signs and Symptoms
1. hyperglycemia; 2. hypoglycemia; 3. polydipsia; 4. polyuria; 5. adrenomegaly

Exercise I
Diseases and Disorders
1. endocrinopathy; 2. Addison disease; 3. adrenalitis; 4. Graves disease; 5. goiter; 6. hyperthyroidism; 7. hypothyroidism; 8. adenoma; 9. acromegaly; 10. thymoma; 11. thyroiditis; 12. diabetes mellitus; 13. metabolic syndrome

Exercise J
Diagnostic Tests
1. glycosylated hemoglobin; 2. fasting blood sugar; 3. fine needle aspiration

Exercise K
Surgical Procedures
1. adrenalectomy; 2. thymectomy; 3. thyroidectomy

Exercise L
Specialties and Professions
1. endocrinologist; 2. endocrinology

Exercise M
Medical Terms Related to the Endocrine System
1. endocrine; 2. glycemia; 3. thymic

Exercise N
Use Medical Terms in Clinical Statements
1. fine needle aspiration; endocrinologist; 2. FBS; HbA1c; 3. Polydipsia; polyuria; 4. hyperthyroidism; goiter; 5. Thymic; 6. adenoma; acromegaly; 7. adrenalitis; Addison disease

Exercise O
Apply Medical Terms to the Case Study
Answers will vary but may include polydipsia, polyuria, endocrinologist, fasting blood sugar, and their corresponding definitions

Exercise P
Use Medical Terms in a Document
1. polyuria; 2. polydipsia; 3. Graves disease; 4. diabetes mellitus; 5. fasting

blood sugar; 6. glycosylated hemoglobin; 7. hyperglycemia; 8. hypoglycemia; 9. endocrinology; 10. Answers will vary but may include nocturia, cyanosis, urinalysis; 11. Dictionary exercise.

Exercise Q
Interpret Language Used in a Medical Record
1. c; 2. a; 3. b; 4. b; 5. answers vary

Exercise R
Use Medical Language in Electronic Health Records Online
Complete with online resources

Exercise S
Online Review of Lesson Content
Complete with online resources

Exercise T
Lesson Content Quiz
1. b; 2. a; 3. b; 4. c; 5. a; 6. b; 7. c; 8. a

Copyright © 2024 by Elsevier, Inc. All rights reserved.

Illustration Credits

LESSON 1

Fig. 1.2, iStock.com/Marco VDM

Fig. 1.5, Callen JP, Paller AS, Greer KE et al: *Color atlas of dermatology*, ed 2, Philadelphia, 2000, WB Saunders.

Fig. 1.7, Mace JD, Kowalczyk N: *Radiographic pathology for technologists*, ed 4, St. Louis, 2004, Mosby/Elsevier.

Case Study Profile, iStock.com/natalie_board

Exercise E, #1, iStock.com/SciePro; **#2**, iStock.com/ktsimage; **#3**, Wilson S, Giddens J: *Health assessment for nursing practice*, ed 9, St. Louis, 2009, Mosby; **#4**, Habif T: *Clinical dermatology: A color guide to diagnosis and therapy*, ed 6, Philadelphia, 2016, Elsevier; **#5**, iStock.com/FatCamera; **#6**, iStock.com/JCPJR; **#8**, iStock.com/Charday Penn; **#9**, iStock.com/Natali_Mis; **#10**, iStock.com/angelp

Exercise O, iStock.com/XiXinXing

LESSON 2

Fig. 2.2, iStock.com/shironosov

Fig. 2.5, 2.15 Bontrager KL: *Textbook of radiographic positioning and related anatomy*, ed 5, St. Louis, 2001, Mosby.

Fig. 2.11, Ballinger PW, Frank ED: *Merrill's atlas of radiographic positions and radiologic procedures*, ed 10, St. Louis, 2003, Mosby/Elsevier.

Fig. 2.18C, iStock.com/Mabdelrazek

Fig. 2.19B, iStock.com/wenht

Case Study Profile, Thinkstock.com/Siri Stafford

Exercise O, iStock.com/pablohart

LESSON 3

Fig. 3.1, Thinkstock.com/AlexRaths

Fig. 3.3, Frazier M: *Essentials of human disease and conditions*, ed 3, St. Louis, 2004, Mosby.

Fig. 3.5 (left), Shiland B: *Mastering healthcare terminology*, ed 2, St. Louis, 2006, Mosby/Elsevier.

Fig. 3.7, Courtesy Dr. Dale M. Levinsky

Figs. 3.8A, Dinulos JGH: *Habif's Clinical Dermatology: A Color Guide to Diagnosis and Therapy*, ed 7, Philadelphia, 2021, Elsevier; **C,** Habif TP, Skin disease: *Diagnosis and Treatment*, ed 4, 2018, Elsevier; **D,** Cohen BA: *Pediatric dermatology*, ed 3, St. Louis, 2005, Mosby; **E,** Kamal A, Brockelhurst JC: *Color atlas of geriatric medicine*, ed 2, St. Louis, 1991, Mosby.

Fig. 3.9A, Cohen BA: *Pediatric dermatology*, ed 3, St. Louis, 2005, Mosby; **B,** iStock.com/PeterTG; **C,** Haught JM et al: Xanthoderma: A clinical review, *Journal of the American Academy of Dermatology;* December 2007, 57(6), Elsevier, 1051-1058.

Fig. 3.10A, Habif TP, Skin disease: *Diagnosis and Treatment*, ed 4, 2018, Elsevier. **B**, Kamal A, Brockelhurst JC: *Color atlas of geriatric medicine*, ed 2, St. Louis, 1991, Mosby.

Case Study Profile, Thinkstock.com/Hemera Technologies

Exercise E, #1, James WD et al: *Andrews' diseases of the skin*, ed 12, Philadelphia, 2016, Elsevier. **#2**, Callen JP et al: *Color atlas of dermatology*, ed 2, Philadelphia, 2000, Saunders; **#3**, Zitelli BJ, Davis HW: *Atlas of pediatric physical diagnosis*, ed 4, St. Louis, 2002, Mosby; **#4**, Wilson S, Giddens J: *Health assessment for nursing practice*, ed 4, St. Louis, 2008, Mosby; **#5**, *Dorland's illustrated medical dictionary*, ed 32, Philadelphia, 2012, Saunders/Elsevier; **#6**, Bork K, Brauninger W: *Skin diseases in clinical practice*, ed 2, Philadelphia, 1998, Saunders; **#7**, *Dorland's illustrated medical dictionary*, ed 32, Philadelphia, 2012, Saunders/Elsevier; **#8**, iStock.com/Plougmann. **#9**, iStock.com/happyfoto; **#10**, iStock.com/aniaostudio

Exercise Q, Thinkstock.com/Medioimages/Photodisc

LESSON 4

Fig. 4.2, iStock.com/pixelfit

Figs. 4.5A and B, Used with permission from Nonin Medical, Inc.; **C,** iStock.com/agrobacter

Fig. 4.13A, iStock.com/Devilkae; **B**, Robertson B et al: *Polysomnography for the sleep technologist*, ed 1, St. Louis, 2014, Mosby/Elsevier.

Fig. 4.14A, Ruppel GL: *Manual pulmonary function testing*, ed 7, St. Louis, 1998, Mosby; **B**, Paulino A: *PET-CT in radiotherapy treatment planning*, ed 1, Philadelphia, 2008, Saunders/Elsevier.

Case Study Profile, iStock.com/kolinko_tanya

Exercise E, #1, Paulino A: *PET-CT in radiotherapy treatment planning*, ed 1, Philadelphia, 2008, Saunders/Elsevier; **#2**, Ruppel GL, *Manual pulmonary function testing*, ed 7, St. Louis, 1998, Mosby; **#6**, getty.com/Ca-ssis

Exercise J, iStock.com/BakiBG

LESSON 5

Fig. 5.2, iStock.com/saengsuriya13

Fig. 5.4A, Ballinger PW, Frank ED: *Merrill's atlas of radiographic positions and radiologic procedures*, ed 10, St. Louis, 2003, Mosby.

Fig. 5.5, Bontrager K, Lampignano J: *Textbook of radiographic positioning and related anatomy*, ed 6, St. Louis, 2005, Mosby.

Fig. 5.9, Damjanov I: *Pathology for the health professions,* ed 3, Philadelphia, 2006, Saunders/Elsevier.

Fig. 5.13, Rollins JH, et al: *Merrill's Atlas of Radiographic Positioning & Procedures,* 15e, St. Louis, 2023, Elsevier

Case Profile, Thinkstock.com/viafilms

Exercise E, #3, James S, Ashwill J: *Nursing care of children,* ed 3, Philadelphia, 2008, Saunders; **#4,** Wein A et al: *Campbell-Walsh urology,* ed 10, Philadelphia, 2012, Saunders; **#5,** Thinkstock.com/belchonock

Exercise R, Thinkstock.com/belchonock

LESSON 6

Fig. 6.1, Thinkstock/John Foxx

Fig. 6.6, Patton K, Thibodeau G: *Anthony's textbook of anatomy & physiology,* ed 19, St. Louis, 2010, Mosby/Elsevier.

Fig. 6.8, Bontrager K, Lampignano J: *Textbook of radiographic positioning and related anatomy,* ed 6, St. Louis, 2005, Mosby.

Exercise E, #6, iStock.com/rudi_suardi

Case Study Profile, ThinkStock/Mike Watson Images

Exercise R, iStock.com/Monkeybusinessimages

LESSON 7

Fig. 7.4, Thinkstock/Keith Brofsky

Fig. 7.6, Patton KT, Thibodeau GA: *Anatomy and physiology,* ed 7, St. Louis, 2010, Mosby.

Fig. 7.7, Bontrager K, Lampignano J: *Textbook of radiographic positioning and related anatomy,* ed 7, St. Louis, 2010, Mosby/Elsevier.

Fig. 7.8, Figs. 7.10B and C, Fig. 7.12A, Ballinger PW, Frank ED: *Merrill's atlas of radiographic positions and radiologic procedures,* ed 10, St. Louis, 2003, Mosby.

Fig. 7.12B, Ignatavicius D, Workman ML: *Medical-surgical nursing,* ed 6, Philadelphia, 2010, Saunders/Elsevier.

Fig 7.15, *Dorland's illustrated medical dictionary,* ed 32, Philadelphia, 2012, Saunders/Elsevier.

Case Study Profile, Thinkstock/KatarzynaBialasiewicz

Exercise E, #1, iStock.com/Zilli; **#3,** Weiss RA: *Sclerotherapy: Treatment of varicose and telangiectatic leg veins,* ed 5, St. Louis, 2011, Elsevier; **#4,** iStock.com/Sukanya082; **#6,** iStock.com/Pixel_away; **#7,** Getty.com/Darrin Klimek; **#8,** iStock.com/PeopleImages

Case Study Profile, Thinkstock/KatarzynaBialasiewicz

Exercise S, Thinkstock/eans

LESSON 8

Fig. 8.2, iStock.com/IPGGutenbergUKLtd

Fig. 8.4, Neville BW et al: *Oral and maxillofacial pathology,* ed 3, Philadelphia, 2009, Saunders/Elsevier.

Fig. 8.5, Kowalczyk N: *Radiographic pathology for technologists,* ed 6, St. Louis, 2014, Mosby/Elsevier.

Fig. 8.6, Aspinall RJ, Taylor-Robinson SD: *Mosby's color atlas of gastroenterology and liver disease,* ed 1, St. Louis, 2002, Mosby.

Fig. 8.8B, Ignatavicius D, Workman ML: *Medical-surgical nursing,* ed 6, Philadelphia, 2010, Saunders/Elsevier.

Fig. 8.9, Anderson KN: *Mosby's medical, nursing and allied health dictionary,* St. Louis, 1998, Mosby.

Fig. 8.11, Kowalczyk N: *Radiographic pathology for technologists,* ed 6, St. Louis, 2014, Mosby/Elsevier.

Fig. 8.12, Hagen-Ansert S: *Textbook of diagnostic ultrasonography,* ed 5, St. Louis, 2001, Mosby.

Fig. 8.14, Bontrager K, Lampignano J: *Textbook of radiographic positioning and related anatomy,* ed 8, St. Louis, 2014, Mosby/Elsevier.

Exercise E, #1, Frank ED, Long BW, Smith BJ: *Merrill's atlas of radiographic positions and radiologic procedures,* ed 12, St. Louis, 2012, Mosby; **#2,** Shiland B: *Mastering healthcare terminology,* ed 2, St. Louis, 2006, Mosby/Elsevier; **#4,** Kowalczyk N: *Radiographic pathology for technologists,* ed 6, St. Louis, 2014, Mosby/Elsevier; **#9,** iStock.com/OGphoto; **#10,** iStock.com/Phynart Studio

Case Study Profile, Thinkstock/Christopher Robbins

Exercise R, Ignatavicius D, Workman ML: *Medical-surgical* **nursing,** ed 6, Philadelphia, 2010, Saunders/Elsevier.

LESSON 9

Fig. 9.3, iStock.com/FlamingoImages

Fig. 9.4, iStock.com/AlexRaths

Figs. 9.6A and B, Jarvis C: *Physical examination and health assessment,* ed 5, Philadelphia, 2008, Saunders; **C,** Zitelli BJ, Davis HW: *Atlas of pediatric physical diagnosis,* ed 4, St. Louis, 2002, Mosby.

Fig. 9.7A, Scheie HG, Albert DM: *Textbook of ophthalmology,* ed 9, Philadelphia, 1977, WB Saunders; **B,** Batterbury M, Murphy C: *Ophthalmology: An illustrated colour text,* ed 4, St. Louis, 2018, Elsevier.

Fig. 9.8, Stein HA, Skatt BJ, Stein RM: *The ophthalmic assistant: Fundamentals and clinical practice,* ed 5, St. Louis, 1998, Mosby.

Fig. 9.10, Jarvis C: *Physical examination and health assessment,* ed 5, Philadelphia, 2008, Saunders.

Fig. 9.11, Barkauskas VH et al: *Health and physical assessment,* ed 3, St. Louis, 2002, Mosby.

Fig. 9.16, Śliwa LS et al: A comparison of audiometric and objective methods in hearing screening of school children: A preliminary study, *International Journal of Pediatric Otorhinolaryngology;* April 2011, 75(4), Elsevier, 483-488.

Case Study Profile: iStock.com/diego_cervo

Exercise E, #1, Seidel H et al: *Mosby's guide to physical examination,* ed 5, St. Louis, 2003, Mosby; **#4,** iStock.com/bubaone. **#5,** iStock.com/DragonImage; **#6,** gettyimages; **#7,** gettyimages/Tetsu/amanaimagesRF

Exercise R, gettyimages/Huntstock

LESSON 10

Fig. 10.1, Thinkstock/BakiBG

Fig. 10.6, Jacob S: *Human anatomy,* ed 1, Edinburgh, 2007, Churchill Livingstone.

Fig. 10.9, iStock/com/StockPhotosArt

Fig. 10.11, Mourad LA: *Orthopedic disorders,* St. Louis, 1991, Mosby Yearbook.

Fig. 10.13, Yousem D, Grossman R: *Neuroradiology: The requisites*, ed 2, Philadelphia, 2003, Mosby.

Figs. 10.14, 10.16, Frank ED, Long B, Smith B: *Merrill's atlas of radiographic positions and radiologic procedures,* ed 11, St. Louis, 2007, Mosby/Elsevier.

Fig. 10.17, Canale ST, Beaty JH: *Campbell's operative orthopaedics*, ed 11, Philadelphia, 2008, Mosby/Elsevier.

Fig. 10.18, Shiland B: *Mastering healthcare terminology,* ed 1, St. Louis, 2003, Mosby.

Case Study Profile, Creatas, Thinkstock: 76753512

Exercise E, #4, iStock.com/MediaProduction; **#6,** Patton K, Thibodeau G: *Anthony's textbook of anatomy & physiology,* ed 19, St. Louis, 2010, Mosby/Elsevier; **#9,** Taylor J, Resnick D: *Skeletal imaging: Atlas of the spine and extremities*, ed 1, Philadelphia, 2000, Saunders; **#11**, iStock.com/SDI Productions; **#12**, Seidel H et al: *Mosby's guide to physical examination,* ed 7, St. Louis, 2011, Mosby.

Exercise R, Ferri F: *Ferri's color atlas and text of clinical medicine,* ed 1, Philadelphia, 2009, Saunders/Elsevier.

LESSON 11

Fig. 11.2, Thinkstock/Keith Brofsky

Fig. 11.4, Adam A et al: *Grainger and Allison's diagnostic radiology*, ed 5, Edinburgh, 2008, Churchill Livingstone.

Fig. 11.5, *Dorland's illustrated medical dictionary*, ed 32, Philadelphia, 2012, Saunders/Elsevier.

Fig. 11.8, Kowalczyk N: *Radiographic pathology for technologists*, ed 6, St. Louis, 2014, Mosby/Elsevier.

Fig. 11.9, Ballinger PW, Frank ED: *Merrill's atlas of radiographic positions and radiologic procedures*, ed 10, St. Louis, 2003, Mosby/Elsevier.

Case Study Profile, Thinkstock/sot

Exercise E, #4, iStock.com/monkeybusinessimages; **#5,** images in left column, Shiland B: *Mastering healthcare terminology*, ed 2, St. Louis, 2006, Elsevier/Mosby; **#9,** iStock.com/Juanmonino; **#10,** iStock.com/Wavebreakmedia

Exercise S, Eisenberg R, Johnson N: *Comprehensive radiographic pathology,* ed 5, St. Louis, 2011, Mosby.

LESSON 12

Fig. 12.1, Thinkstock

Fig. 12.3, From Mendeloff A, Smith DE: Acromegaly, diabetes, hypermetabolism, proteinuria and heart failure, *The American Journal of Medicine;* 1956, Elsevier; 20(1):133.

Case Study Profile, iStock.com/Pichunter

Exercise E, #1 Forbes CD, Jackson WF: *Color atlas and text of clinical medicine,* ed 3 (p. 309, **Figure 7.55**), St. Louis, 2003, Mosby; **#3,** Swartz MH: *Textbook of physical diagnosis: History and examination,* ed 3, Philadelphia, 1998, Saunders.

Exercise P, iStock.com/mycan

Page numbers followed by "*f*" indicate figures; "*t*"
indicate tables; and "*b*" indicate boxes.

ERCP. *See* Endoscopic retrograde
  cholangiopancreatography (ERCP)
Erectile dysfunction (ED), 178*t*, 184*t*
Erythema, 72*t*
Erythr/o, 61*t*
Erythrocytes (RBCs), 70, 70*b*, 71*f*, 71*t*, 77*t*, 197
Erythroderma, 68, 71*t*
Esophageal, 239, 244*t*
Esophagitis, 239, 244*t*
Esophag/o, 234*t*, 239
Esophagogastroduodenoscopy (EGD), 246,
  253*t*, 260*t*
Esophagus
  anatomic structure of, 231*t*, 232
  function of, 232, 233*f*
ESWL. *See* Extracorporeal shock wave lithotripsy
  (ESWL)
ET. *See* Endotracheal (ET)
Eustachi, Bartolomeo, 272*t*
Eustachian tube, 272*t*
Excision, 94*b*
Exfoliative dermatitis, 68
Exhalation, 89*f*, 90
External auditory canal, 272*t*, 273*f*
External ear, 272*t*, 273*f*
Extracorporeal shock wave lithotripsy (ESWL),
  144*t*, 148*t*
Eye(s)
  abbreviations related to, 292, 292*t*
  anatomic structures of, 271*t*-272*t*, 276, 276*f*
  disorders of, 278-279, 279*b*, 287*t*-288*t*, 289
  functions of, 272*f*, 273
  medical terms related to, 280*t*-281*t*, 287*t*-288*t*,
    289, 300*t*
    by clinical category, 292-294
    in case study, 296
    in clinical statements, 295
    in electronic health records, 298
    in medical document, 296-298
    quiz on, 299
  pathway of light through, 272*f*
  professionals who work with, 274*b*, 274*f*
  pronunciation and spelling of terms related
    to, 281, 291
  word parts related to, 275*t*, 276-281, 277*b*, 300*t*

F
Fallopian tubes, 159*b*, 159*t*. *See also*
    Uterine tubes
Falloppio, Gabriele, 159*b*
Farsightedness. *See* Hyperopia
Fasting blood sugar (FBS), 386*t*, 390*t*
FBS. *See* Fasting blood sugar (FBS)
Female reproductive system
  abbreviations related to, 184*t*, 184-185
  anatomic structures of, 159*t*-160*t*, 163, 165*f*
  disorders of, 164-165, 165*f*, 170, 177*t*
  functions of, 160-161
  medical terms related to, 171*t*-172*t*, 177*t*,
    179-180, 194*t*
    by clinical category, 185-188
    in case study, 189
    in clinical statements, 189
    in medical document, 190, 191*f*
    quiz on, 192-193
  pronunciation and spelling of terms related to,
    172-173, 183
  word parts for, 162*t*-163*t*, 163-172, 164*b*, 167*b*,
    169*b*, 193*t*
Femoral, 314*t*
Femoral artery palpation, 53, 53*f*
Femor/o, 303*t*
Fine needle aspiration (FNA), 386*t*, 390*t*
Fissures, anal, 252
Flu. *See* Influenza (flu)
Fluoroscopy, 168*b*
FNA. *See* Fine needle aspiration (FNA)
Fowler position, 42*b*, 43*t*
Fractures (Fx), 326*t*, 331*t*, 339
Frontal plane, 41*f*, 41*t*
Fungal infections, 66, 66*f*
Fx. *See* Fractures (Fx)

G
Gallbladder, 232*t*, 248, 248*b*
Gallstones, 248
Garcia, Manuel, 95*b*
Gastrectomy, 241, 244*t*
Gastric, 241, 244*t*
Gastric ulcers, 241*f*, 255*t*
Gastritis, 241, 244*t*
Gastr/o, 234*t*, 240-241
Gastroenteritis, 241, 244*t*
Gastroenterologists, 241, 244*t*
Gastroenterology, 244*t*
Gastroesophageal, 241, 244*t*
Gastroesophageal reflux disease (GERD), 255*t*, 260*t*
Gastrointestinal, 260*t*
Gastrointestinal (GI) tract, 232, 233*f*
Gastroscope, 242, 244*t*
Gastroscopy, 242, 244*t*
Gastrostomy, 242, 244*t*, 246
Genetic testing, 19*t*
-genic, 8*t*, 14, 346*t*
GERD. *See* Gastroesophageal reflux disease (GERD)
GI tract. *See* Gastrointestinal (GI) tract
Gingivalgia, 237, 244*t*
Gingivitis, 237, 244*t*
Gingiv/o, 234*t*, 237
Glauc/o, 71*t*
Glaucoma, 287*t*
Glossitis, 238, 244*t*
Gloss/o, 234*t*, 238
Gluten enteropathy, 254*t*. *See also* Celiac disease
Glycated hemoglobin (A1c), 386*t*
Glycemia, 383, 385*t*
Glyc/o, 380*t*
Glycosylated hemoglobin (A1c), 386*t*, 390*t*
Goiter, 386*t*
Gout, 326*t*
-gram, 91*t*, 129*t*, 162*t*, 199*t*, 201*b*, 304*t*, 346*t*
-graph, 199*t*, 201*b*, 346*t*
-graphy, 91*t*, 129*t*, 162*t*, 199*t*, 201*b*, 235*t*, 346*t*
Graves disease, 386*t*
Greek and Latin word parts, 1, 2*f*, 3
Guillain-Barré syndrome, 351
Gums, 232*t*
Gynec/o, 162*t*
Gynecologists, 166, 171*t*
Gynecology, 172*t*

H
Hair, 59-60, 62*f*
Hair follicles, 62*f*
Hard of hearing (HOH), 292*t*
HbA1c. *See* Glycated hemoglobin (A1c)
HD. *See* Hemodialysis (HD)
Headache, 358*t*. *See also* Cephalalgia
Hearing, 273*f*, 274
Heart
  anatomic structure of, 195*t*, 200*f*, 207*f*
  functions of, 197
Heart attack, 215*t*. *See also* Myocardial infarction (MI)
Heart failure (HF), 4, 214*t*, 221*t*
Hematemesis, 266
Hemat/o, 128*t*, 199*t*, 212
Hematologists, 212, 213*t*
Hematology, 212, 213*t*
Hematoma, 212, 213*t*
Hematuria, 132, 133*b*, 135*t*
Hemi-, 346*t*
Hemiplegia, 356, 358*t*
Hem/o, 128*t*, 199*t*, 212
Hemodialysis (HD), 144*b*, 148*t*
Hemoglobin A1c, 386*t*. *See also* Glycated hemoglobin
  (A1c)
Hemolysis, 212, 213*t*
Hemorrhage, 215*t*, 217*b*
  intracranial, 317
Hemorrhagic stroke, 365*f*
Hemorrhoids, 255*t*
Hemostasis, 212, 213*t*
Hepatitis, 247, 253*t*
Hepat/o, 234*t*, 247
Hepatoma, 247, 253*t*

Hepatomegaly, 247, 253*t*
Hernia, 162*b*, 326*t*
Herniated disk, 326*t*
Herpes, 72*t*
HF. *See* Heart failure (HF)
HHD. *See* Hypertensive heart disease (HHD)
High Fowler position, 42*b*
Hist/o, 8*t*, 10
Histology, 10, 10*b*, 17*t*
History and physical form, 395*f*-396*f*
Hodgkin lymphoma, 211
HOH. *See* Hard of hearing (HOH)
Horizontal plane, 41*t*
Hormones, 378*t*, 379
Horny tissue, 62*f*
HPV. *See* Human papillomavirus (HPV)
HSG. *See* Hysterosalpingogram (HSG)
HTN. *See* Hypertension (HTN)
Human papillomavirus (HPV), 184*t*
  vaccine for, 182*b*
Hydr/o, 128*t*, 346*t*
Hydrocephalus, 355, 358*t*
Hydronephrosis, 138, 142*t*
Hyper-, 91*t*, 95*b*, 304*t*, 380*t*
Hypercapnia, 96, 97*t*
Hyperglycemia, 383, 385*t*
Hyperopia, 279*b*, 287*t*, 288*f*
Hyperoxia, 96, 98*t*
Hyperpnea, 96, 98*t*
Hypertension (HTN), 215*t*, 221*t*
Hypertensive heart disease (HHD), 221*t*
Hyperthyroidism, 383, 385*t*
Hypertrophic, 310, 314*t*
Hypertrophy, 310, 314*t*
Hypo-, 61*t*, 91*t*, 95*b*, 380*t*
Hypocapnia, 96, 98*t*
Hypochondriac regions, 41*t*, 42*f*
Hypodermic, 64, 65*b*, 65*t*, 67*t*, 77*t*
Hypogastric region, 41*t*, 42*f*
Hypoglycemia, 383, 385*t*
Hypopnea, 96, 98*t*
Hypotension, 215*t*
Hypothyroidism, 383, 385*t*
Hypoxia, 96, 96*b*, 98*t*
Hysterectomy, 168, 172*t*
Hyster/o, 162*t*
Hysteropexy, 166, 168, 172*t*
Hysterorrhaphy, 168, 172*t*
Hysterorrhexis, 168, 172*t*
Hysterosalpingogram (HSG), 168, 168*b*, 172*t*, 184*t*
Hysterosalpingo-oophorectomy, 168, 172*t*

I
-ia, 91*t*, 129*t*, 199*t*, 235*t*, 304*t*, 346*t*, 380*t*
-iasis, 128*t*, 235*t*, 304*t*
Iatr, 254*b*
IBS. *See* Irritable bowel syndrome (IBS)
-ic, 4, 8*t*, 33*t*, 61*t*, 95*b*, 162*t*, 235*t*, 275*t*, 304*t*, 346*t*, 380*t*
Ile/o, 234*t*, 312*b*
Iieostomy, 246, 253*t*
Ileum, 246*b*
Iliac, 314*t*, 338
Iliac regions, 41*t*, 42*f*
Ili/o, 303*t*, 312*b*
Iliofemoral, 312, 315*t*
Ilium, 301*t*
Immunotherapy, 18*t*
Impetigo, 72*t*
Impotence, 178*t*
Incision, 93*b*
Incontinence, 144*t*
Infections, 19*t*
  bladder, 132
  cervical, 164
  kidney, 138
  respiratory, 109*t*, 112*f*
  urinary tract, 144*t*, 148*t*
Inferior, 36, 37*b*, 40*t*, 50*t*
Infer/o, 33*t*
Inferolateral, 40*t*
Inflammation, 19*t*
Influenza (flu), 109*t*, 115*t*

COMMON TERMINOLOGY

Acronym: A term formed from the first letter of several words that can be spoken as a whole word; usually contains a vowel.

EXAMPLE: laser (light amplification by simulated emission of radiation)

Build: Constructing a medical term from its definition using Greek and Latin word parts as a learning exercise.

EXAMPLE: the term meaning "inflammation of the kidney" may be constructed from nephr/o (kidney) and -itis (inflammation) to arrive at the term nephritis.

Combining form: Combination of a word root and a combining vowel.

EXAMPLE: therm/o. Often referred to as a word part.

Combining vowel: Usually an **o**. Used between word parts to ease pronunciation.

EXAMPLE: therm/o/meter

Eponym: Medical term named for a person or a place.

EXAMPLE: Parkinson disease

Etymology: Origin and development of a word.

EXAMPLE: Cadaver, denoting a corpse or dead body, is derived from the Latin word *cadere*, which means to fall. The term literally means fallen and originally described those who fell dead in battle.

Implied meaning: Requires a more precise definition than literal translation.

EXAMPLE: an/emia. The literal translation is without blood; the implied meaning is a condition characterized by the deficiency of red blood cells and hemoglobin.

Literal translation: Translation of the word parts that make up a medical term to arrive at its meaning.

EXAMPLE: therm/o means heat, -meter means instrument used to measure; therefore, thermometer means instrument used to measure heat. In some medical terms literal translation does not define the current use of the term.

EXAMPLE: The literal translation of meta/stasis is beyond control; the implied or current definition is transfer of disease from one organ to another.

Medical language or medical terminology: A professional language made up of medical terms used mostly by those engaged directly or indirectly in health care.

Medical term: Word(s) used to describe anatomic structures, medical diagnoses, diagnostic procedures, surgical procedures, and signs and symptoms of illness and disease. Medical terms originate from Greek and Latin word parts, such as gastr/itis; eponyms, such as Alzheimer disease; acronyms, such as laser; and modern language, such as bone marrow transplant.

Prefix: Attached at the beginning of a word root to modify its meaning.

EXAMPLE: re/play

Suffix: Attached at the end of a word root to modify its meaning.

EXAMPLE: play/er

Translate: Using the meaning of the word parts to define a term.

EXAMPLE: nephr/o means kidney, -itis means inflammation, nephritis means inflammation of the kidney.

Word part: Consists of Greek and Latin prefixes, suffixes, word roots, and combining vowels.

Word root: Core of the word giving the medical term its primary meaning.

COMMON PLURAL ENDINGS FOR MEDICAL TERMS

In the English language, plurals are often formed by simply adding *s* or *es* to the word. Forming plurals in the language of medicine is not so simple. Use the table below to learn common plural endings for medical terms.

SINGULAR ENDING	PLURAL ENDING	EXAMPLE SINGULAR	PLURAL
-a	-ae	vertebra	vertebrae
-ax	-aces	thorax	thoraces
-ex	-ices	cortex	cortices
-is	-es	pubis	pubes
-ix	-ices	cervix	cervices
-ma	-mata	sarcoma	sarcomata
-nx	-nges	pharynx	pharynges
-on	-a	ganglion	ganglia
-sis	-ses	diagnosis	diagnoses
-um	-a	ovum	ova
-us	-i	bronchus	bronchi